THE NEW MASSAGE

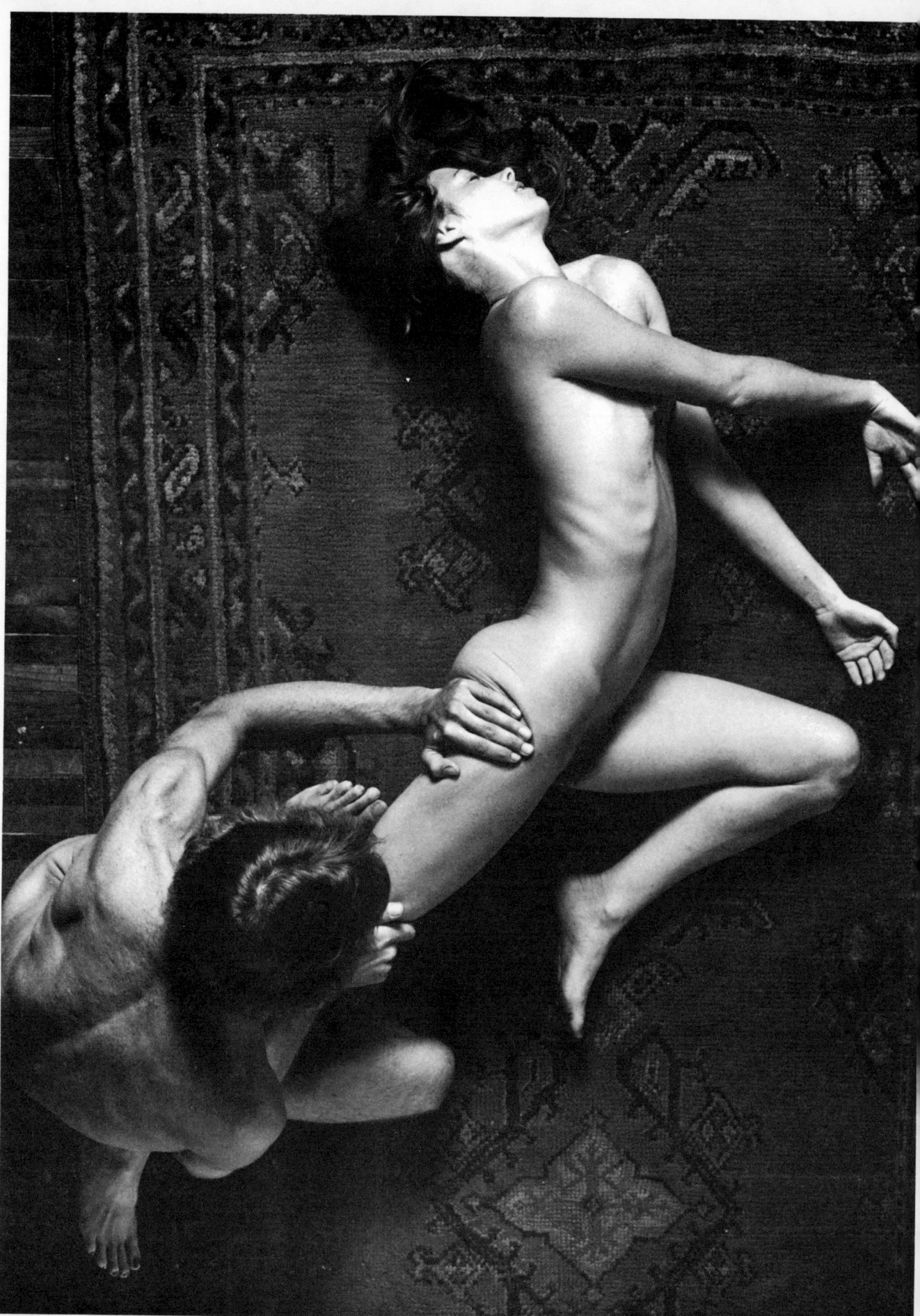

The New Massage

Total Body Conditioning for People Who Exercise

By Gordon Inkeles

Photography by Greg Peterson

G. P. Putnam's Sons   New York

The author wishes to express
appreciation for permission to quote and
reproduce artwork from the following
sources:
Portion of Plate 25 from *The Anatomy
Coloring Book* by Wynn Kapit and
Lawrence M. Elson. Copyright © 1977
by Wynn Kapit and Lawrence M. Elson.

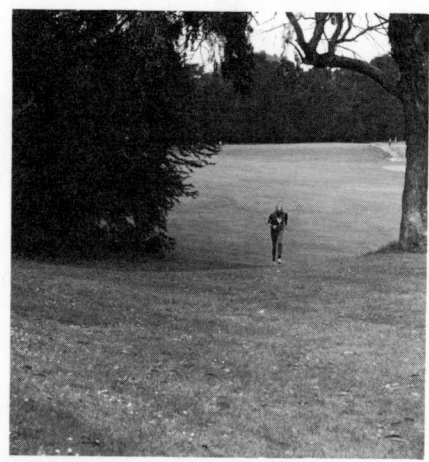 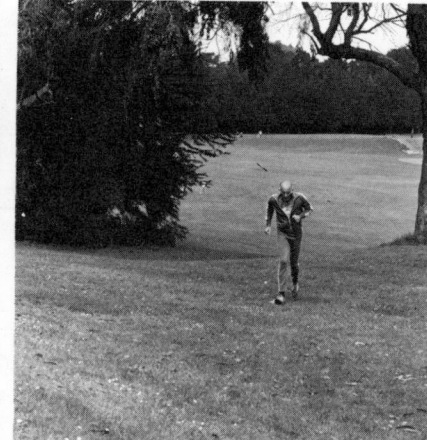 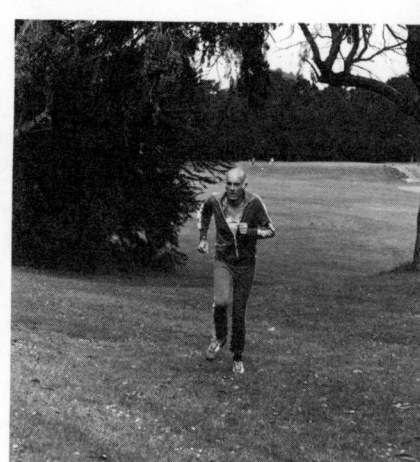

Reprinted by permission of Harper &
Row, Publishers, Inc. Four-part
bandaging illustration from *Functional
Disorders of the Foot* by F. D. Dickson
and R. L. Dively. Copyright © 1939 by
F. D. Dickson and R. L. Dively.
Reprinted by permission of J. B.
Lippincott Company.

Book design and illustration by
Jon Goodchild

Printed in the United States of America

Gratefully to Arthur Giddens,
who believes in almost everything,
and to my son Yuri,
not yet old enough to have beliefs

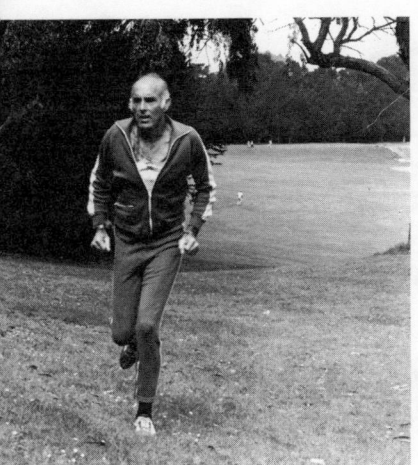 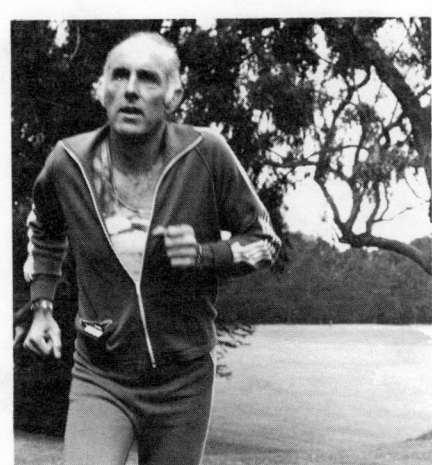 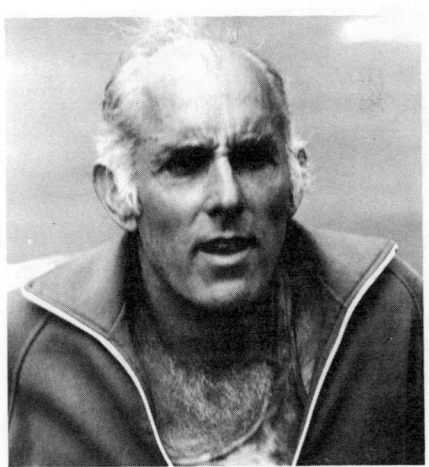

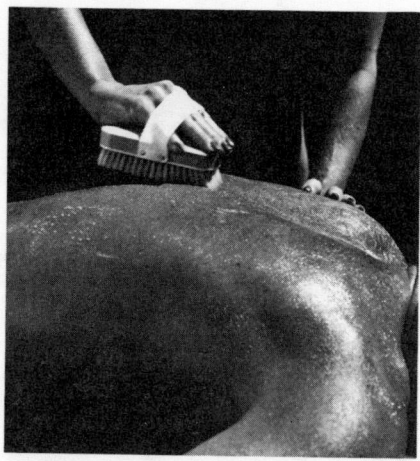

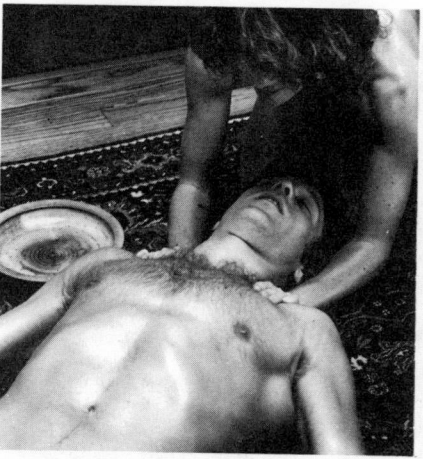

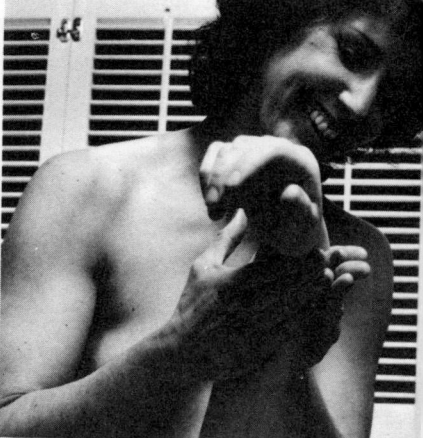

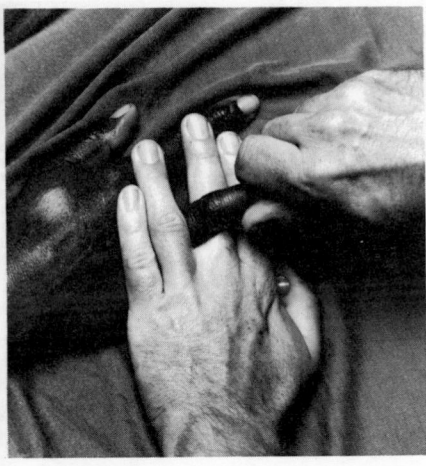
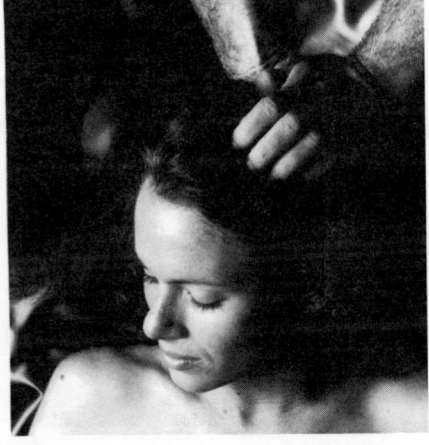
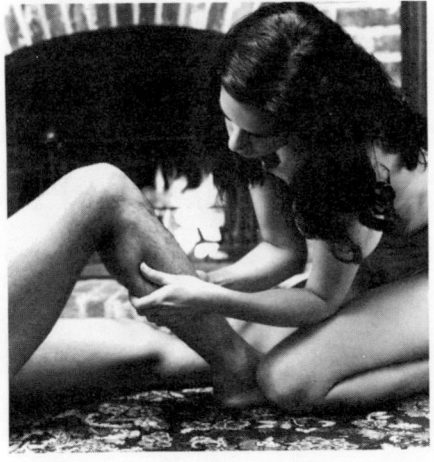

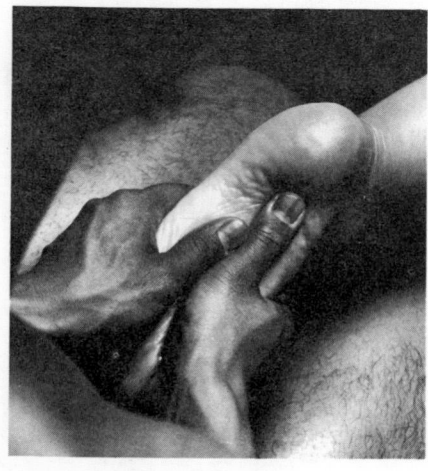 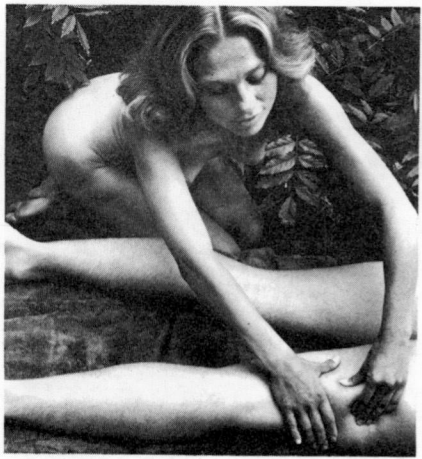 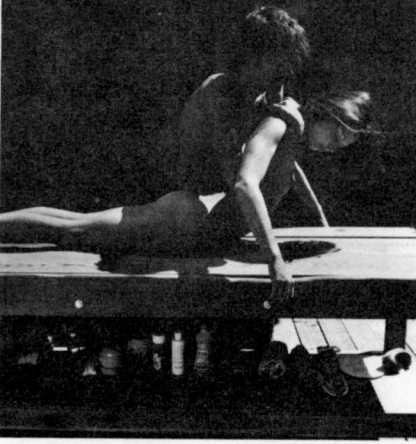

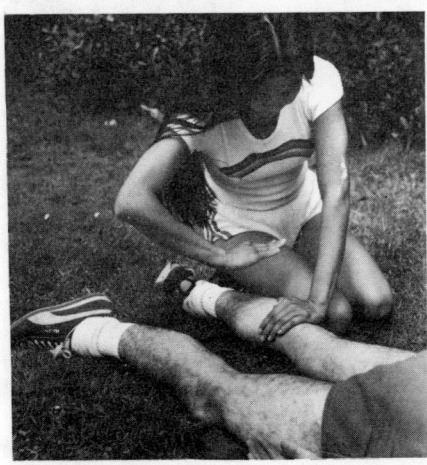
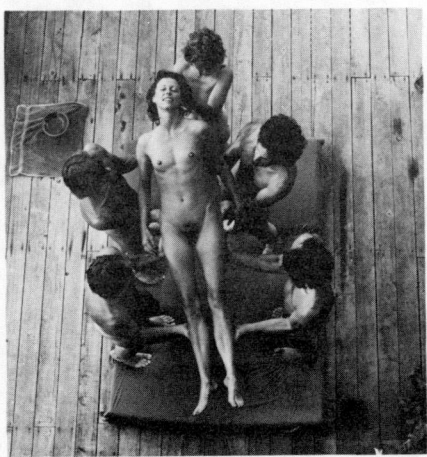

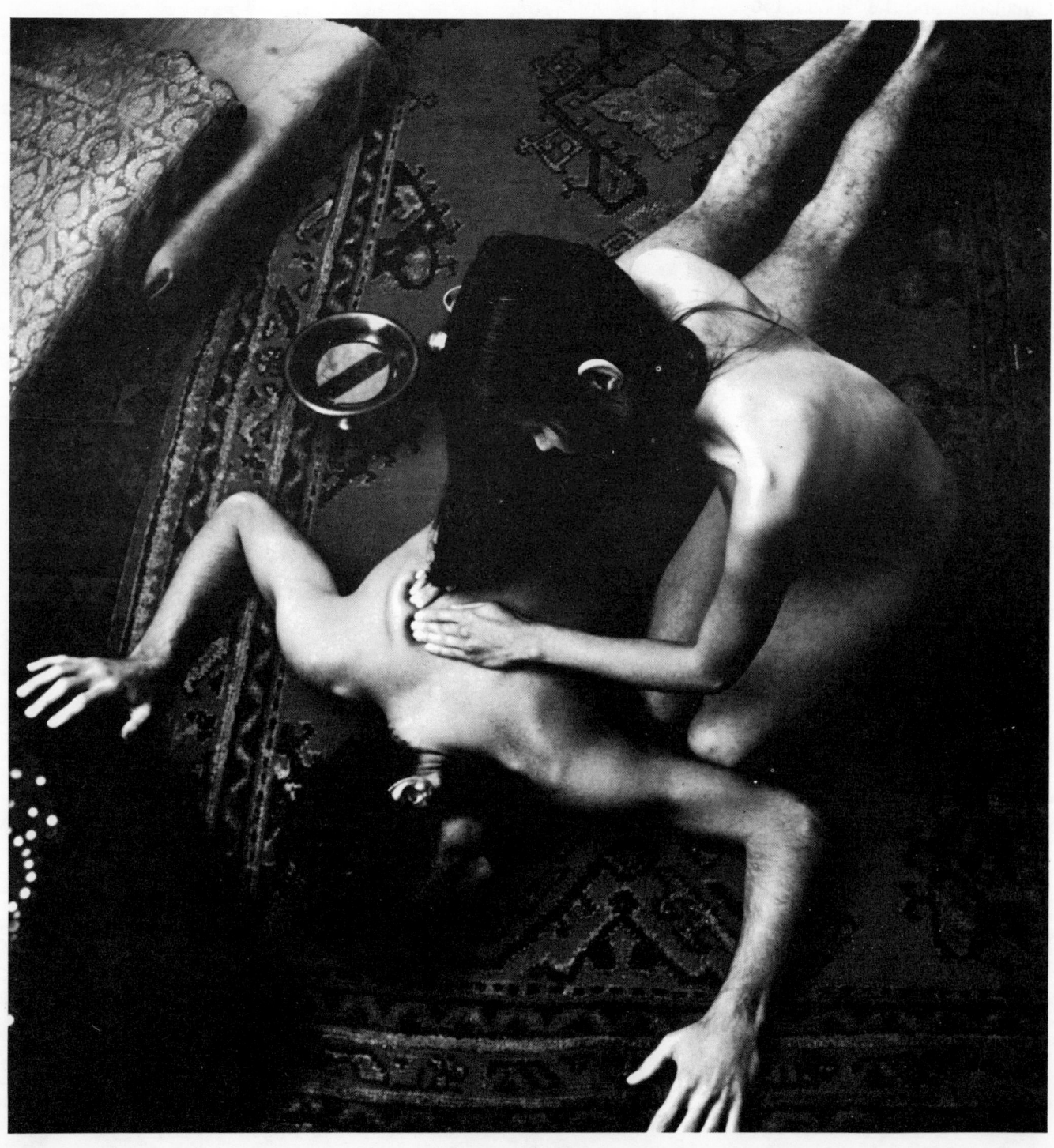

Preface

The Art of Sensual Massage was written to demystify the practice of massage. I wanted to offer people an alternative to dense, unreadable physical therapy texts that further the clinical stereotype of massage as a cold, impersonal experience. The book encouraged readers to get right into massaging each other and to forget about professional training, anatomy, and inhibitions. Many of them did. Over the past few years I have been massaged frequently by readers of that book, and believe me, it still feels great.

You might ask where eight years of massage would lead a writer, and the answer is inside: inside the body, where changes that can take place under a masseur's hands have the most profound importance for people interested in health and body conditioning. Those changes, and the techniques which make them happen, are at the heart of this book. Instead of popping a pill, readers can use massage to mobilize the body's hidden resources. Throughout the book, amateur and professional masseurs will find drugless therapy methods for a wide range of common ailments.

The New Massage provides the beginner with step-by-step comprehensive massage techniques for the entire body. Hedonists who have already sampled massage are encouraged to dig right into the full body massage which will add more pleasure to your partner's life in a single afternoon than most people experience in a month. Massage presents people with a universal truth, and the message is joy, communion, and peace. If exercise is important to your partner, I urge you to learn the techniques in this book very slowly, perhaps three or four movements per session. That way the amazing Fluid Release sequences will come off smoothly, without hesitation, when you're massaging.

The electrifying effects of these sequences on an athlete simply have to be seen and felt to be believed. Although these effects were documented seventy-five years ago, they have been meticulously ignored by athletes, who, like most other Americans, avoid touching each other after the age of six. That regrettable habit is finally disappearing, and athletes have a chance to try a drug-free new training aid. In every sport Fluid Release techniques will improve performance, increase endurance, and lower fatigue levels.

Massage is one of life's most compassionate moments, and yet before 1970 there was no meaningful photographic treatment of the subject. Since then many photographers have responded to this unique artistic challenge. I believe you will find in the work of Greg Peterson some of the most exquisite massage photography that has ever been done. Peterson has finally recorded nuances of expression and mood that were once known only to certain masseurs and their blissful partners.

Jon Goodchild, designer of *The Art of Sensual Massage*, has returned with an elegant concept for this new book. Putnam's incomparable Diane Matthews understood and believed in the project when it was in its infancy. *The New Massage* would not have been possible without her.

Gordon Inkeles
Miranda, California.
March 1980

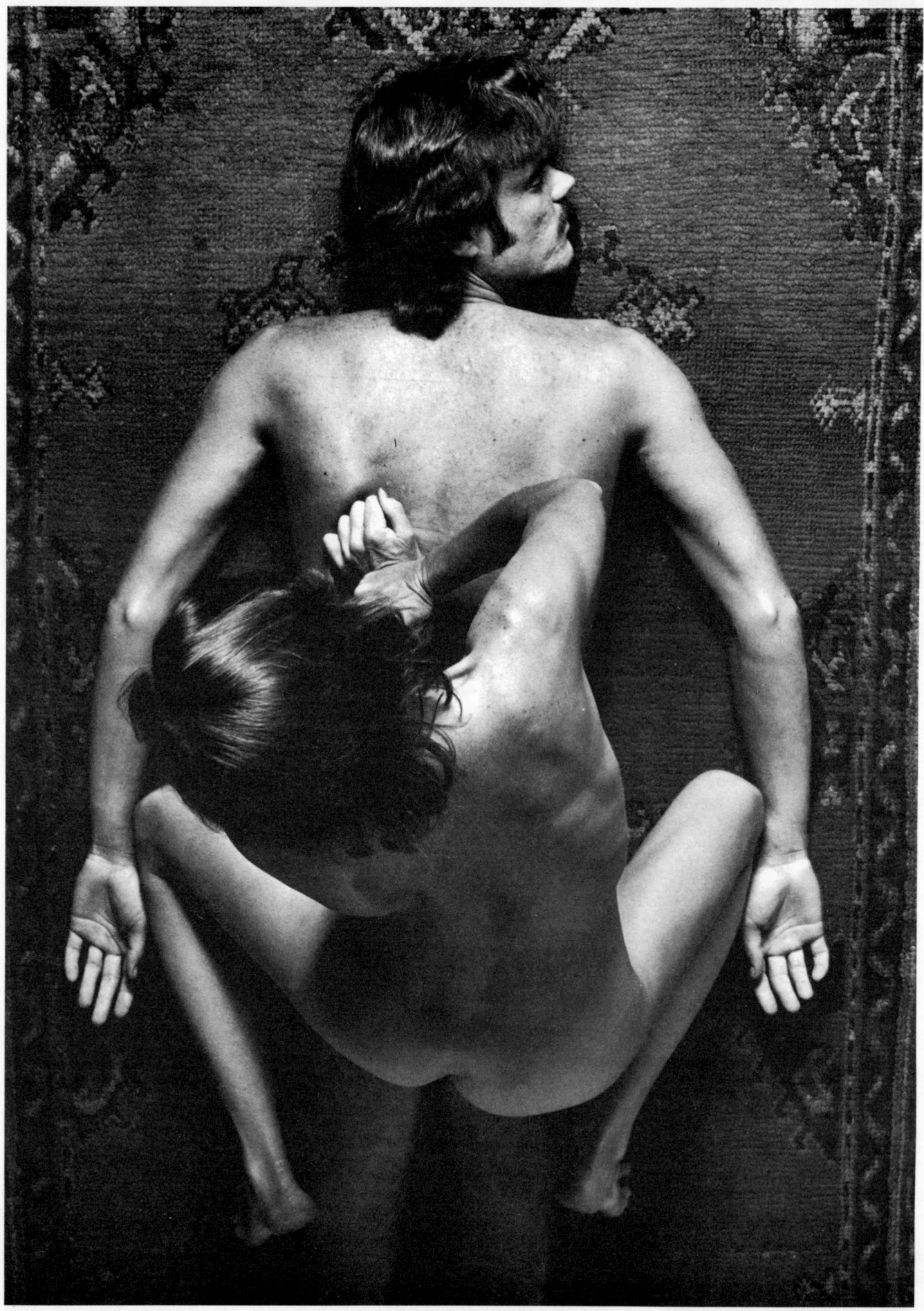

Introduction

. . . That is the substance of re-membering—sense, sight, smell: the muscles with which we see and hear and feel—not mind, not thought: there is no such thing as memory: the brain recalls just what the muscles grope for: no more, no less: and its resultant sum is usually incorrect and false and worthy only of the name of dream.

William Faulkner
Absalom, Absalom

Three thousand years ago citizens of the Mediterranean civilizations began every day with an experience called the bath. For several hours in the early morning these ancients devoted themselves to body care. They either bathed themselves or were bathed by attendants. Intricate exercise programs had been developed to strengthen the body while particularly stiff muscles were rubbed with warm vegetable oil. The experience went on to include a full body massage aimed at awakening the nerves, stimulating the circulation, and freeing the action of the joints. Finally, the entire body was rubbed with a very fine oil to keep the skin elastic and supple all through the day. After about two hours of this heady stuff people felt ready to sit down to a leisurely breakfast. The two-hour morning bath has been replaced, in our advanced civilization, with a five-minute experience called the shower.

The understanding that education involves the parallel development of mind and body was at the heart of the philosophy of ancient societies. Since this concept cannot really be improved upon, it has simply been rediscovered periodically for the past 3,000 years. The current interest in physical fitness represents our society's bid to revive a very ancient philosophy. If good health and good feelings about yourself are your goal, exercise is really not an option; it is an absolute necessity. We all have seen the alternatives: the ever-expanding waistline, the dozens of "minor" medical problems, and, finally, the onset of one of the killer diseases—usually circulatory, usually fatal, and usually preventable if only one had exercised. How many joggers, burdened by this grim thought, rush unsmiling through our streets and parks as though Mr. Death himself were in pursuit?

Any kind of exercise, particularly running, can easily become a grim, tiresome ordeal if performance is the only goal. Even people who love to run must learn to cope with profound levels of exhaustion when the body reaches its limit. It's always hard for beginners to start exercising, and it's difficult to become really proficient; too often the spirit is willing, but the flesh is not. Are fatigue and pain the secret price that physically active people must pay for health and fitness? The puritanical assump-

tion that all progress in life must somehow be accompanied by suffering can be applied to exercise. However, the notion is false and irrelevant because massage can be used exactly the way the Greeks used it: to increase endurance and control fatigue.

By understanding the chemistry of fatigue and learning to alter it, you can dramatically increase your endurance and virtually eliminate the unpleasant side effects of a long run, a hard workout, or grueling tennis match. You can do this by using massage to disperse the accumulated fatigue products that irritate the muscles after exercise.

Lactic and carbonic acids appear in the muscles and surrounding tissues shortly after exercise begins. These acids are waste products that cause the pain and occasional cramping many athletes and dancers suffer after a workout. Lactic acid, the main irritant, is formed when glycogen stored in the muscles and liver is burned during exercise. It must either be reconverted to sugar, stored once again or drained out of the muscles, then sent through

13

the complex lymph system and finally out of the body. Pain will persist until this process of either reconverting or excreting muscle wastes has been completed. That can take hours or even days. Large amounts of acidic wastes place an enormous burden on the muscles that have been exercised. Fluid wastes and poisons saturate the muscles, causing the familiar irritation that often plagues athletes the morning after a workout. To eliminate this irritation, masseurs seek to stimulate the metabolic process, thereby hastening reabsorption and release rate of wastes.

One of the chief benefits of massage is the unique way it can be used to accelerate the flow of blood through the body without straining the heart. Any mammal licking a bruise instinctively understands that enhancing the blood supply diminishes pain. Precisely the same accelerated blood flow coupled with direct pressure disperses accumulations of stagnant toxins throughout the body.

About 100 years ago physicians who were interested in the effects of massage on waste disposal injected India ink into the muscles of two rabbits. Afterward both rabbits resumed the usual hyperactive rabbit life, but the injected leg of one rabbit was massaged regularly. A month later the rabbits were killed and dissected. Ink had stained black the muscles surrounding the injection site in the leg of the rabbit that had not been massaged. As for the rabbit that *had*

been massaged, no trace of India ink could be found *anywhere in the body.* The importance of this nasty little experiment can hardly be exaggerated to anyone interested in fitness.

Removal of wastes, particularly those produced by exercise, can be dramatically accelerated by massage. The specific technique for doing this, called Fluid Release, not only increases your endurance while you exercise but benefits the health of the entire body. Fluid Release movements free the muscles and surrounding tissues of fatigue-causing wastes that might otherwise take weeks to be fully metabolized. Following the initial massage movements toward the heart, wastes concentrated in the muscles begin to disperse. The effect on athletes? When acidic wastes are released from the muscles immediately after exercise, pain disappears, and pleasure takes its place.

Fatigue works directly on the body by slowing muscle recovery rates. Following an exercise session, the muscle recovery rate after five minutes of rest is usually about 20 percent. A person capable of doing fifty push-ups will, after five minutes of rest, be able to do ten more. But if five minutes of Fluid Release massage is substituted for the five minutes of rest, muscle recovery rates are *somewhere between 75 to more than 100 percent!* This astonishing

fact accounts for the extraordinary international record of East German track teams, whose runners are routinely massaged by individuals trained in methods of draining fatigue products from the muscles. For the same reason boxers are massaged, not rested, between rounds. Throughout the book you will find techniques based on the concept of Fluid Release, the basis of muscle recovery after any kind of exertion. When you remove fatigue products from the muscles, your partner comes out of an exercise session relaxed, smiling, and stronger.

You can add an hour of pleasure to an exercise experience you and your partner share by learning the massage technique in this book. In every case movements have been chosen because of their unique ability to enhance a wide range of exercise programs. Even if your partner isn't exercising, the movements will work as an absolutely splendid full body massage. Many of the strokes you will learn go beneath the skin to promote the health of internal organs like the liver and brain. On the most basic level massage is therapeutic simply because it is an intensely pleasurable experience. The idea of pleasure itself as therapy is grounded on the assumption that what most people want out of life is to have a good time. And anyone who has experienced the deliciously sensual haze that envelops one afterward understands that massage is one way of getting there.

---

* Douglas Graham, *Massage* (Philadelphia: Lippincott, 1913), p. 83.

The Pre~Massage Bath

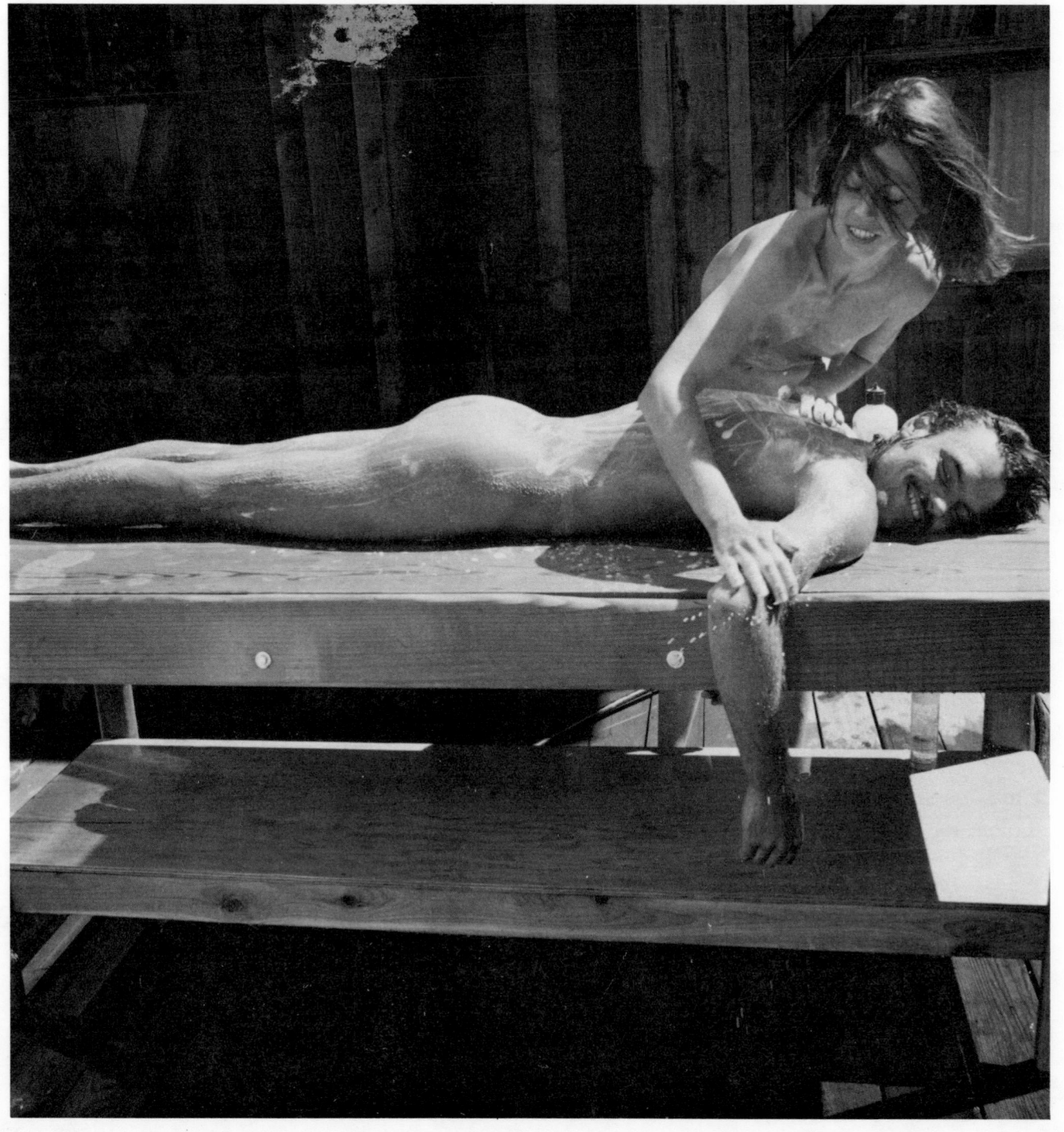

The Pre-Massage Bath

It was well-nigh midday when Petronius awoke, exceedingly wearied, as usual. He said himself that he felt exceedingly benumbed in the morning and had no power to collect his thoughts. But the morning bath and a careful kneading of the body done by the hands of skilful slaves gradually hastened the sluggish course of his blood, refreshed him, and enlivened him and restored his strength.
—HENRYK SIENKIEWICZ, Quo Vadis?

It's no accident that one of the most cherished additions to modern homes is the two- and three-car garage, not the two- and three-person bathroom. What can you say of a culture that takes better care of its cars than of the bodies of its citizens? Modern bathrooms, however lavishly appointed, are designed for the use of one person at a time, usually behind a locked door. These bathrooms operate like garages for the body, where quick efficient service is far more important than pleasure and the body itself is reduced to an object. Despite this depersonalization, bathing, like eating, is best enjoyed in a friendly, relaxed, communal atmosphere. If only because solitary bathers cannot even *see* half of their own bodies, the easiest way to bathe is together.

Despite centuries of antisensual conditioning, the joys of communal bathing are so irresistibly wholesome it's hard to believe there are still laws prohibiting this delicious experience in several states. Ordinary hot-water bathing cleans the body in a superficial way. Visible dirt is removed and, if you're lucky enough to have a full-size (read antique) bathtub, you can go part of the way toward actually relaxing your body. It's possible that biological engineers of the future will find a way to fit the human race into compact cars, truly stylish shoes, and minibathtubs. Until that time modern bathtubs will remain somewhat difficult for those of us who have not had gymnastics and happen to be more than four and a half feet tall. If you want to double your partner's enjoyment of an ordinary massage, you have to help clean his or her body totally before you begin. To do this, you must go far beyond the confines of minibathtubs and mere soap and water.

The tactile sense is the original sense, the first sense developed by the most ancient single-celled creatures on earth. For 3 billion years they have lived in a dark, utterly silent world where every-thing that is known is felt. In human beings the tactile sense is the primary sense.

Apart from the brain itself, the skin is the body's most complex organ. Any square inch of it contains hundreds of pleasure, pain, pressure, heat, and cold receptors. In the same square inch you can find fifteen feet of blood vessels and about seventy-two feet of nerves. Skin is the

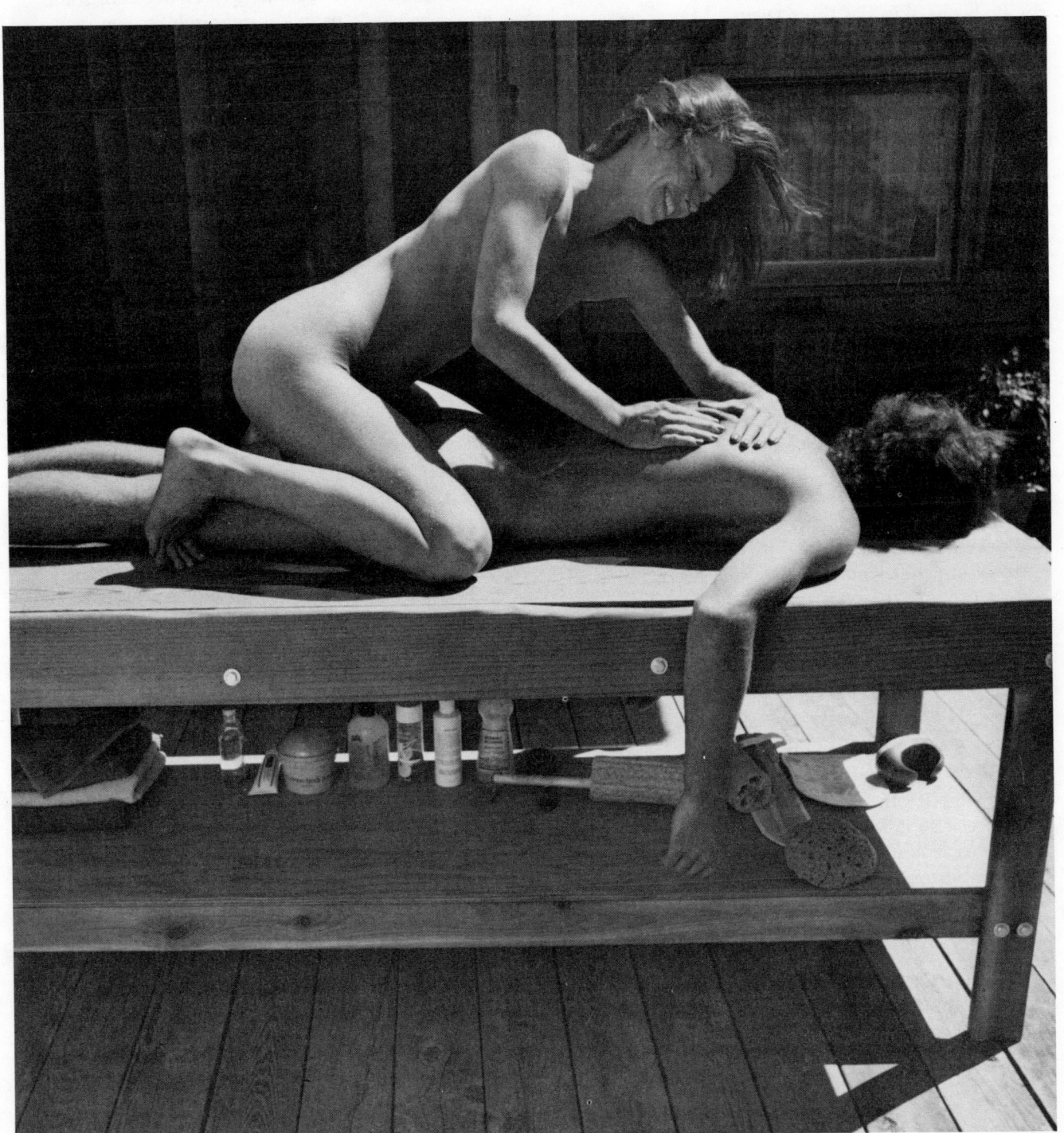

"eye" of the nervous system. Every massage movement will contact it directly. Its thickness can vary from about one-fiftieth of an inch on the eyelids to as much as one-third of an inch on the palms and soles. Throughout the body the skin has three layers which fit together snugly via countless ridges and valleys. The two inner layers are covered with a rich carpet of blood vessels, glands, nerves, and fat lobules. Part of the exposed top layer is made of a horny material that is actually dead skin cells. These dead cells can clog the pores and keep the skin from feeling and breathing naturally. Part of the exhilaration that follows a good bath comes from discarding some of this dead, horny layer of skin.

Puritanical attitudes toward the body are nowhere more apparent than in the bathing habits common to most Americans. People bathe merely to remove dirt from their bodies, not to feel anything. We have a nation obsessed with gratification that ignores the most basic sense and the body's largest organ.

Since all massage movements affect the skin, the aim of the premassage bath is to clean the skin far more thoroughly than ordinary soap-and-water bathing. The idea is to bring the skin to a point where it can feel and then stimulate it so it will feel. By doing this, you increase the tactile possibilities for the entire massage, and no matter how much massage your partner has experienced, he will notice a difference after a premassage bath. Even before the massage begins, your partner becomes relaxed and totally aware of his body.

Studies of very old people all over the world reveal one factor common to all of them: Throughout their lives they sweat copiously every day. This curious fact, often cited by sauna enthusiasts, would seem to imply that the oceans of sweat generated after fifteen minutes in a sauna can actually extend one's life. But the kind of sweating these old folks do is usually the result of good old-fashioned manual labor, still popular in those parts of the world where leisure time is scarce and exercise for its own sake has not yet become fashionable. The idea that it is healthful or even generally beneficial to roast your body, which is mostly water, at temperatures very near the boiling

point of water is certainly debatable. Many people bolt from the sauna in four or five minutes, hearts racing, feeling slightly dizzy, and doubting their own senses. Wasn't this supposed to be a relaxing experience? For some people it definitely is; you may not be one of them. One of the most important considerations in any bath is the way one feels afterward.

Saunas, Jacuzzis, and hot tubs are expensive to set up and use huge amounts of energy. (If you already have one and want to use it with massage, please see "How Bath Temperatures Affect the Body," page 26). A body shampoo costs practically nothing and uses less energy than a shower. It

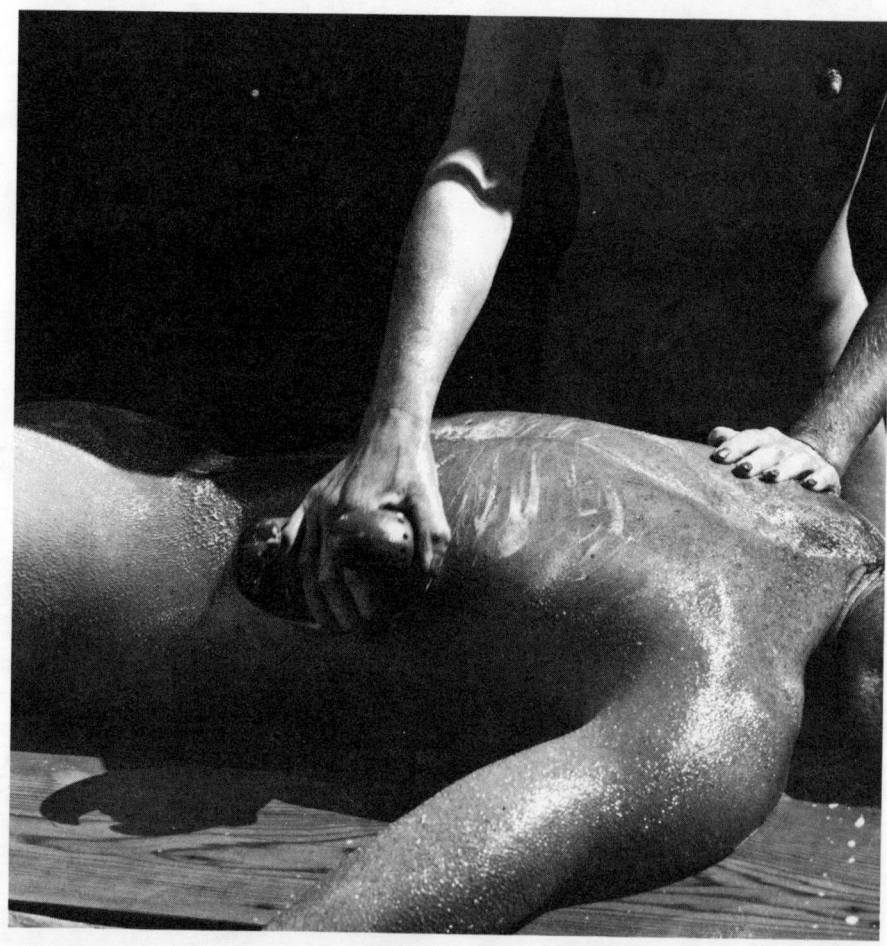

will leave your partner feeling absolutely wonderful without using 800 gallons of hot water, a specially designed redwood room, or high-speed electrical devices. During a body shampoo, you become directly involved with the bath by using your own hands, thus establishing the kind of close physical contact you will be sharing during the massage. The body shampoo will do even more for your skin than a sauna, without taxing the heart or making you sweat. If massage is your aim, it's better to sweat and exercise your heart when you exercise your body. Use the body shampoo to get your partner cleaner than he's ever been in his life. It's the ideal introduction to the world of massage—you can lie back and do absolutely nothing but feel. For most people the experience of being bathed becomes a dreamy sort of return to early childhood, the last time anyone touched or bathed their entire body.

The most important aspect of communal bathing is simply the experience of being bathed by another person. This is easiest on a bath table, but if you don't have space, you can certainly improvise in your own bathtub or shower. Use soap and a flexible

shower spray to direct water to specific parts of your partner's body. A shampoo brush, loofah, or bath mitt will loosen the dead surface layer of skin and stimulate the growth of new cells. These simple tools leave your partner's skin relaxed and glowing the first time you use them. Cover the whole body with soft round strokes. You can use pressures on the back and legs which are virtually impossible for an individual bathing alone.

Almost as delightful as being bathed by another person and equally foreign to the experience of most Americans is the exotic sensation of being oiled. A very light bath oil can be prepared simply by mixing one part almond with two parts sesame seed oil. Add a bit of lemon to restore the skin's slightly acidic pH. Bath oil replaces natural skin oils that are always lost to soap and water. Oil the skin after a bath and salt rub.

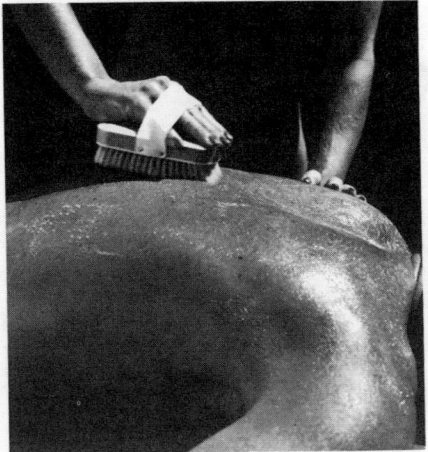

Salt rubs are not for the timid or extremely sensitive. They are massively stimulating and, for those who enjoy them, absolutely indispensable. If your partner has a lot of body hair, this is one way to amplify the cleansing action of a body shampoo substantially. The effects of a brief salt rub are immediately apparent and visible. Skin reddening all over the body gives direct evidence of the enormous potential this treatment has as a circulation stimulant. Beyond that, the salt rub acts as a kind of general tonic for the entire body. The salt's mildly abrasive effect will remove all the skin debris you may have missed during the body shampoo and leave your partner tingling.

You need to moisten your partner's body slightly with a damp washcloth to temper the abrasive action of the salt on skin. For the same reason it's best to dampen the salt a bit before you begin. Use coarse salt if possible.

Take a moment to be sure there are no cuts or tender spots anywhere on your partner's body. Salt will irritate them and spoil the effect of the rub. Go easy on the face. Avoid the area around the eyes and mouth.

Once you've moistened the whole body, cover your washcloth with a moderately thick layer of salt. Salt, like massage oil, is more easily controlled when you add it to your hand and avoid dumping it onto the skin. Any rubbing that precedes a massage should imitate the rhythms of massage. Try to avoid jerky scrubbing motions on broad expanses of the body like the torso and back. The salt rub will be far more effective if you work over your partner's body with vigorous, even, circular strokes. Use the entire flat surface of your hands. Press down and circle with the washcloth while your free hand circles against the skin. Pressures should be about equal. When you've covered every part of the body with at least three vigorous circles, wash the salt off with warm water, and dry your partner.

One sad consequence of living with high stress levels is that a great many people walk around with cold hands and feet. The best way to warm them up along with the rest of the body is with large soft hot towels. You can warm towels by placing them inside a large paper bag and putting it in the oven for ten minutes at 200 degrees. As long as the paper bag isn't exposed to an open flame, it will not burn and your towels will be warm and perfectly dry. If you are fortunate enough to have a towel large enough to reach from head to toe, you can cover your partner's body with a single movement. Working with smaller towels, begin at the feet and overlap the

towels until the body is covered. Whatever size, the towels should go down with one long sweeping motion. Everything that touches your partner during the massage, whether it be your hands, your hair, your knee, or a hot towel, becomes a part of the massage. Because your partner will experience the massage with his eyes closed, the tactile sense is exquisitely sensitized. To help establish the mood, use the same speed and rhythm in laying down the hot towels that you will use later on the legs and arms.

When your partner's entire body is covered, from scalp to toes, pat the towel gently so that it conforms to the outlines of the arms, legs, and torso. This luxurious sensation of being pressed and patted prepares your partner for the warm, infinitely relaxing experience that is about to begin.

Leave the towels on for about five minutes. When you're ready to remove them, pull the bottom edge of the towel slowly and evenly until the top of the towel gradually breaks contact with your partner's toes.

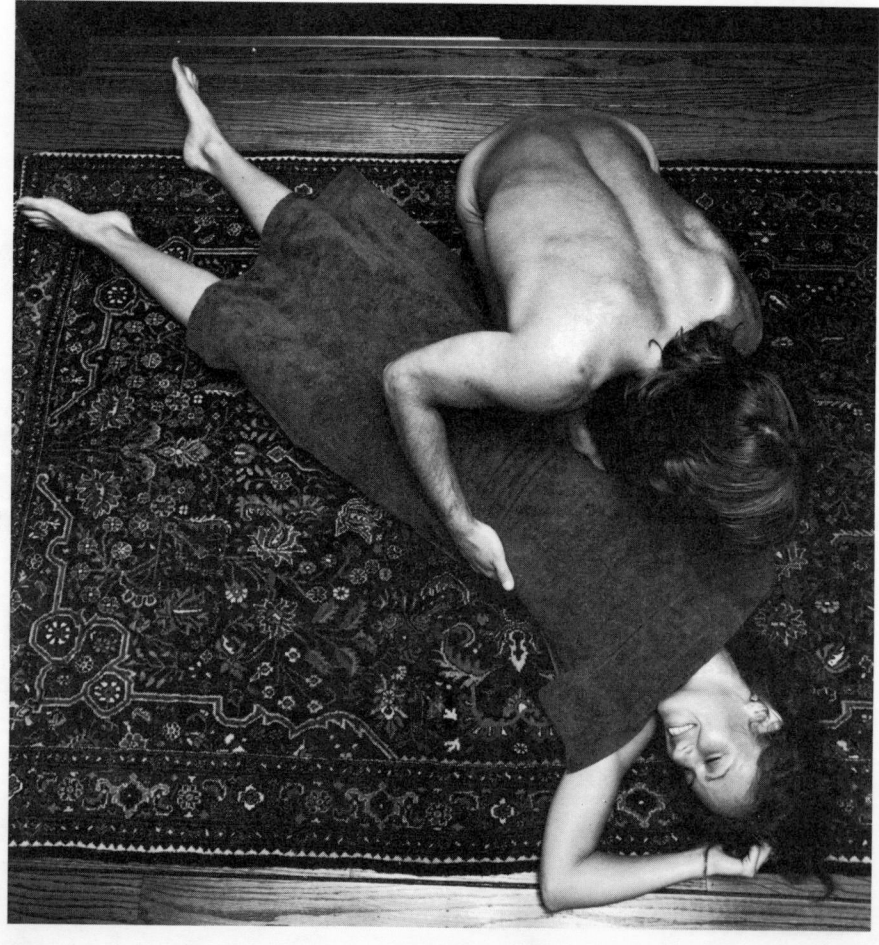

Hair Brushing the Body

In the dark the hair rules.
—ROBERT DUNCAN

After the bath, just before you oil for the first time, your partner's skin is intensely sensitized. If you have long hair, this is the time to use it. Considering the fact that your partner may have just run several miles or played a game of squash, it may seem rather superficial merely to brush your hair across the back and legs. Remember, though, that the point of

exercise is not only to strengthen but to awaken the body. Begin by slowly covering your partner's head with your hair. This wordless gesture will help him to relax even more and to take the first step toward receiving a massage: closing his eyes.

Hair brushing is a little like dance. You must learn to move your body smoothly as you descend so that the hair flows across your partner's body in a single, long, uninterrupted motion. When you reach the feet, turn slowly, without breaking contact, and return to the head.

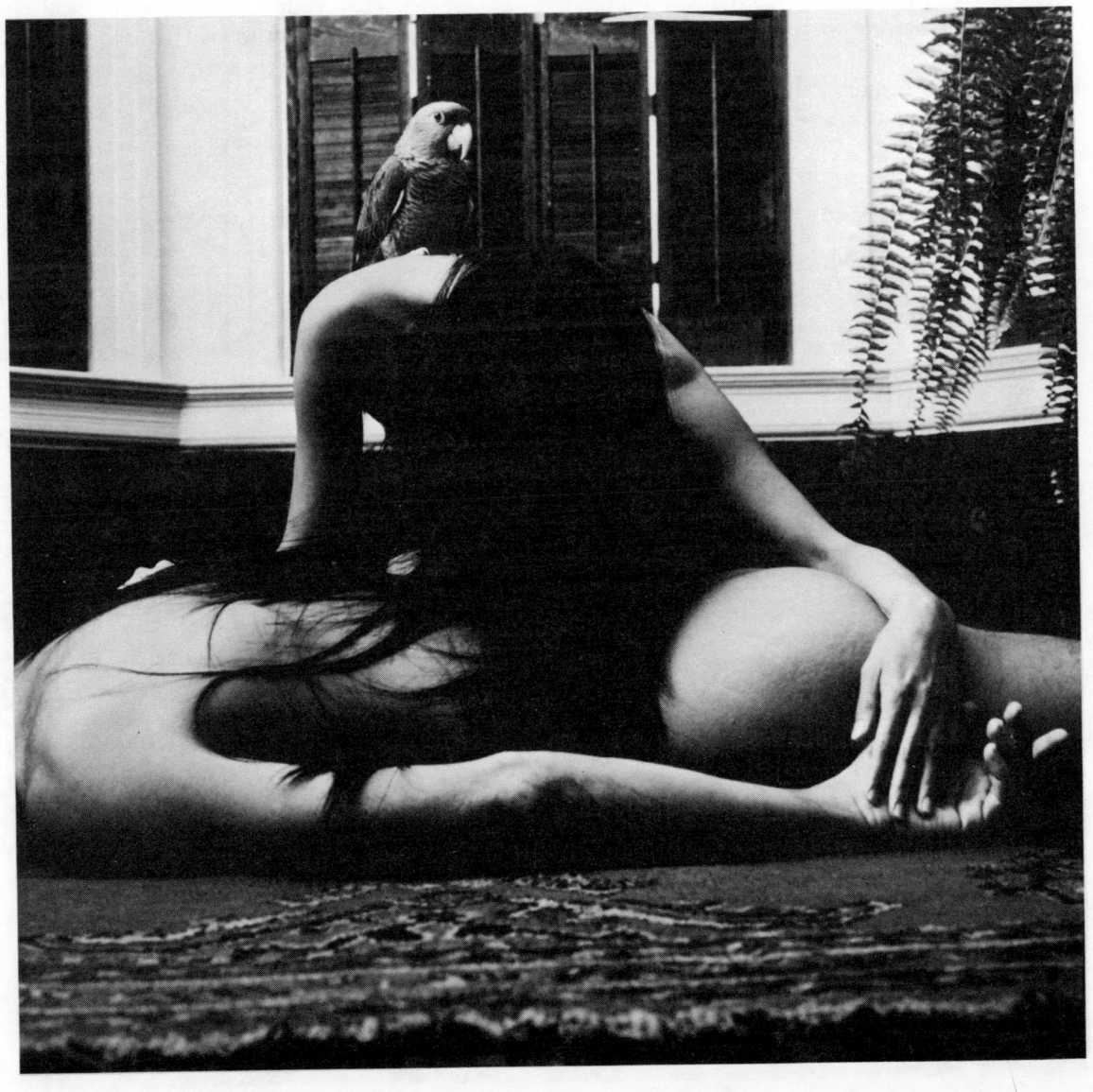

Like massage itself, premassage bathing works best on a surface where no muscles are used to support any part of the body. On a bath table the body shampoo experience is so close to massage that it's always fun to go ahead and blend the two. With the addition of a four-inch foam pad a bath table can double as a massage table, or if your partner doesn't mind the extra stiffness of soft wood, it can serve as is.

Bath tables do require a certain amount of drainage. A deck, yard, pool, or even a flat rooftop will do. In a natural setting with a temperature warm enough for swimming, you can use your bath table and continue with massage on the spot.

Here is a bath table that will double as a very fine massage table. One person can build it in a weekend. It can be left outdoors throughout the warm months or, when the hex bolts are removed, can be taken apart for storage in less than an hour. You can set it up in the outer room of a sauna or in a warm corner of your living room. Wherever you put it, this table seems to invite people to collapse onto it for hours at a time. A surprising number of people have always wanted to do that on a table.

All the pieces in the plans are cut to a size that will comfortably accommodate most adults. If much of your massaging involves small children, you may want to

vary the table width to support your partner's arms at the elbows when they are folded over the sides. You can also shorten or lengthen the legs as necessary, so that the actual massage surface is just below your waist. If you make changes in the height of the table, be sure to compensate for the optional foam pad which, when compressed, adds about two extra inches.

Remember that every part of the table will be exposed to water. Discuss this question with your lumber supplier, and choose a soft wood that can be adequately sealed against moisture.

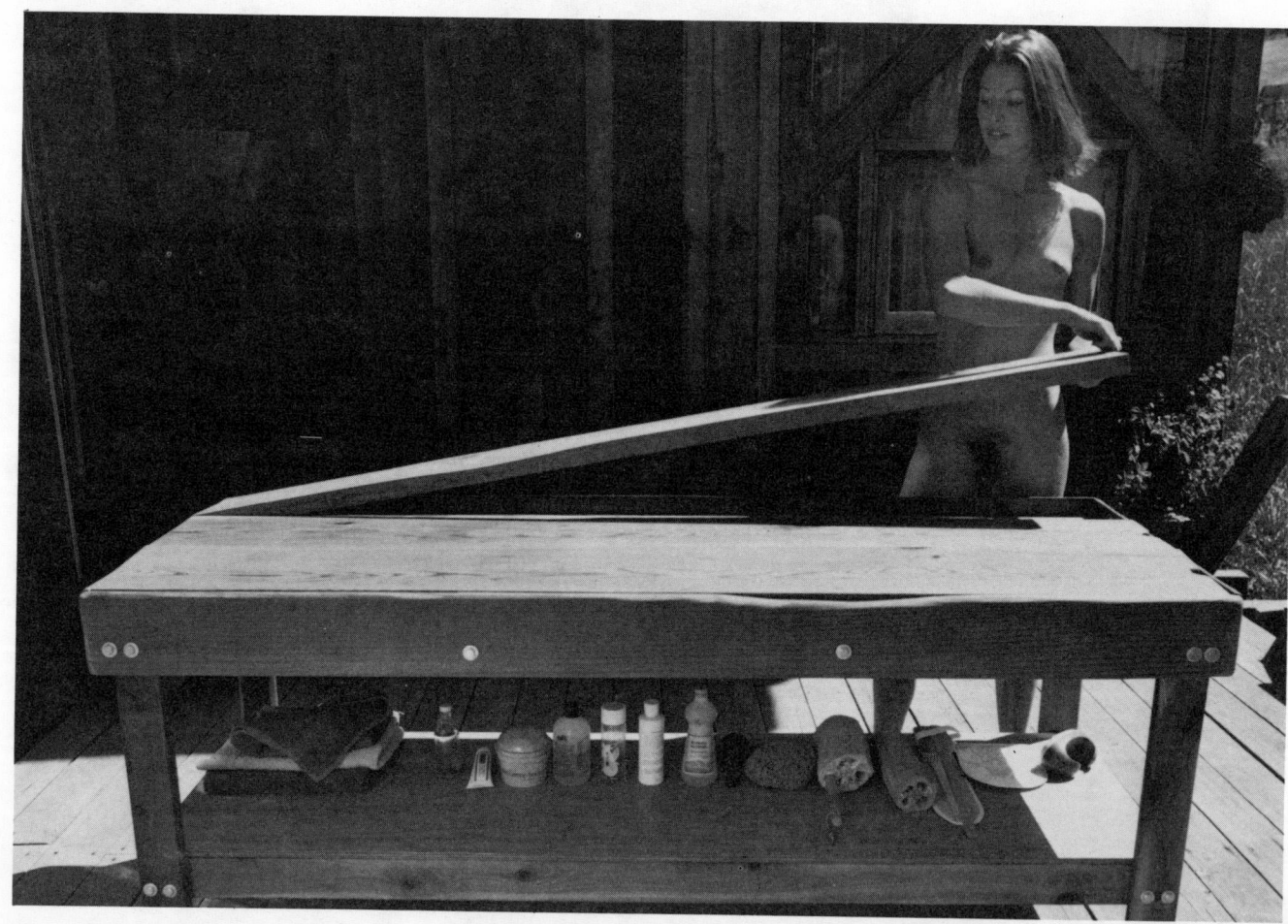

Cut a four-inch piece of foam rubber to the exact size of your tabletop. Covered with a bed pad and sheet, this cushion provides a nearly perfect surface for massage. The lower table can be used for storage of oils, towels, a vibrator, alcohol, or even clothes. If you decide to use the table "as is" without adding a foam pad, expect a bit of oil to get on the body support boards. These boards can easily be removed and washed after the massage.

Small people can do things with big people on a massage table that just aren't possible on the floor. Don't give up on the body lifts you'll be learning throughout the book until you have tried them on a table; you'll be surprised by how much easier massage becomes.

Elevate the legs opposite your drainage holes with one-inch shims. This will allow most of the water to flow out the drainage end. Water sources can vary, but they must include a way to rinse your partner with warm water. If you're improvising, a shower extension connected to a bathtub or sink will work, or you can haul warm water to the table in a bucket. Remove towels and anything else on the lower table that might be affected by water. After the bath you can rinse the body support boards and set them up to dry.

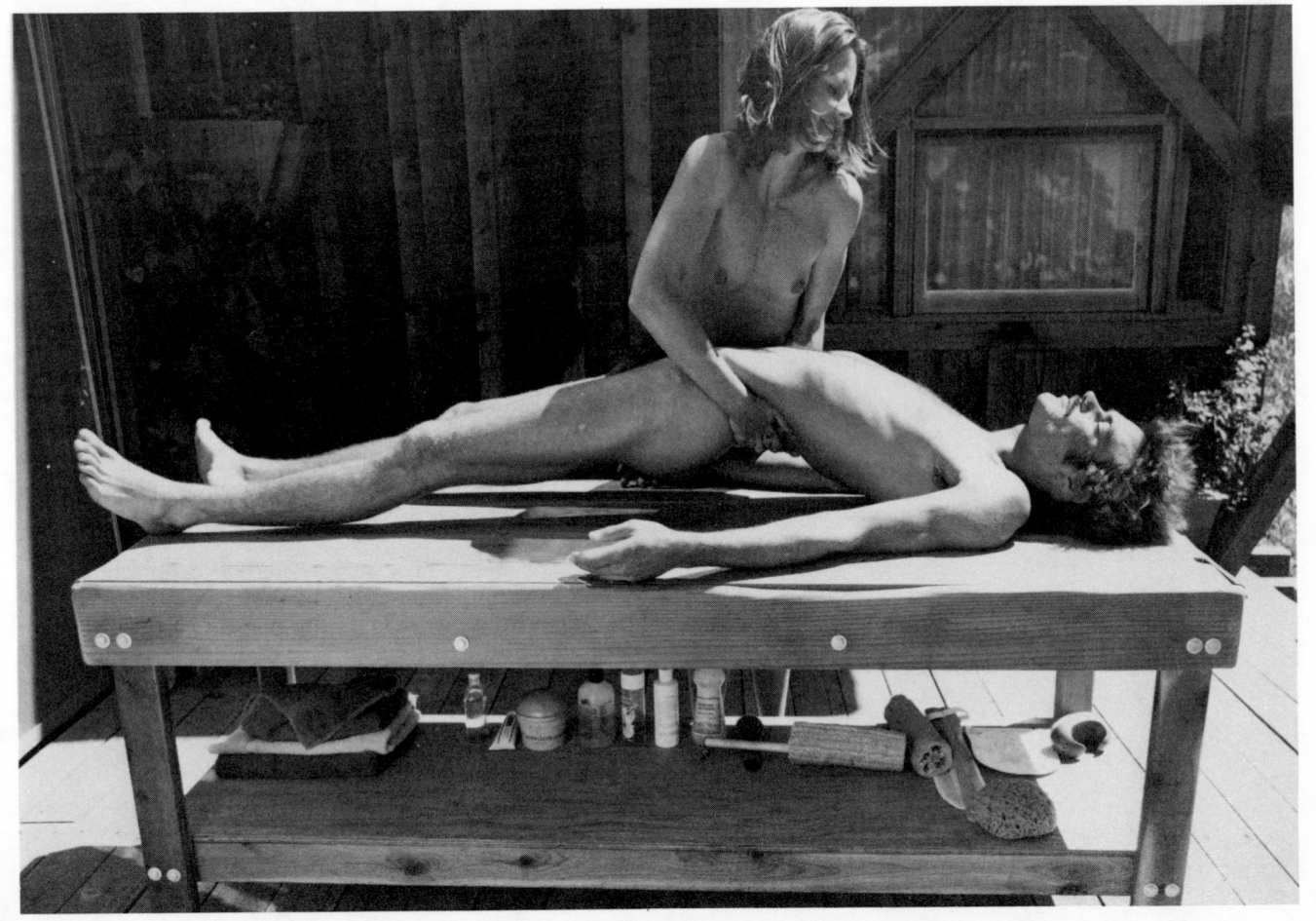

Dimensions: 76″ long × 30″ wide × 30″ high

Materials

2 sheets ½″ shopgrade plywood
38 linear feet soft wood 2 × 4
19 linear feet soft wood 1 × 6
21 linear feet soft wood 2 × 10
8 ⅜″ hex bolts 4½″ long with flat and lock washers and nuts
8 ⅜″ hex bolts 3½″ long with flat and lock washers and nuts
4 ⅜″ hex bolts 3″ long with flat and lock washers and nuts
8 #10″ flathead screws with washers
1 pint latex paint
1 quart clear resin sealer
1 pound 1½″ finishing nails
miscellaneous sandpaper and steel wool

Read all the way through these instructions once before beginning to work on your table.

1. Out of a 2 × 4 cut 4 legs 28″ long.

2. Out of a 2 × 4 cut 4 table supports 74½″ long.

3. Cut the upper plywood table to 74½″ × 28½″.

4. Cut the lower plywood table to 74½″ × 22¼″.

5. Out of the 2 × 10, cut 3 pieces to 74½″. These are the body support boards.

6. Out of the 1 × 6, cut 2 pieces 74½″ and 2 pieces to 30″. These are your table supports.

7. Pencil in two squared-off lines at each end of your table supports. The first line should be 1⅛″ from the end, and the second line should be 2⅜″ from the end.

8. Find and mark the center of each line. At that point drill a ⅜″ hole.

9. On two of the table legs select one end to be the bottom. Square off a line 12″ from that end. Now lay these legs on a flat surface so they are parallel to each other and 74½″ apart.

10. Lay one of the table supports along these 12″ lines, and be sure that each end of the table support is flush with the outer edge of the leg. The leg and the table support should form a perfect 90-degree angle. Once you've lined up the legs and the table support, mark the legs for drilling by inserting a pencil through the ⅜″ holes drilled in the table support.

11. Repeat this process with two other legs and another table support. Once you have all four legs marked, go ahead and drill the 8 new holes with a ⅜″ bit.

12. Attach the smaller tabletop to the upper part of the two table supports with glue and finishing nails.

13. Match up the legs with their supports by lining up the holes you've drilled in them. Insert the 4½″ hex bolts with washers and nuts. Tighten them just a bit.

14. Attach the larger upper table to its supports using the same procedure you followed in No. 12.

15. Hold one of the 74½″ 1 × 6's flush against the bottom and ends of an upper table support. With a pencil make a mark on the 1 × 6 through the holes of the support.

16. Do the same thing on the other side, and drill all eight holes in the 1 × 6.

17. Place the upper table so that the plywood rests on top of the legs and the supports are on the outside. Adjust the legs so they are flush with the ends of the upper table. Once you've done this, tighten up the lower table bolt assembly, and drill holes into the legs by inserting the drill through the upper table support holes.

18. Insert the bolt assemblies through the 1 × 6 and corresponding holes in the table supports and legs. Tighten them.

19. Place the 30″ 1 × 6's flush against the ends of the upper table supports. Drill for 2″ #10 screws, and tighten down the screws.

20. Finish the upper tabletop and inside of 1 × 6 to protect against moisture.

21. Lay the 2 × 10 body supports inside the 1 × 6 frame.

22. Sand all sharp edges that can contact the body and the tops of your 2 × 10 body supports. Buff with steel wool. Seal all exposed surfaces of the table with several coats of preserva-tive. After the final coat of preservative, buff the whole surface one more time until all the stickiness is gone.

23. (Optional.) Insert 2½" plywood shims lengthwise at the joints between the outside and inside 2 × 10 body supports. This will slightly raise the center of the table, make it more comfortable for some folks, and facilitate drainage.

24. Drill small holes at one end of the plywood upper table for drainage.

25. Notch the ends of the body support boards so they can be lifted easily. Color code the three boards by dabbing a bit of color on the ends to match a color on the inside of the 1 × 6 frame.

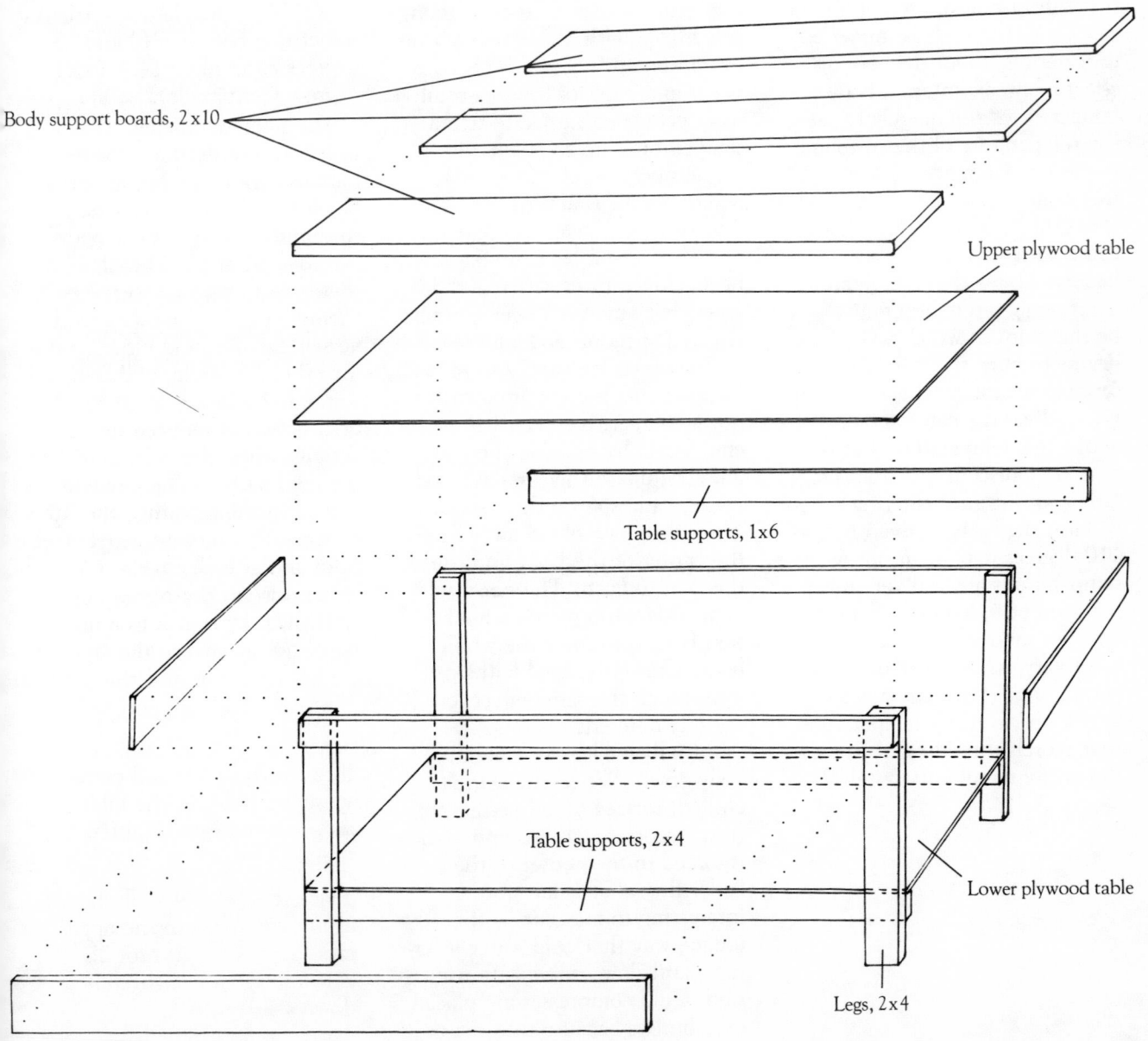

Body support boards, 2 x 10

Upper plywood table

Table supports, 1x6

Table supports, 2 x 4

Lower plywood table

Legs, 2 x 4

How Bath Temperatures Affect the Body

If after a cold bath or shower the patron comes out chilly, shivering, blue-lipped or goose fleshed, it indicates that her body reaction is not good.
—FRANK NICHOLS, Theory and Practice of Body Massage

The difference between a hot bath that strains the body and one that leaves you feeling great may be just a degree or two. The 2 million sweat glands that cool the skin in hot air are neutralized as soon as the body is immersed in water. Without the cooling effect of sweat, internal body temperatures rise quickly to meet the temperature of the surrounding water. Commercial fever thermometers are not calibrated above 110 degrees Fahrenheit because patients are not expected to be alive above that temperature. That temperature also happens to be the point at which water begins to burn the skin and seriously to tax the heart. Certain rare individuals can tolerate baths above this temperature, but they should be discouraged from bragging about it and tempting others to burn themselves. Even below 110 degrees maximum hot-water temperatures are still very much a question of individual tolerance. Because internal body temperatures vary, as do metabolic rates, people should not attempt to "work up" to water temperatures that scorch the skin and strain the entire circulatory system.

Sauna and hot tub enthusiasts who want to combine their favorite bath with massage should consider investing in a good (submersible for hot tubs) thermometer. Overheated bathers usually cannot stand any further stimulation, and massage becomes difficult or impossible. Bath fans who simply cannot take the extreme temperatures their hot-tubbing friends relish may find relief in a steam bath. Whether the steam is in a cabinet or room, it is mixed with air, which acts as insulation and allows the body to sweat and cool itself. As a result, most people can tolerate steam temperatures up to about 140 degrees Fahrenheit. In saunas, where the air is almost totally dry, tolerance levels rise even higher. Some folks can take dry heat temperatures above 200 degrees, but saunas can certainly be enjoyed at more moderate levels.

Trust your feelings, and remember that a communal bath is not a competitive event. In general, warm baths relax the muscles, dilate the surface blood vessels, and soothe the nerves. They also draw blood away from the center of the body and cause the skin to flush. The net result of all this warm gentle stimulation is relaxation of the whole body. Curiously, cold baths can have much the same effect for entirely different reasons.

Initially cold baths slow the body down. When the skin is chilled, surface blood vessels contract, muscles tighten, and blood is forced to the center of the body. But what is far more interesting to masseurs is the unique way that cold water interrupts and slows nervous transmission. Cold compresses are placed over bruises because they act as a natural painkiller. This simple analgesic effect can readily be extended to the whole body when it is immersed in cold water for three to five minutes. If a cold-water bath isn't available, a cold shower with good pressure will do almost as well. Cold water will, of course, absorb body heat, and it's wise to experiment with temperatures that are bearable. The range of tolerable cold-water temperatures is wider than that of hot water. Most people will settle on something between 40 and 65 degrees Fahrenheit (4.4 and 18.3 degrees Centigrade).

The immediate effect of cold water is to tense the surface muscles, contract the surface blood vessels, and drive the blood toward the center of the body. But as soon as a cold bath is over, these reactions tend to reverse themselves. The surface blood vessels expand, and blood rushes into them. Muscles and skin feel warm and relaxed. Even so, the brief period of reduced nerve activity while the body is still *in* the cold bath can be absolutely crucial in the relaxing of a jittery personality. Nervous people feel calm and at ease after a cold bath because when the nerves reawaken, they return to a normal state, not an overstimulated one.

Preparing for Massage

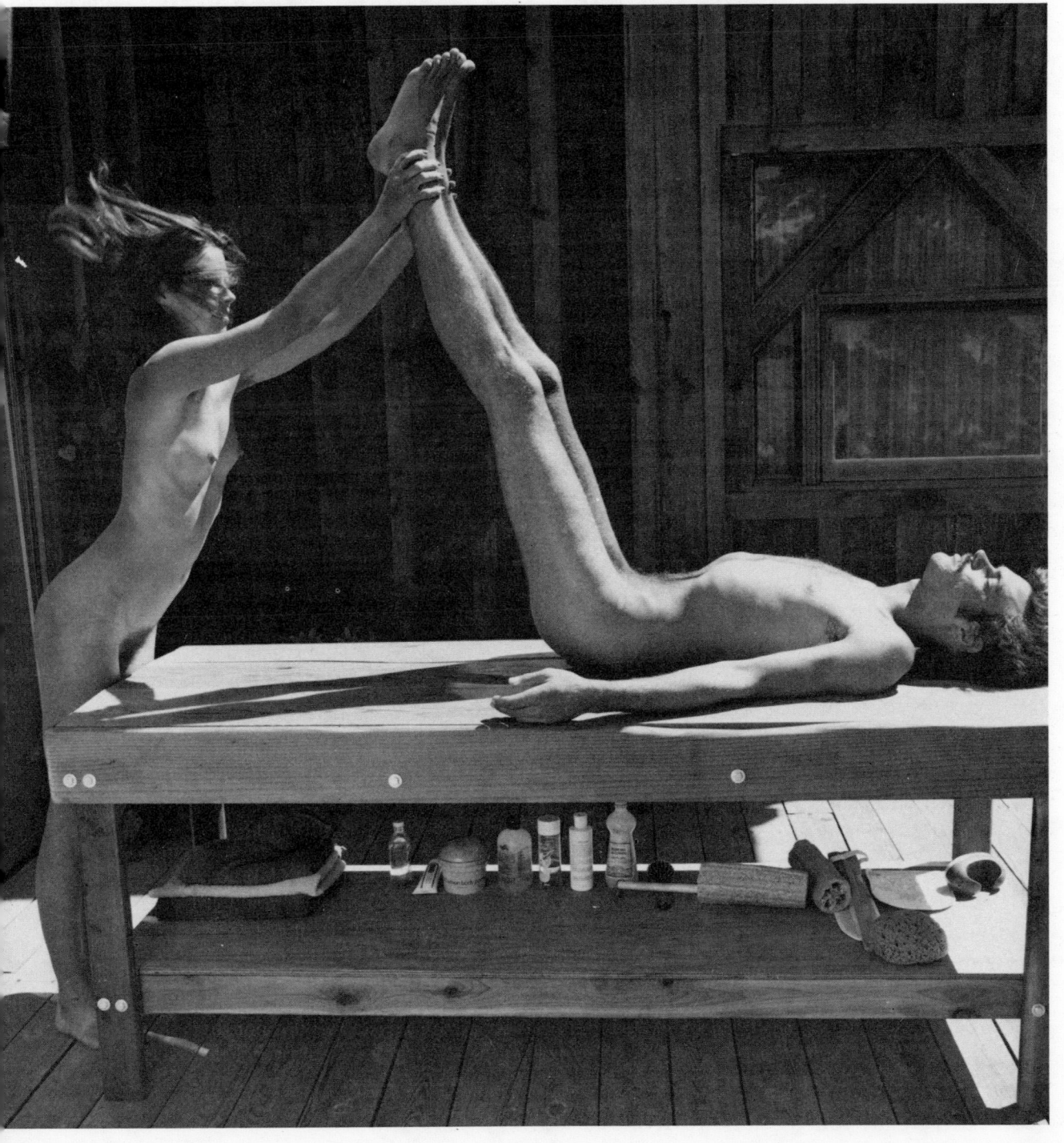

Preparing for Massage

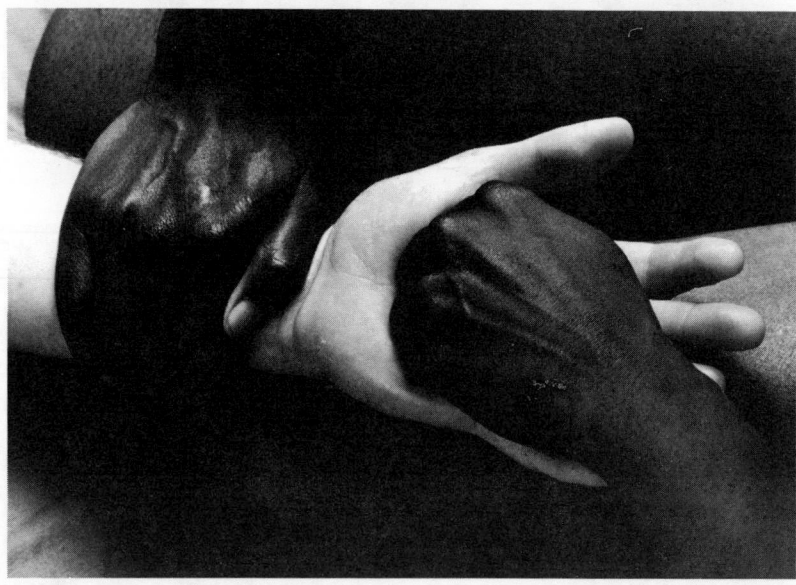

Since massage reaches so many of the senses at once, there should be no interruptions or distractions while you work. The experience is so relaxing and pleasurable that your partner has the chance to yield and become utterly sensitized. Something similar happens to audiences during any serious theatrical effort, and that's why actors don't interrupt a performance to rearrange sets or accept phone calls.

If you view massage as a theatrical situation, you can arrange your place so that very little will distract you or your partner during the experience. Of course, it's not always possible to massage where there are no distractions at all. It's worthwhile, though, to make every effort to quiet things down around your massage area. The obvious distractions to consider right away are ones that might force you to abandon the massage altogether. Make sure that children are cared for and that you're not expecting company. Can you manage to live without phone calls for a few hours? Do you have demanding pets that are likely to bound into the massage area without warning? Your partner will experience the massage with eyes closed, and this, of course, intensifies all the other senses. You may take for granted automatic appliances that switch on and off, television programs in the next room, and the smell of food cooking. Don't expect your partner to miss any of this. Sounds and smells that are routinely shut out can dominate your partner's consciousness during massage. If you're working in a crowded environment where it's difficult to control all these factors, you can provide your own sounds and scents. Choose sounds that your partner likes. You might want to look through a record collection, choose a radio station, or merely open a window to let in the sound of falling rain. Scents are discussed on page 29.

The area where you massage should be warm and inviting. The temperature on the massage surface must be at least 70 degrees Fahrenheit. If you're working on the floor the room temperature will have to be somewhat higher. You may be sweating after the massage, but remember that your partner will be very sensitive to drafts and cold air. Chilled muscles will contract and completely ruin the massage. Warm your hands by pressing them under your armpits before you touch your partner.

You don't need bright lights to learn these movements or do massage. Brilliant overhead lighting will serve to remind your partner of his last stay in a hospital. Long-burning candles and oil lamps are great favorites.

You do need some padding under your partner, but a sleeping bag will do as well as a Persian rug. In fact, ordinary bed sheets will smooth out the massage surface and are easily cleaned if oil staining occurs. Whatever you decide on, be sure your massage area is very clean.

Most of the massage movements in the book are cycles that move across the body and return to the spot where they begin. Each cycle should be repeated at least three times. The long ones, like the circulation movements for the limbs and back, will easily stand ten repetitions.

Even while you're learning the movements, everything you do is going to feel very good. People love to be touched, and no machine, surface, or material has ever been devised to improve upon human hands.

The familiar resistance to physical contact, so common in the United States, merely reinforces old puritanical fears that the body is dirty and animalistic. These same nervous fears probably control and inhibit the sense of smell. The fact that life is full of very pleasant fragrances is not always apparent to many Americans [until they have visited countries where markets smell like produce and small towns are scented by wild flowers.] Your partner's office, school, bedroom, and car all may smell suspiciously like the same cleanser, but there is no reason why a massage area must follow suit.

So many dreams and memories are associated with forgotten scents that the specific scent of your massage area is very important. Incense has probably been used to make people feel good as long as massage itself. One stick or cone will scent most rooms for the duration of a massage. Your partner may have a preference; if not, you may want to experiment with the exquisitely delicate Japanese perfume incenses or a stronger natural wood scent like piñon or juniper from New Mexico.

LEONATO: *Indeed, he looks younger than he did, by the loss of a beard.*
DON PEDRO: *Nay, a' rubs himself with civet. . . .*
WILLIAM SHAKESPEARE, Much Ado About Nothing

After tailfins, power windows, air pots, remote digital TV tuning, instant breakfast, and plant growth hormones, you can't say that America does not deserve commercial massage oils which sell for more than a dollar an ounce. These oils are not brought up from deep wells in Saudi Arabia; they're purchased wholesale from cooking oil distributors for something less than a dollar a quart. Once the oil is saturated with an overwhelming scent, it is bottled in chic little glass or plastic containers and *named*. One hopes a poor writer was well paid for dreaming up these awesome names. They suggest some ancient forgotten culture or fabulously rare perfume, an obscure religious ceremony or the essence of unimaginably rare flowers. Somehow, it is hoped, these exotic names will manage to justify the horrifying odors which are blithely tacked onto ordinary vegetable oils. Or perhaps the point is merely to intimidate the buyer enough to justify the unbelievable price that appears next to the name on the label. Either way, the fact that your massage oil bears a name evoking Hindu mythology does not give you license to spread a fluid across your partner's body which would offend the Board of Health.

29

Anyone who is capable of finding the way to a food market can bring home a quart of massage oil for less than two dollars. Safflower, coconut, almond, any of the clear light vegetable oils are wonderful for massage. A quart can be scented with six drops of lemon extract or your partner's favorite essence. An ordinary bowl can be used to hold oil. Better yet, put your blend in a narrow-spout plastic squeeze bottle recycled from ketchup, Vaseline, or shampoo. Squeeze bottles don't spill all over your massage area (and your partner) the way bowls do when you hit them with your knee. Some squeeze bottles have shutoff valves built into the cap, a handy feature that ensures against oil spill if the bottle is knocked over. If you're using one of these bottles, be sure not to break contact with your partner when you shut off the valve.

Massage oil should always be warm. If you warm it in a glass bottle set in simmering hot water before you begin the massage, you will not need to warm it again once the oil is transferred to a plastic bottle.

Oiling lubricates the skin and makes stroking and kneading smooth and comfortable. You'll use it on every part of the body. Always add the oil to your hands, and then stroke it onto your partner's body, using the whole flat surface of your hands. The sensation of being oiled is immediately relaxing and will serve as your partner's introduction to massage on most parts of the body. Add more oil whenever your hands begin to pull against the skin. Oil can be removed with a warm towel after you massage each part of the body. Some people enjoy the way it feels on their skin and like to live with it for a few hours.

Like lovemaking and yoga, massage is a kind of primal dance. It's very important that your rhythms be consistent throughout. Tiny movements like kneading the ball of the thumb should have the same speed as a circulation stroke on the back or legs. Consistent rhythms have a soothing, almost hypnotic effect on the nervous system. It's easy to establish your rhythm as soon as you begin working on your partner, then to maintain the same speed as the strokes flow into one another. Every contact, no matter how inconsequential, becomes a part of the experience because the tactile sense is exquisitely sensitized during massage. Try to avoid random, jerky motions.

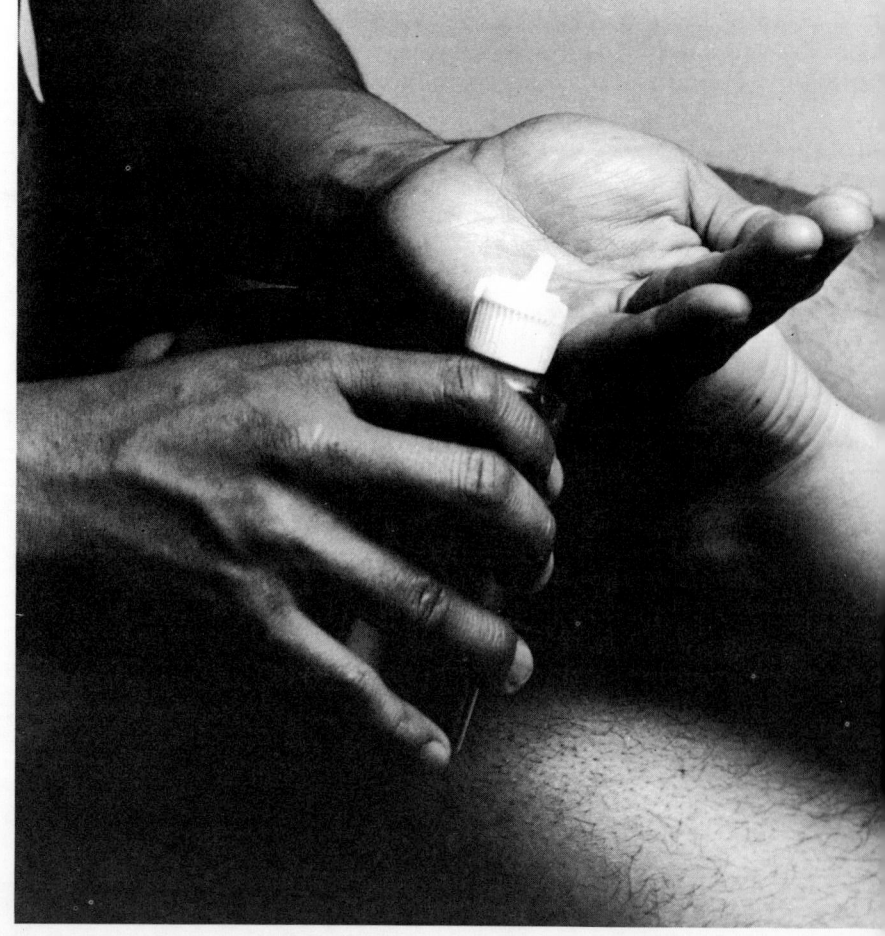

Even though massage will eventually bring peace to the most nervous personality, some people get very tense just before you lay hands on them. If you find that your partner is lying rigidly on the massage surface as though awaiting the approach of a surgeon, a few simple preliminary relaxation techniques will help make the transition to that special place where the body will surrender all tension.

Generally it's best not to use the word "relax" when you want someone to relax. Far too many people remember that word delivered as a terse command while some bored nurse swabbed alcohol on the left buttock. Whenever you want to help your partner experience movements more fully, make suggestions instead of giving orders. You might suggest that the head will be more comfortable if it's turned slightly. Pick it up gently and begin to turn it as you make the suggestion. If premassage relaxation is your goal, you might suggest that your partner make himself as heavy as possible: let the weight of his body sink through the table or floor. To help your partner get into that utterly relaxed "heavy" state, he can intentionally tense up his body and then, while breathing very deeply, allow all the tension to leave the muscles. This allows a tense individual to *feel* the difference between tension and relaxation.

Many people feel a great deal of tension simply because they are constantly preoccupied with personal problems. Since massage animates the tactile sense, the body's primary sense, the experience has a remarkable way of bringing people into the here and now. But the exhilarating trans-

formation that occurs during almost any full body massage will not take place if your partner is encouraged to dwell on problems, plans, dreams, or ambitions. Certainly he must trust you to begin a massage. But that trust need not compel him to pour out his most personal secrets.

Whatever you choose to say before the massage begins should be light and positive. Since the tone you use is far more important than concepts or words, it's useful to remember that there's something pleasing about every body and every day of the year.

Try to eliminate noise and finally conversation itself. Words come between your partner and the feeling.

Where does your body end? Does the skin really mark the boundary between you and the rest of the universe? It may not after a full body massage in a quiet natural place. The body seems to melt, and people feel intimately connected to earth, sky, and the living things around them. To prepare your partner for this incomparable moment, think about some of the preparations you made before indoor massage. Is the massage area clean and soft? Will there be sudden interruptions? Are the towels and oil close by? Is there enough room to move around your partner comfortably? Outdoor massage does call for a few unique preparations, and most of them have to do with

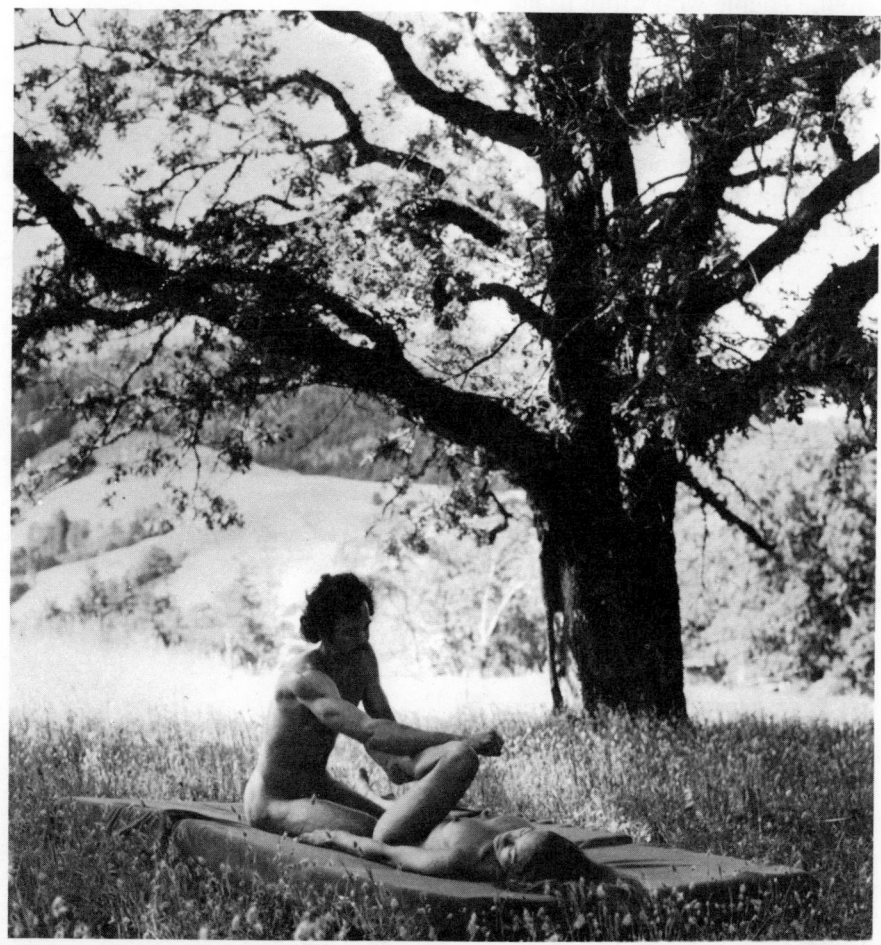

temperature. It's important to remember that your massage *surface* should be at least 70 degrees Fahrenheit. If the sun is intense, you may want to stay out of the direct rays. Who knows how much time will pass from the beginning of the massage to the moment when your partner will actually get up and move? Begin outdoor massage early enough in the day so the temperature will not drop precipitously while you're working. One more thing on the natural approach: To E. F. Dilray of St. Louis, Missouri, I would like to award the Arnold Schuster medal for eternal vigilance.* Thanks to Mr. Dilray, police were able to apprehend and later to convict a certain young couple who wrote to me from jail. They were practicing massage in a remote wooded area near the Mississippi River. Carefully concealing himself behind some rocks on a nearby bluff, Dilray had observed their naked bodies.

Just a few words before you begin will determine whether your partner has any problems which would prohibit massage. These problems include fever, skin eruptions, large bruises, inflamed joints, sensitive veins, and tumors. In all these situations massage can spread the condition to surrounding tissues. If you intend to massage the eyes, be sure your partner removes contact lenses before you begin.

During the actual massage, any movement that causes pain should be abandoned immediately. Go on to another movement or a different part of the body.

The astonishing effectiveness of acupuncture as demonstrated recently in China leaves little doubt that Western medical specialists have erroneously ignored this healing art. There is still considerable resistance to it simply because almost nobody in the West understands acupuncture. By way of explanation, Chinese acupuncturists have offered detailed "meridian" charts which do not seem to correspond to the way the nervous system or any other system actually works. The way out of all this confusion may finally be at hand.

Recent neuroanatomy research conducted by Dr. Steven Colwell of the University of California suggests that Western scientists have simply been looking in the wrong place to confirm the existence of the mysterious acupuncture meridians. Instead of examining the nerves of the hands and legs, Dr. Colwell and his colleagues have gone directly to the center of the brain. There they have located tiny maps which may correspond quite precisely to acupuncture meridian charts. The points on the body that activate these inner brain circuits are so precise that they can be triggered only by instruments no larger than the point of a needle. Although the study of acupuncture is outside the scope of this book, it is also outside the scope of casual study groups and weekend workshops. It must be regarded as a medical specialty that requires a thorough knowledge of anatomy, neuroanatomy, and physical medicine. Those willing to make this sort of commitment may eventually

* In the fall of 1952 an alert citizen named Arnold Schuster spotted Willie Sutton, the notorious bank robber, at a Brooklyn gas station. Arnold notified the authorities, who promised him protection and a big reward. A few hours later Willie was cornered and surrendered without a fight. Not too long after that Arnold moved to a local cemetery.

change the course of Western medical thought by incorporating ancient Chinese health principles.

Elsewhere in the East shrewd businessmen have adroitly capitalized on the West's imperfect understanding of acupuncture. They insist that the human body is a living machine which is covered with exotic little pressure points. Once these points are pushed (by fingertips which are several hundred times wider than the point of an acupuncture needle), magical things begin to happen all over the body. Developed and refined in Japan a few years ago, this concept has found a huge audience with Western button lovers, who secretly believe all things Eastern must be 4,000 years old and shrouded in a peculiar mystical aura that cannot be penetrated by the logic-bound Western mind.

Immensely successful pressure point schools have already been franchised throughout Japan and are beginning to catch on here in the United States. Graduates of these schools combine basic massage techniques with aggressive finger poking to the soft, relaxed inner tissues. The resulting pain levels around vital organs are often so great that speech is momentarily impossible. But if speech were possible, the victim might remind his smug tormentor that the human body is not, alas, covered with ubiquitous little push buttons like the dashboard of a Toyota.

Influencing the health of internal organs with massage requires only a basic understanding of how the nervous system operates. The entire body is controlled by the brain via the nerves. Virtually all the beneficial effects of massage are directly related to changes in the nervous system. Soothe the nerves that supply the liver, and the arteries of the liver dilate.

Most of the internal organs are supplied by nerves that branch at the spinal cord and surface just above the organ itself, but there are a few notable exceptions you should deal with in the course of a complete body massage. Although the heart is primarily supplied by nerves from the spine, heart trouble is usually signaled by pain radiating down the left arm. This phenomenon is called referred pain, and it marks an important nervous connection. Masseurs recognize that because pain from the heart is felt in the left arm it's worthwhile to massage that arm whenever you're working on the heart. The same nerves that carry pain can be used to transmit pleasure. Referred pain centers will be discussed periodically throughout the text. Use them to reach inside the body and soothe the vital organs.

Occasionally, someone will surprise you by falling asleep. One of the most unfortunate effects of accumulated stress is that people eventually reach the point where total relaxation becomes a fond memory. Even during sleep itself, back and shoulder muscles remain somewhat tense and exhaustion takes the place of relaxation. For these people, getting through the long days and nights becomes a kind of grim ordeal, one that often ends abruptly five minutes after massage begins, when they fall into a deep, blissful sleep. This sudden drifting away can be somewhat disconcerting if you're not ready for it because it seems as though your partner has abandoned the massage altogether. On the contrary, sleep is a sign that you have broken through what may be years of accumulated tension.

Since absolutely nothing is required of your partner during a massage except relaxation, you can continue what you were doing because it's working. You're not massaging the conscious mind; you're massaging the body. As you stroke and knead, you'll notice that people rarely move at all during massage sleep. If you finish at the end of the day, you might want to let your partner sleep on until the next morning. (See "Insomnia," page 177.)

Many Americans, citizens of the world's most abundant food supplier, are seriously worried that they may not be getting their money's worth at the market. So many diet books have attacked modern food processing that all canned, refined or frozen products suddenly appear dangerous and wholly lacking in nutritive value. Nervous purists go even further and deplore the use of anything sweet, salty, spicy or fattening until nearly every dish is regarded with the same dismay that Socrates must have felt for his final cup of hemlock.

How many "health conscious" Americans are afraid of their food when they sit down to the dinner table (while half the world has no dinner or table)? You are what you eat, argues the purist, as he rejects yet another sumptuous dish and begins the familiar lecture on poisons and toxins. Guilt masquerading as health awareness brings stress to the dinner table and guarantees an utterly joyless meal. For thousands of years human beings have demonstrated how easily they can prosper on a wide range of foods. The right diet for you is an important and very personal choice, but no matter how carefully you choose, diet is only a small part of the total health equation.

In massage, diet and nutrition are considered separately. "You are what you eat." This mechanistic concept of nutrition might work if health were merely a question of consumption, but you can fill your stomach with the most nutritious food and do very little for your body.

The body receives no nutrition at all until food is digested and enters the bloodstream. At that point the nutritional requirements of the left foot depend on the quality of blood circulation to that foot and throughout its tissues. The most carefully planned diet will do almost nothing to develop important veins and arteries if it is not combined with vigorous exercise.

Unfortunately most exercise programs concentrate on a fraction of the body's 600 muscles. A tennis player will favor his racket arm. A runner may forget to develop his arms, and weight lifters often lack aerobic capacity. In every case when blood supply to the neglected area is reduced, *nutrition* is limited. Internal nutrition measures all the real benefits blood can bring to the body's tissues, including oxygen itself.

Massage can be used to boost internal nutrition rates that diet and exercise cannot affect. Masseurs can bring oxygen to overexercised muscles which are about to cramp or triple the blood supply to muscles that haven't been exercised at all. (See "Exercise and Massage," page 153.) Throughout the book you will find movements which are specifically designed to increase nutrition to parts of the body that most exercise programs ignore.

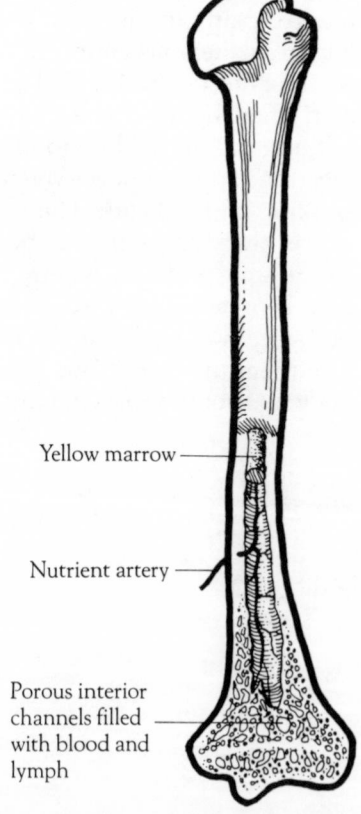

Yellow marrow

Nutrient artery

Porous interior channels filled with blood and lymph

Blood-soluble nutrients penetrate to all parts of a bone

How to Use the Book

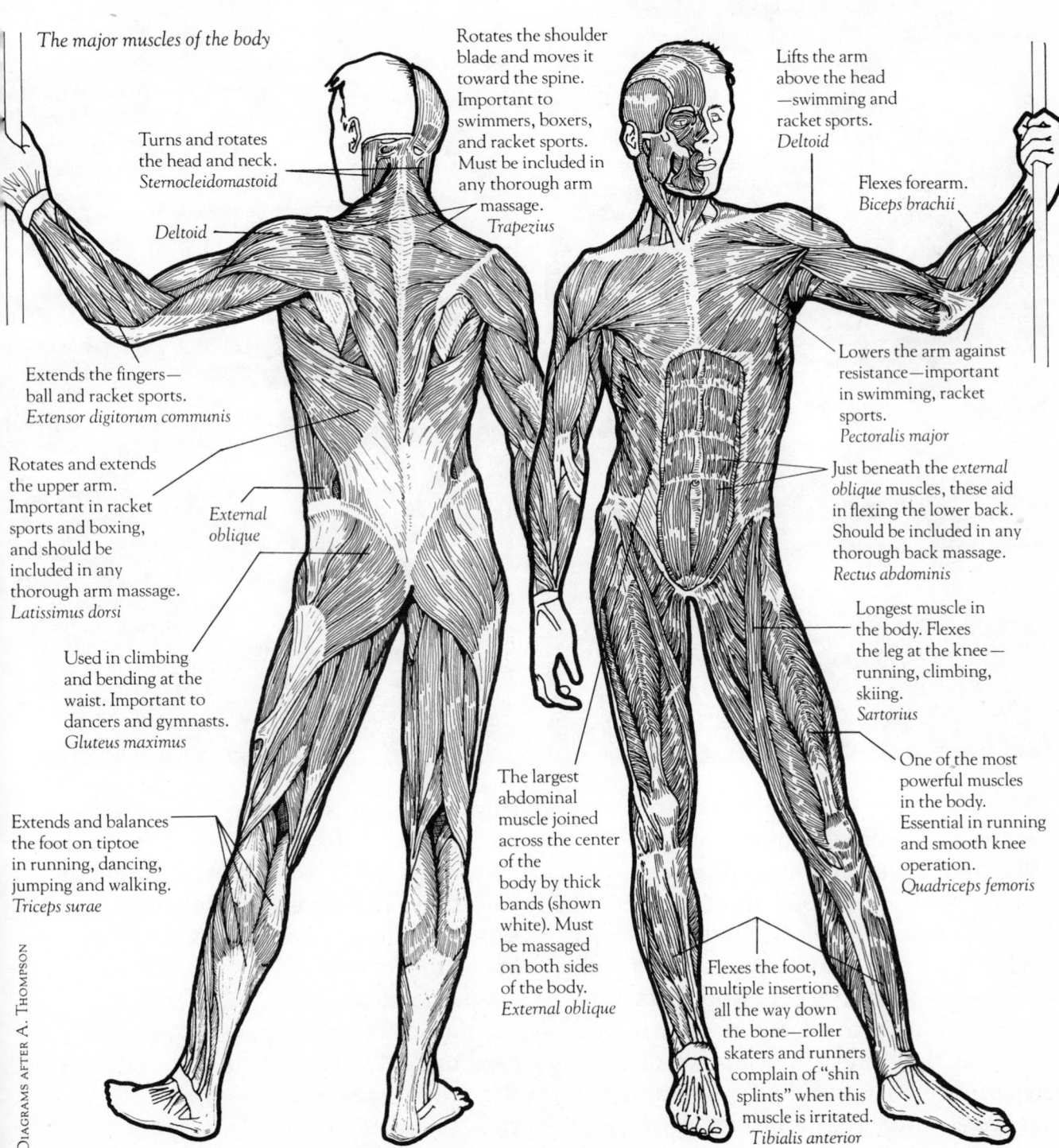

The major muscles of the body

Turns and rotates the head and neck.
Sternocleidomastoid

Deltoid

Rotates the shoulder blade and moves it toward the spine. Important to swimmers, boxers, and racket sports. Must be included in any thorough arm massage.
Trapezius

Lifts the arm above the head —swimming and racket sports.
Deltoid

Flexes forearm.
Biceps brachii

Extends the fingers— ball and racket sports.
Extensor digitorum communis

Rotates and extends the upper arm. Important in racket sports and boxing, and should be included in any thorough arm massage.
Latissimus dorsi

External oblique

Lowers the arm against resistance—important in swimming, racket sports.
Pectoralis major

Just beneath the *external oblique* muscles, these aid in flexing the lower back. Should be included in any thorough back massage.
Rectus abdominis

Used in climbing and bending at the waist. Important to dancers and gymnasts.
Gluteus maximus

Longest muscle in the body. Flexes the leg at the knee— running, climbing, skiing.
Sartorius

The largest abdominal muscle joined across the center of the body by thick bands (shown white). Must be massaged on both sides of the body.
External oblique

One of the most powerful muscles in the body. Essential in running and smooth knee operation.
Quadriceps femoris

Extends and balances the foot on tiptoe in running, dancing, jumping and walking.
Triceps surae

Flexes the foot, multiple insertions all the way down the bone—roller skaters and runners complain of "shin splints" when this muscle is irritated.
Tibialis anterior

DIAGRAMS AFTER A. THOMPSON

How to Use the Book

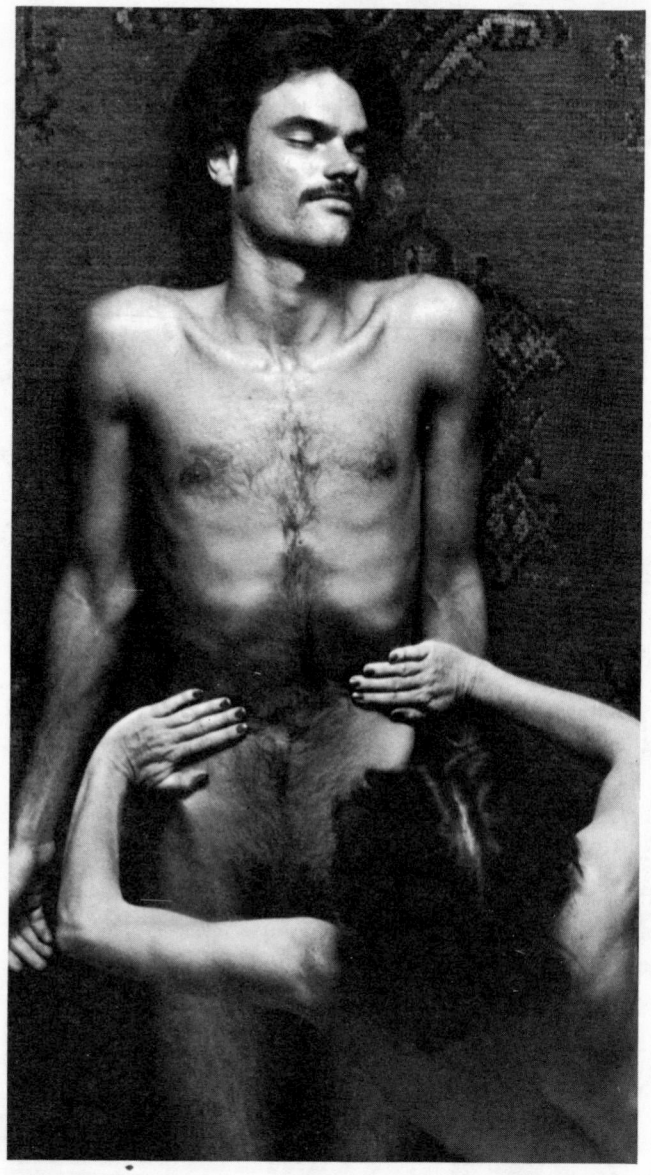 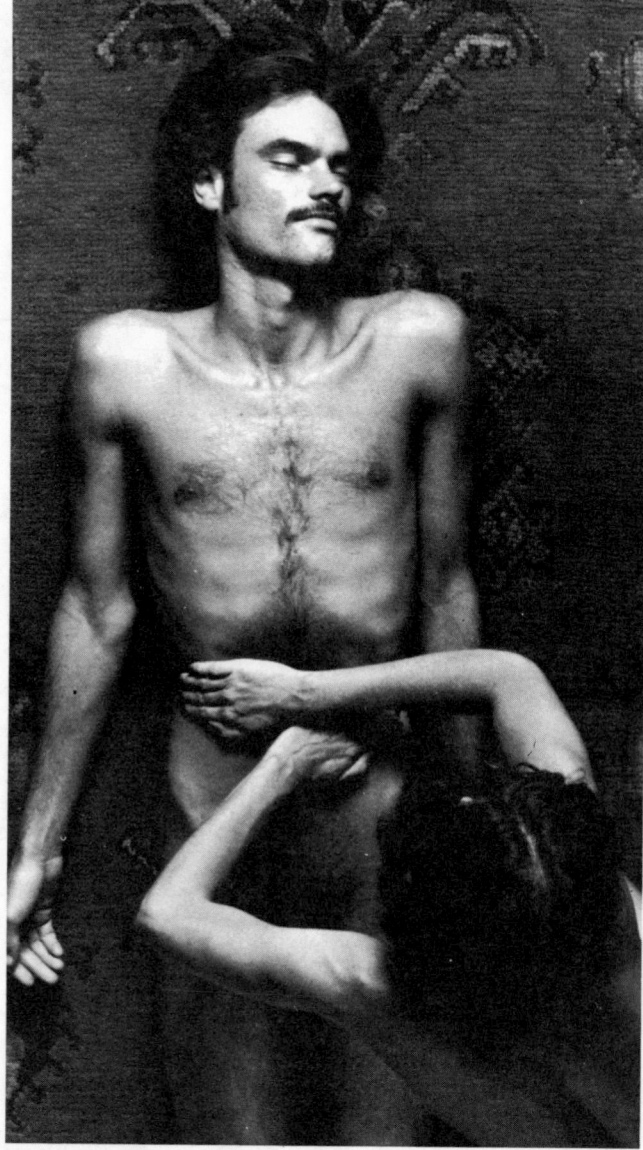

The full body massage section of the book contains more than 130 different movements. All have been chosen for their unique ability to benefit specific muscles, nerves, blood vessels, and other body tissues. All of them feel very, very good. Readers who learn the entire 130-movement repertoire will have, at their fingertips, an awesome experience guaranteed to please almost any one of the 4 billion human beings who live on this planet.

Much of the technique in the full body massage involves a wide range of variation on six basic movements. Variations can range from styles using just the fingertips to strokes that employ the whole hand and forearm. Generally, exceptions to these basic movements are used to deal with parts of the body (like the knees, toes, eyes, and spine) that call for special kinds of attention.

Friction: Rapid oscillating pressure over a specific area. Promotes deep arterial tissue circulation, aids lymph flow. Especially useful at the joints, over major lymph nodes and certain internal organs.

Percussion: Light-cushioned blows over well-muscled parts of the body. Soothes the nerves, tones the skin. Limited applications on the front of the body; very useful on the back of the legs and back.

Kneading: Rhythmic lifting and squeezing the flesh. Pumps nutrients through the muscles, drains wastes. Useful on the soft, fleshy parts of the body and over most muscles.

Stroking: Constant pressure while both hands glide over the skin. Stimulates venous circulation. Used on every part of the body; particularly important on the extremities.

Passive Exercises: Pulling and rotating parts of the body to exercise the joints. Increases the mobility of joints, strengthens ligaments and tendons, and boosts production of synovial fluid. Used on all of the body's mobile joints.

Brushing: Light fingertip contact. Transfers sensation from one part of the body to another. Used at the end of massaging each part of the body.

Since Fluid Release begins when tensed muscles relax, every movement in this book can benefit an athlete. All the first 4 basic movements help relieve muscle fatigue. Several variations on each of these movements appear in every chapter. Use them to create a full body massage that will leave an athlete feeling refreshed and invigorated. You can heighten their effect by adding more massage on any part of the body.

Once you've learned these 4 movements on the torso, you'll be able to use them anywhere on the body. Generally, the text will focus on the most important muscles to knead, the exact spot to apply friction to a crucial joint, or the best areas for percussion. Even so, if Fluid Release is your only aim in doing massage, you can broaden the scope of all these movements. All of the arm's muscles can be effectively kneaded. Friction can extend from shoulder to wrist, and percussion can include the entire fleshy surface of a limb. The effect on specific nerves, blood vessels, and joints discussed throughout the book will be diminished because you'll be spending less time on them. Still, a basic 4-movement Fluid Release sequence will drain wastes from the body's main muscle groups. If your partner is measuring his performance in a sport, he will notice an immediate change in muscle recovery rates as fatigue-causing chemicals are metabolized during and after massage. With generalized versions of these 4 movements a simple full body massage can be completed in about thirty minutes.

Once you've learned the basic Fluid Release sequence, you are halfway to a one-hour body massage. Simply add 4 more movements for each of the eight parts of the body. Choose movements that can easily be generalized to include a whole section of the body. Full-hand compression movements, forearm strokes, and the full stroking movements all can be spread easily across a part of your partner's body. The hour will pass quickly for both of you.

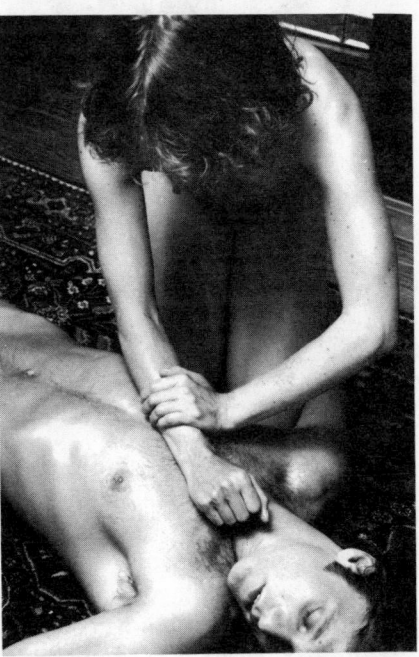

Its five senses, delicate and vibrant, communicate the whole delight and glory of the world at the price of being equally receptive to its agony and horror. For the body is sensitive because it is soft, pliant, and impressionable, but it lives in a universe which is for the most part rock and fire.

ALAN W. WATTS
Nature, Man and Woman

A complete full body massage can last for the better part of an evening. Once you've learned all the techniques in this book, it's easy and natural to invent movements of your own that fit the rhythm. Watch your partner closely, and repeat movements that he likes. There is no reason why ten relaxing movements on the back cannot become thirty. Or fifty. Your partner is not likely to object because most people have *never* experienced this much

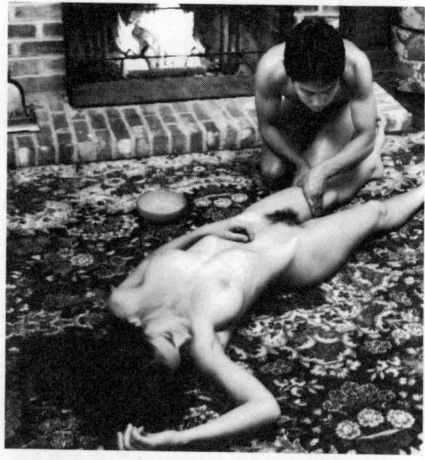

continuous physical attention. As your massage technique improves, the continuous physical attention will become continuous sensuality. Everything your partner feels during massage lingers for hours, and that's why the best time for a complete full body massage is the evening. The two of you should forget about the demands of clocks, phones, friends, and family. That leaves just your hands and the body beneath them.

There are many ways to move around your partner's body while you massage. Getting from an arm to a leg is easy enough as long as you maintain contact with your partner while you're repositioning your body. But unless you're using a massage table, the longer moves (from an arm to the opposite foot, for example) can be awkward. The sequence below is easy to remember and lets you move around the edge of your partner's body without ever having to cross over the center. Use it while you're learning massage. As you work with massage, it's fun to improvise new sequences. Whatever you decide on, try to have the total body in mind when you begin. It's always embarrassing to complete a full body massage and find out later that you managed to skip an entire arm.

This sequence follows the chapter progression in the "Full Body Massage" section (page 38). Use it one step at a time as you complete each chapter.

1. The torso: End on a shoulder.

2. The first arm: End with the hand next to your partner's head (page 73).

3. The palm side of the first hand: End by picking up the arm above and below the elbow and laying it at your partner's waist.

4. The back of the first hand: End with ten general circulation movements on the arm. Stop on your partner's shoulder at the top of the tenth movement. Press your hands lightly on the shoulder while you move from the waist to the top of your partner's head.

5. The head and neck: Hold one hand lightly against the center of your partner's forehead, and move the other down the arm you have not yet massaged. Once you have good contact with the arm, reach down and lift it with both hands above and below the elbow.

6. The second hand: Begin massaging the second hand with the palm side next to your partner's head. This hand should be massaged exactly the same way as the first hand. Use your general circulation movement to begin massage of the arm.

7. The second arm: End by brushing down the arm to your partner's fingertips. As you break contact there with one hand, take hold of the nearby leg with the other.

8. The first leg: Position your body down toward the foot as you do your first movements here. End by moving onto the top of the first foot.

9. The first foot: End by moving to the middle of the second leg.

10. The second leg: End by moving onto the top of the second foot.

11. The second foot: End by having your partner turn over.

12. The bottom of the feet: Do one after the other.

13. The back of the legs: Do one after the other. Keep contact with one leg while you move around the feet to do the other.

14. The back: Finish by brushing the entire body with your fingertips (page 152).

The Torso

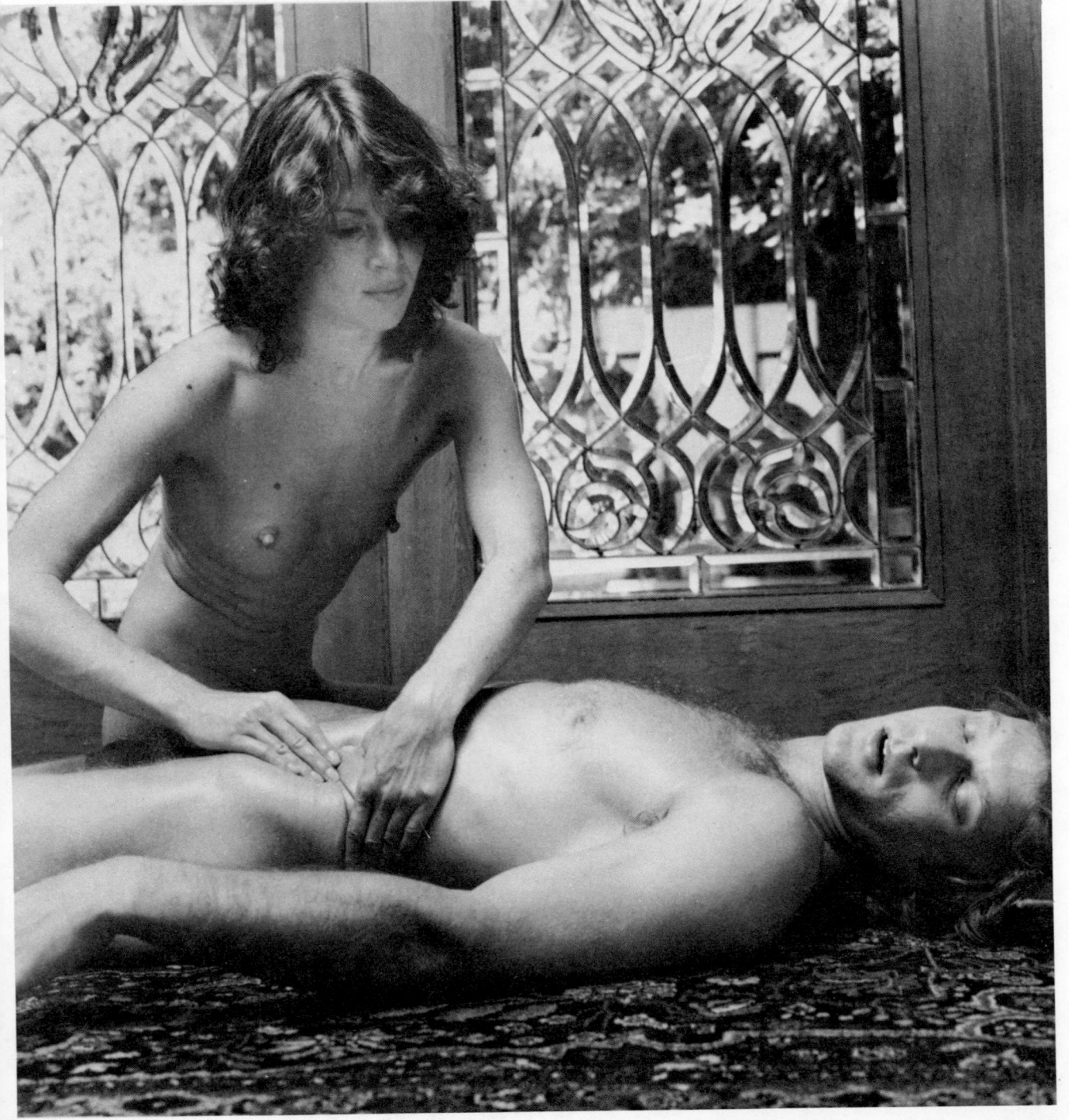

The Torso

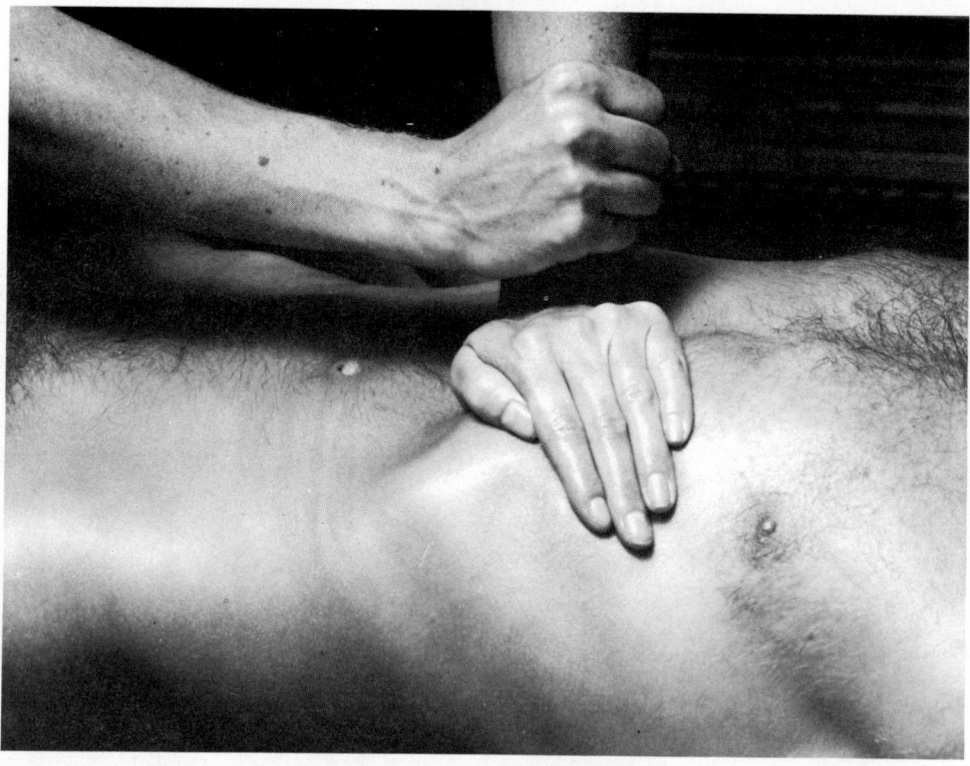

The torso contains all of the body's vital organs except the brain. Since so many of the internal muscles around the organs are involuntary, your partner may not feel the immediate effects of massage. Nevertheless, the liver, lungs, and stomach all will benefit from movements in this chapter. The heart alone can be reached more effectively via certain nerves on the back. (see "Heart Massage," page 51). Massaging abdominal muscles, which are often underexercised, will definitely aid the digestive process. The kings of the Sandwich Islands were aware of this beneficial effect. They had themselves massaged after *every meal* to aid digestion. Do write if you find a restaurant that offers this delightful service. In the meantime, gourmet readers are encouraged to try light abdominal massage no more than one hour after a meal. Be sure to elevate your partner's torso with large pillows because lying flat just after eating puts a strain on the heart.

Massaging the abdomen stimulates blood circulation along the entire network of gastrointestinal veins and plays an important role in dispersing all body wastes. These wastes range from imperfectly digested food and lactic acid to the extremely fine tissue debris that is found throughout the body. The wastes serve as irritants until they are fully metabolized. Intestinal wastes that collect in the appendix are sometimes never properly metabolized. Perhaps someday the frequency of appendicitis in people who have received regular massage will be studied. I've never heard of a single such case.

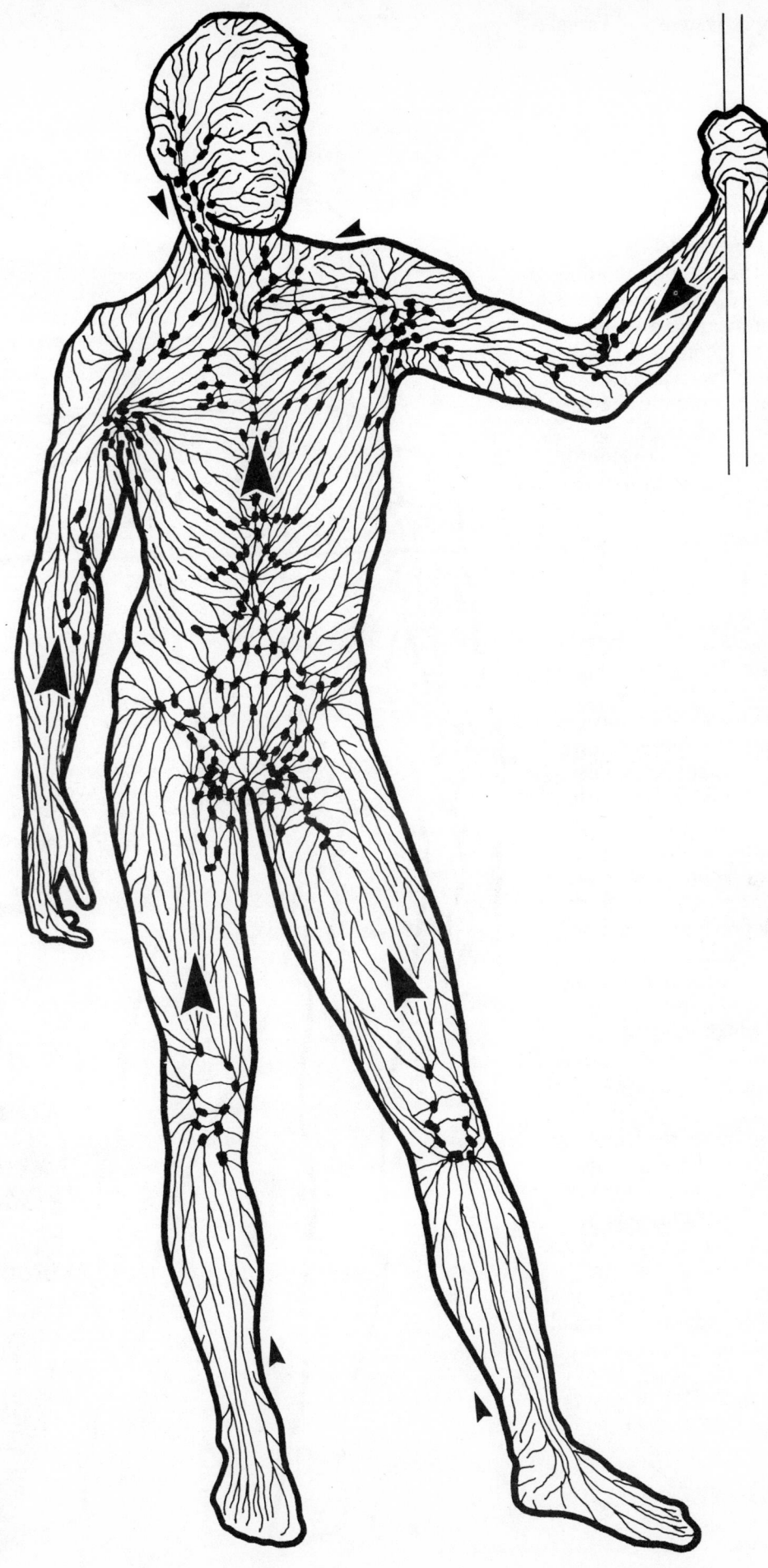

Diagram shows the major
nodes and the direction of
lymphatic flow

Whether you're dealing with lactic acid, nerve debris, or intestinal toxins, it's important to realize that all these wastes not only irritate your partner but actually block complete metabolism. Exercising for an hour when the muscles are so thoroughly blocked with lactic acid that they are not being properly supplied with nutrition is self-defeating. By stimulating circulation in the chest and abdomen, you drain wastes from the external muscles and, at the same time, supply nutrition to all the internal organs, the interior muscles, and finally the skeleton itself.

Extra muscle and tissue wastes (discussed in the introduction) that are generated during exercise are one of the main factors that cause unnecessary fatigue in runners and other athletes. Wastes that are not reconverted to sugar in the muscles pass through the exquisitely fine filtering action of the lymph system. Within this system a milky white fluid called lymph carries impurities and excess fluids which have been extracted from the body's tissues. Throughout the body, lymph collects in dozens of nodes or glands. Inside these nodes the lymph is pumped through screening devices which are used to filter out impurities. This filtering action is so thorough that individual bacteria and *parts* of dead cells are effectively trapped. Once trapped in the lymph nodes, the harmful bacteria stimulate production of white blood cells which destroy similar bacteria at the source of infection and throughout the body.

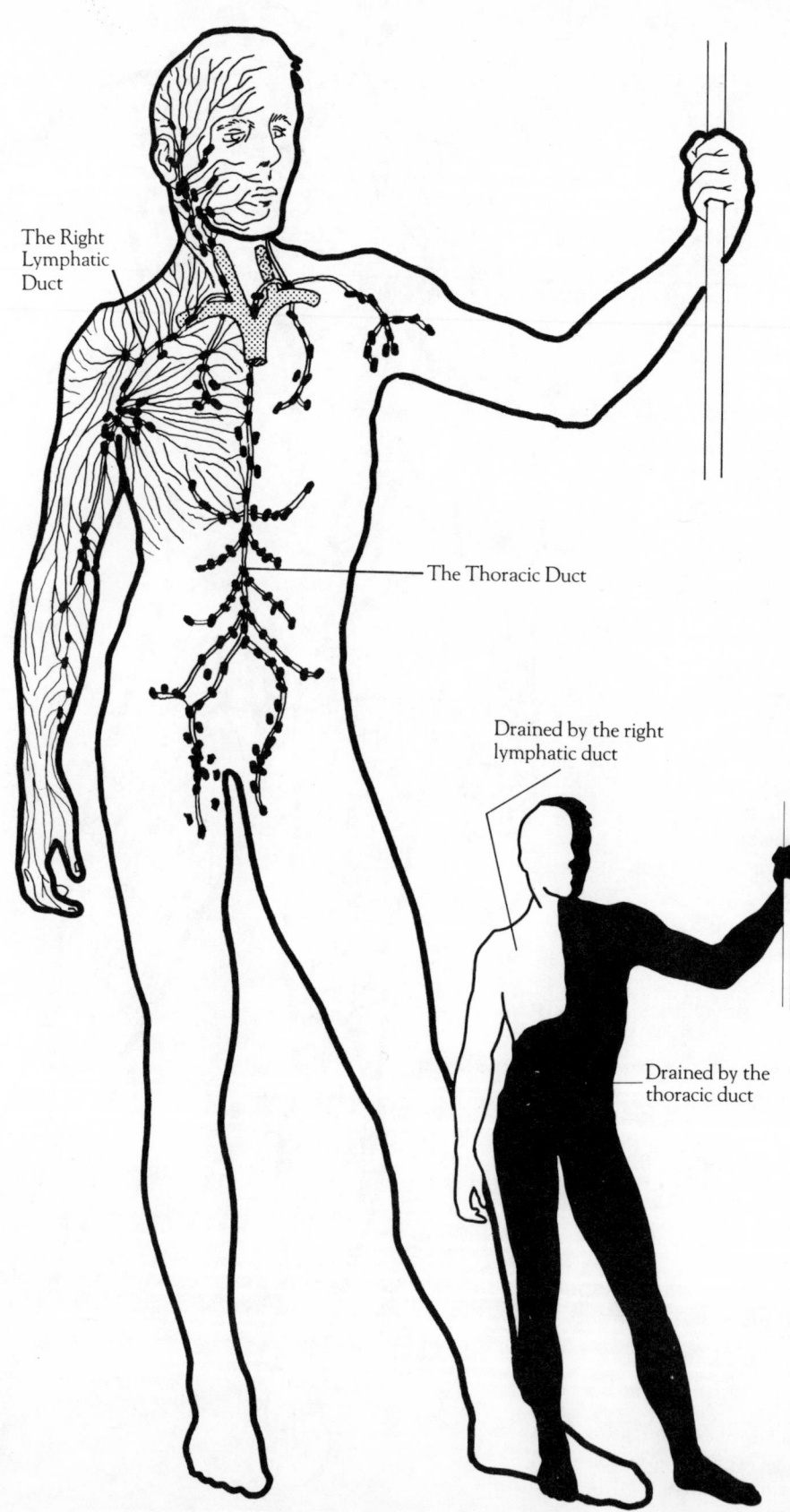

The Right Lymphatic Duct

The Thoracic Duct

Drained by the right lymphatic duct

Drained by the thoracic duct

Since there are always harmful bacteria and impurities in the body, the lymph system is usually kept quite busy. Large amounts of lactic acid and tissue wastes, generated during exercise, must be expelled from the system.

Completing this massive filtering process, tiny lymph vessels reach every part of the body and form a kind of secondary circulatory system. In twenty-four hours, the system circulates two liters of lymphatic fluid throughout the body. Since it has no heart of its own to pump, the lymph system depends instead on the natural massagelike action of surrounding muscles. Valves in the lymph system are stimulated during breathing and whenever the body is moved. Even though this natural stimulation is accelerated during exercise, it is far outstripped by waste production. You can use massage to control this imbalance and literally press wastes through the entire lymph system. The results are immediate and apparent: Fatigue seems to evaporate and is replaced by a serene sense of well-being. The Greeks and Persians recognized this function and incorporated massage into their daily exercise routine. You can do the same thing.

The Fluid Release techniques used by East German track teams whenever they compete are easy to learn and use. Once you have integrated them into your exercise routine, you'll wonder how you could have gotten along without them. Perhaps the reason you haven't heard about the crucial relationship between massage and exercise is that many people in this society are still afraid of massage because it involves close physical contact. This fear is finally starting to evaporate, and simple massage techniques are already being used as a formidable "secret weapon" by college swim teams here in the United States.

With a precise understanding of how massage works every athlete can use Fluid Release techniques to improve performance and dramatically reduce fatigue levels after exertion.

There are two parts to Fluid Release massage. You begin by stimulating and draining the lymph system, then go on to drain lactic acid and wastes from the muscles of the arms and legs.

You can reach all five of the body's most important lymph node centers when you massage the chest and abdomen. Concentrating on these areas will speed the removal of wastes from muscles all over your partner's body. Since lymph movement involves an entire system, not

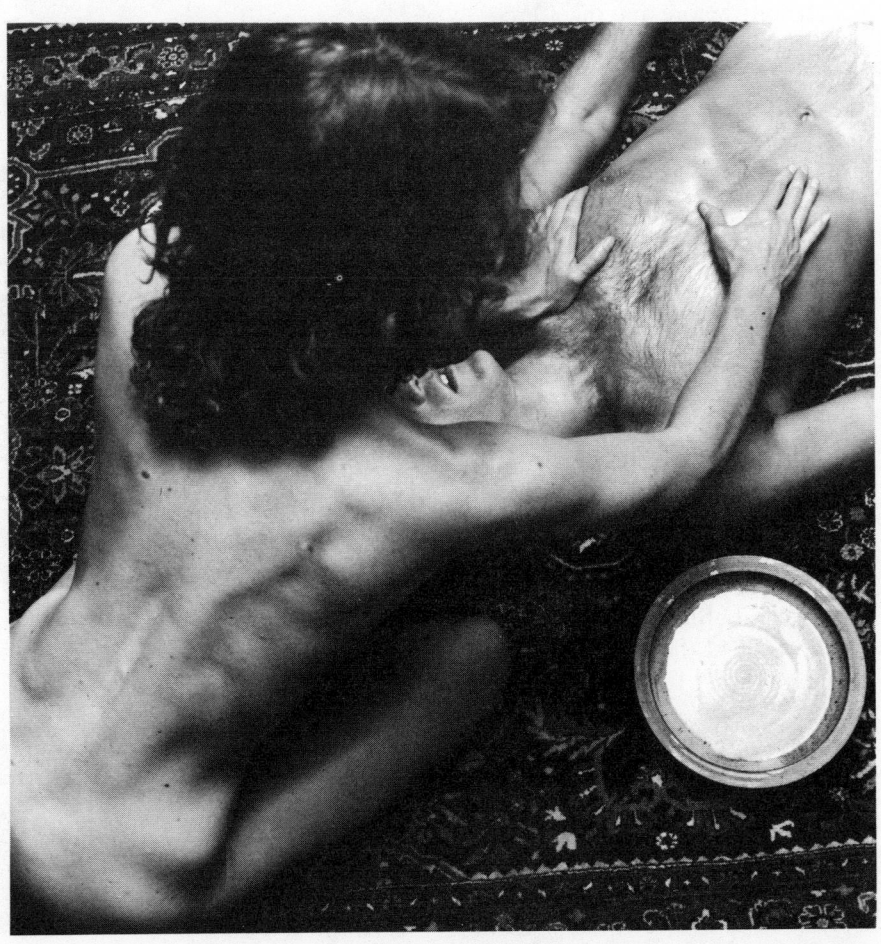

just specific points on the body, direct stimulation of the five lymph centers should be combined with a complete body massage. If you begin with the chest and abdomen, you are effectively clearing the central lymph nodes so that muscle wastes generated during exercise will have somewhere to go when you massage the legs, feet, and back (see diagram).

There's a four-stroke sequence that you can use all over the lymph centers of the chest and abdomen. The idea is to stimulate specific lymph glands and then press fluid out of the area. The first two movements—vibration and friction—can be done without oil. Occasionally you may want to add a light percussion movement before you oil. Once you've oiled the area, you can knead it thoroughly and finally press the lymph along with a hand-over-hand circulation movement. Smaller lymph glands, like the ones in the neck and behind the knee, will respond to the same sequence. Once you've learned the sequence, it's easy to incorporate it as part of a complete body massage anywhere in the body. When you reach the arms and legs, you may want to go back and work once again on the lymph nodes on the top of those limbs. All the stagnant toxins that you move out of the lymph nodes will be rapidly metabolized and eliminated. People will often feel the results of a thorough Fluid Release massage for most of a week.

The friction movement marks the beginning of your massage. The rate and pressure used in this movement have a great deal to do with its effect on your partner. Light frictions, especially over the

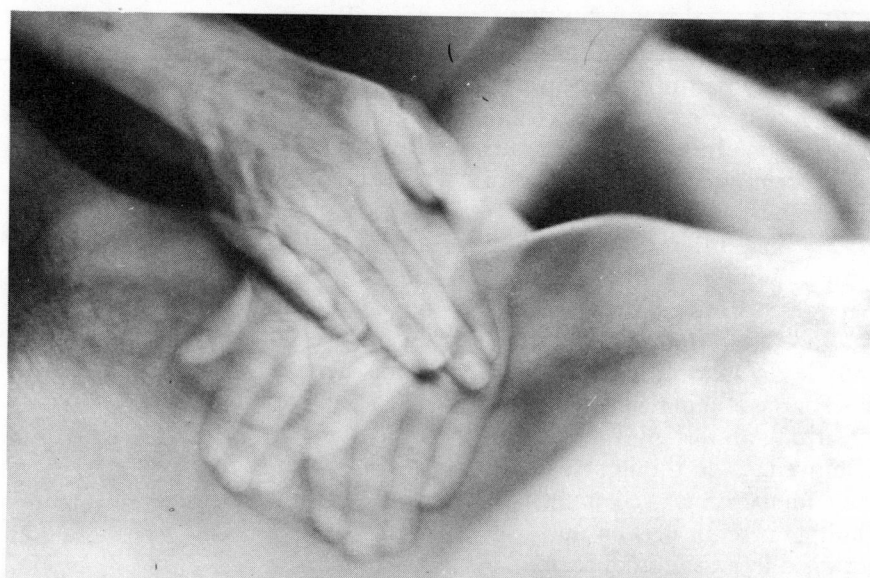

nerve centers discussed throughout the book, have a soothing effect. If you increase your rate and pressure, friction begins to anesthetize the local nerves providing masseurs with a

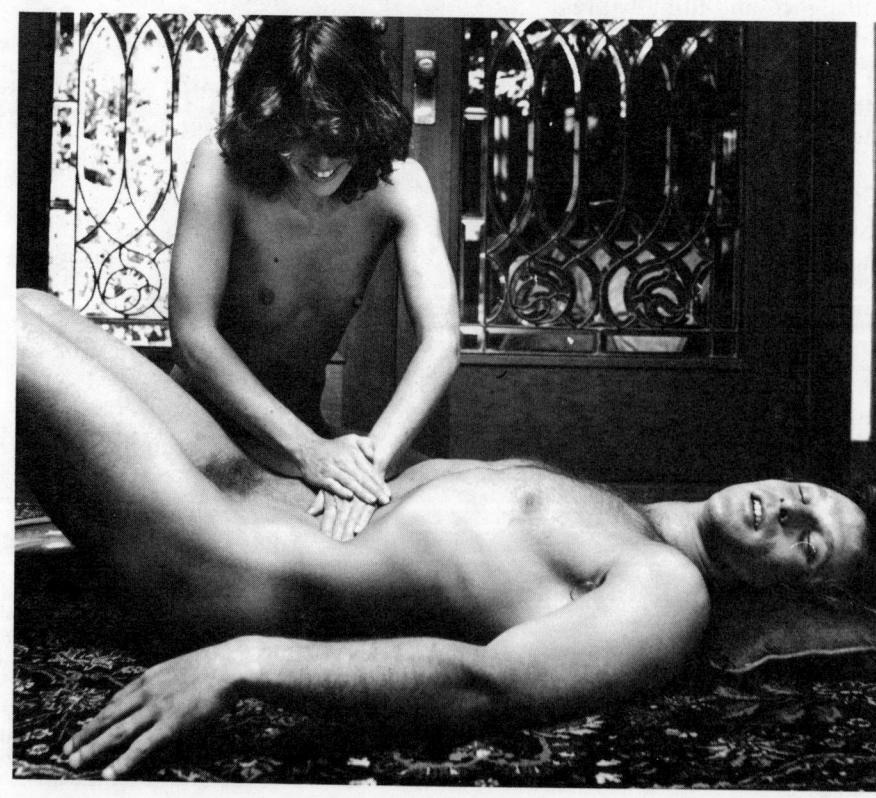

natural, drug-free sedative (See "Insomnia," page 177). For athletes, the friction movement offers a simple way to begin clearing toxins from the lymph system. On the torso you'll use it on all five of the major lymph centers.

In union there is strength, and the fingers should be kept close together in doing friction and manipulation. But it is astonishing how persistently they are sometimes held out straight and spread far apart, reminding one of the feet of a frightened duck in a thunderstorm and the sound of quack suggests itself as appropriate for the one as the other. During every friction movement your hands and your partner's skin must move as one. For that reason this is one of those massage movements that can work well *without* oil. Since you'll be leading with it on the torso, rub your partner down twice with a warm towel to ensure the best possible skin contact.

Don't break contact with your partner's body for any reason until you finish the entire body (if you've decided to do just the torso, maintain contact over that part of the body). This constant contact allows your partner to experience the entire massage as a single, smooth, uninterrupted motion. Remembering this as you move from one lymph center to another, keep contact with your partner's body with at least one hand.

Generally there are two variations on the friction movement: one for firm tissues like the shoulders and skull and another for soft tissues like the stomach and kidneys. The firm tissues will accept more pressure and a greater rate of vibration than soft tissue will. There are opportunities for both kinds of friction movement when you massage your partner's torso.

Perhaps more than any other movement friction allows you to reach beneath the surface tissues and to affect the internal organs. You can often actually feel them rippling under your fingers. A few minutes of friction to the liver and heart immediately before exercise will greatly increase nutrition to these organs and ease the strain on them when you begin to exercise.

The general rule in friction, as in all massage, is to use as much of the hand as possible. If you're working around the abdomen or on the back, you'll be able to use the whole of your hand, but if you're using friction on the forearm or neck, just the fingertips will work best. Friction frequently should begin at speeds that you feel comfortable maintaining for at least a couple of minutes. Keep in mind that you may want to use it for longer periods of time under certain circumstances. This movement does not rely on muscle power; pressures should remain light and even. If your arm gets tense, it's usually a sign that you're going too fast, so slow down.

*Graham, *op cit.*, p. 52.

Kneel next to your partner's chest (as shown). Many of the friction and vibration movements work best if you "anchor" or hold still an adjoining part of your partner's body. Use whichever hand you favor to deliver the vibration while the other hand anchors on your partner's arm or rib cage (as shown). Press down on your anchor hand just hard enough so there is no friction under it. The hand you actually use for the friction movement will move in

Friction movements start working on the tissues just beneath the skin. If your partner wishes to increase the capacity of the lungs through an exercise program, these friction movements over the chest will substantially increase blood supply to both lungs. This not only helps the lungs combust oxygen, but tones all of the surrounding muscles. (See "Exercise and Massage," page 153).

On the soft tissues of the abdomen a gentle circular friction movement will stimulate circulation. Because it increases the blood supply, abdominal friction will aid the digestive process. This movement will also bring nutrients to the internal abdominal muscles and strengthen them. You can work hand over hand (as shown). Begin by anchoring one hand against your partner's rib cage, and press down with the other hand on the center of the abdomen. Pressing down lightly, shake this hand from side to side. As you shake, slowly work outward in a corkscrew pattern from the center of the abdomen. As you approach the outer borders, your circles will get larger and larger. Remember that your pressure throughout should be light but steady. When you reach the upper limits of the abdomen where you can begin to feel the lower ribs, return to the center, and begin again. Even when returning to begin the movement again, your hands should never break contact with your partner's body. Work on the whole abdominal area by making three complete circles like this, and then move over to the lymphatic cluster at the top of one of the legs. The best way to reach those clusters is to flatten your friction hand slightly so that a broader section of your fingers comes in contact with your partner's body as shown. Anchor your other hand on the rib cage or side of the thigh, and work on the lymphatic cluster on the top of the leg for two minutes. Keep the pressure on your partner even.

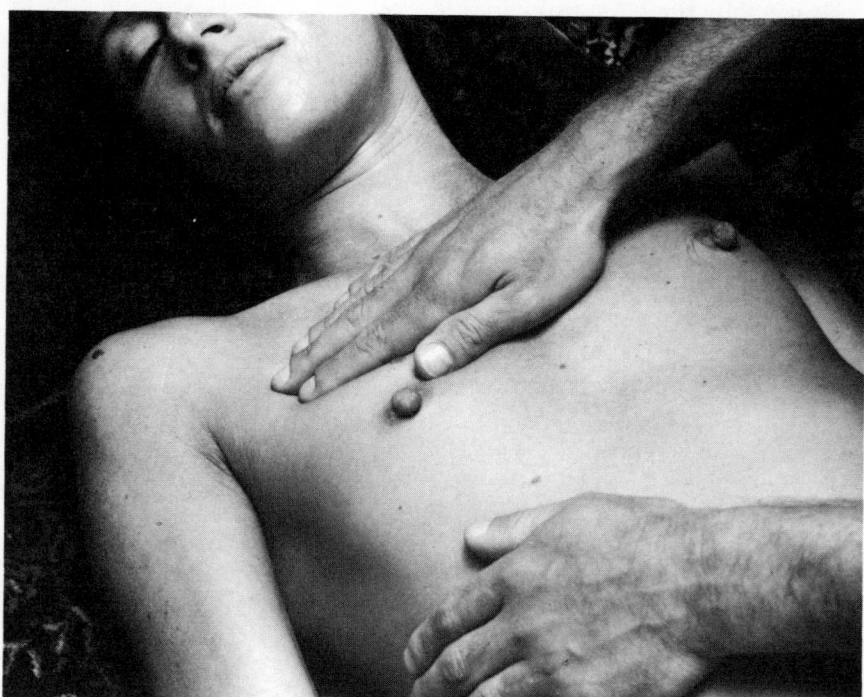

short circles across the chest, focusing on the lymphatic clusters (see diagram). Press down on the skin just hard enough to move the underlying tissues when you rotate your hand. Move your hand in a very small circle; feel the muscles ripple beneath it.

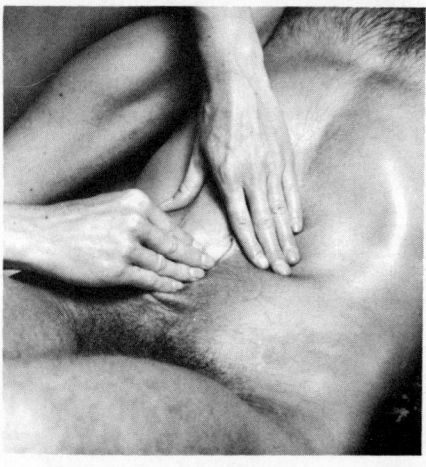

While most massage movements concentrate on manipulating interior muscles, vibration strokes focus on the skin itself. Skin, the body's largest organ, is routinely starved for the better part of a lifetime. Vibration movements liberate skin from the tyranny of fashion designers, detergent manufacturers, and shoe salesmen and allow it to do what it was intended to do: feel. When you liberate your largest organ, the

effects are immediately apparent. Tiny subcutaneous muscles all over the body begin to relax, perhaps for the first time since childhood, simply because the skin is no longer resisting an unpleasant environment. As you move across the chest, glance at your partner's face. You may notice that infinitely relaxed smile so familiar to experienced masseurs.

Thumb vibration is done with the entire surface of the thumb from the fingertip to the base of the hand. Your other four fingers remain spread (as shown) and make superficial contact throughout the movement. To stimulate the skin effectively, friction movements travel back and forth across the body in a pattern of overlapping circles. Begin thumb vibration at your partner's shoulders with your hands as far

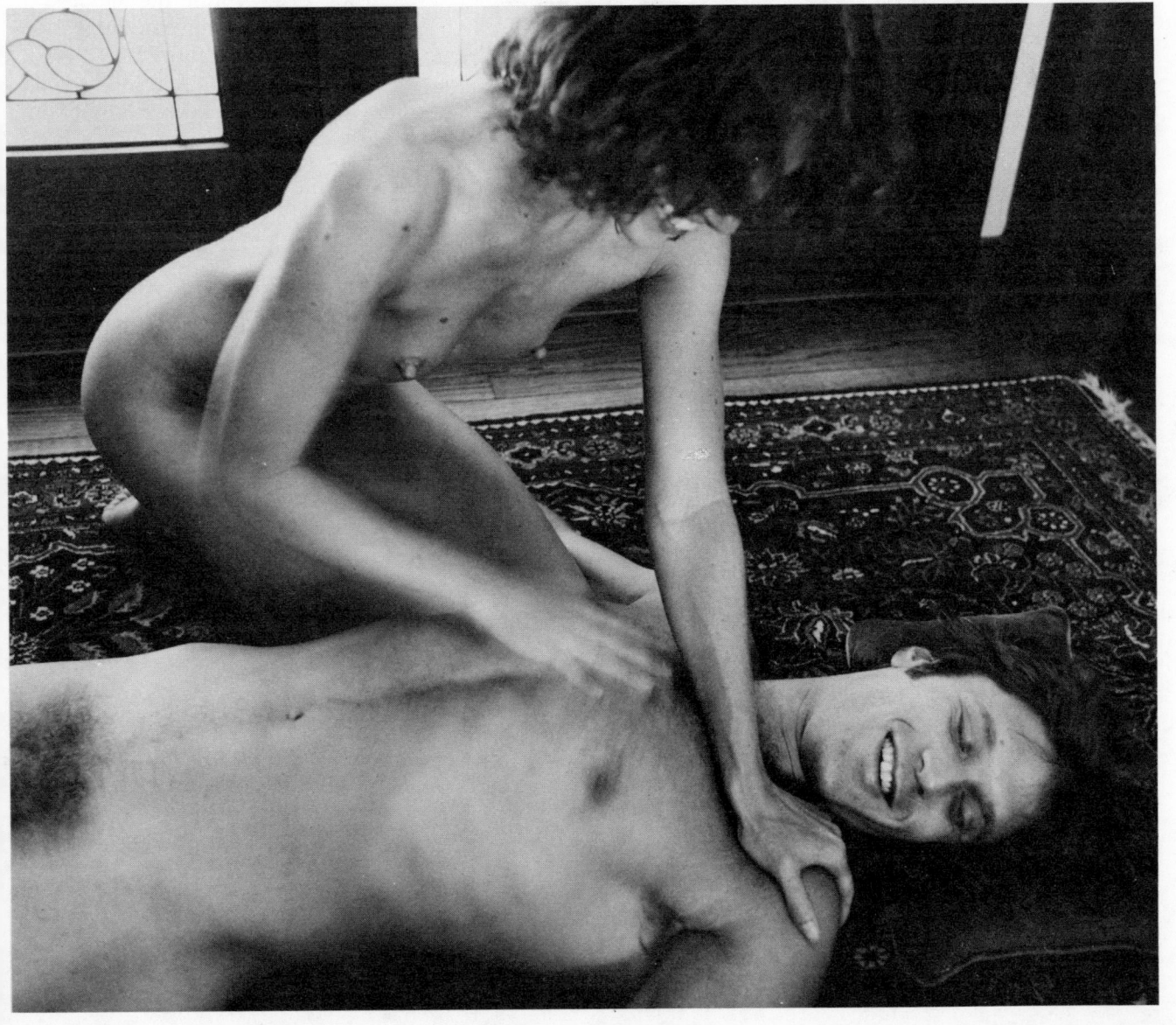

apart as they will be during any part of the massage. Moderate pressures are fine because in vibration movements your hands should slip along the surface of the skin instead of pressing down. Since vibration deals with the skin, not with a specific muscle group, you'll want to cover the entire surface of your partner's chest and abdomen. The best way to do this is to work up and down the chest in parallel lines. When you reach the waist on your first

Full-hand vibration operates almost the same way as thumb vibration. The difference here is that you make contact with your entire hand from fingertips to wrist. This movement gives you more contact and works best if you allow your hand to relax at the wrist. That way you're vibrating with your hand, not with your entire arm.

It's useful for masseurs to view the body as a river. Veins, arteries, and the vast capillary system are the watercourses that carry the blood to and from the heart. They also carry fatigue products or wastes away from the muscles. Vibration and friction movements free the wastes trapped in the muscles all over your partner's chest. The next stroke, a simple circulation movement, will stimulate subsurface venous and capillary systems and will pump wastes away from the muscles.

Begin this movement by oiling your partner's entire torso. All the movements that follow will require oil. Whether or not you work from a plastic squeeze bottle, be sure to maintain contact with your partner, using your forearm or knee throughout the oiling process. If you're beginning with massage and are still a bit hazy on oiling, this is a good time to review the Massage Oil section of the book (see page 29).

Because the heart is so near the center of the torso, stroking movements on this part of the body focus on stimulating the blood vessels rather than actually pressing the blood in a specific direction (as you will be doing later on the arms and legs). Begin fan stroking with your hands together just below your partner's neck, fingers pointed slightly outward (as shown). Keep your fingertips together, and press down to the edge of the rib cage. When you reach that point, turn your hands, and begin moving up your partner's side with your fingers pointed down. Allow your fingers to mold to the form of your partner's body as you come up over the shoulders and return to your starting position. Although this movement involves

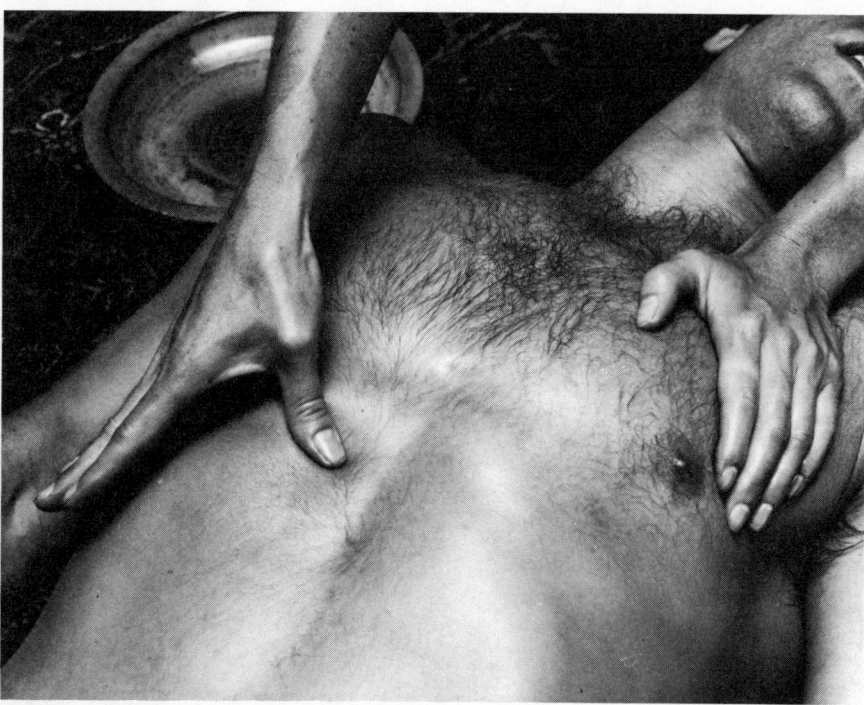

descent, begin working back up toward the head in a line parallel to your descent. Cover the entire chest and abdomen three times, but go easy over the breasts and ribs. Remember it's the skin you want to reach, not the tissues below.

turning and repositioning your hands, you'll find that when you've tried it a few times, it will flow as a single uninterrupted motion. Once you've reached that point, you can begin the fan part of the movement, which simply involves ending the bottom part of the movement a bit higher each time (see diagram).

After you have covered the top or the rib cage part of the torso ten times, you're ready to go on to the abdominal portion of the torso. This involves moving to your partner's waist so you can work up toward the head. Put one hand flat on the center of

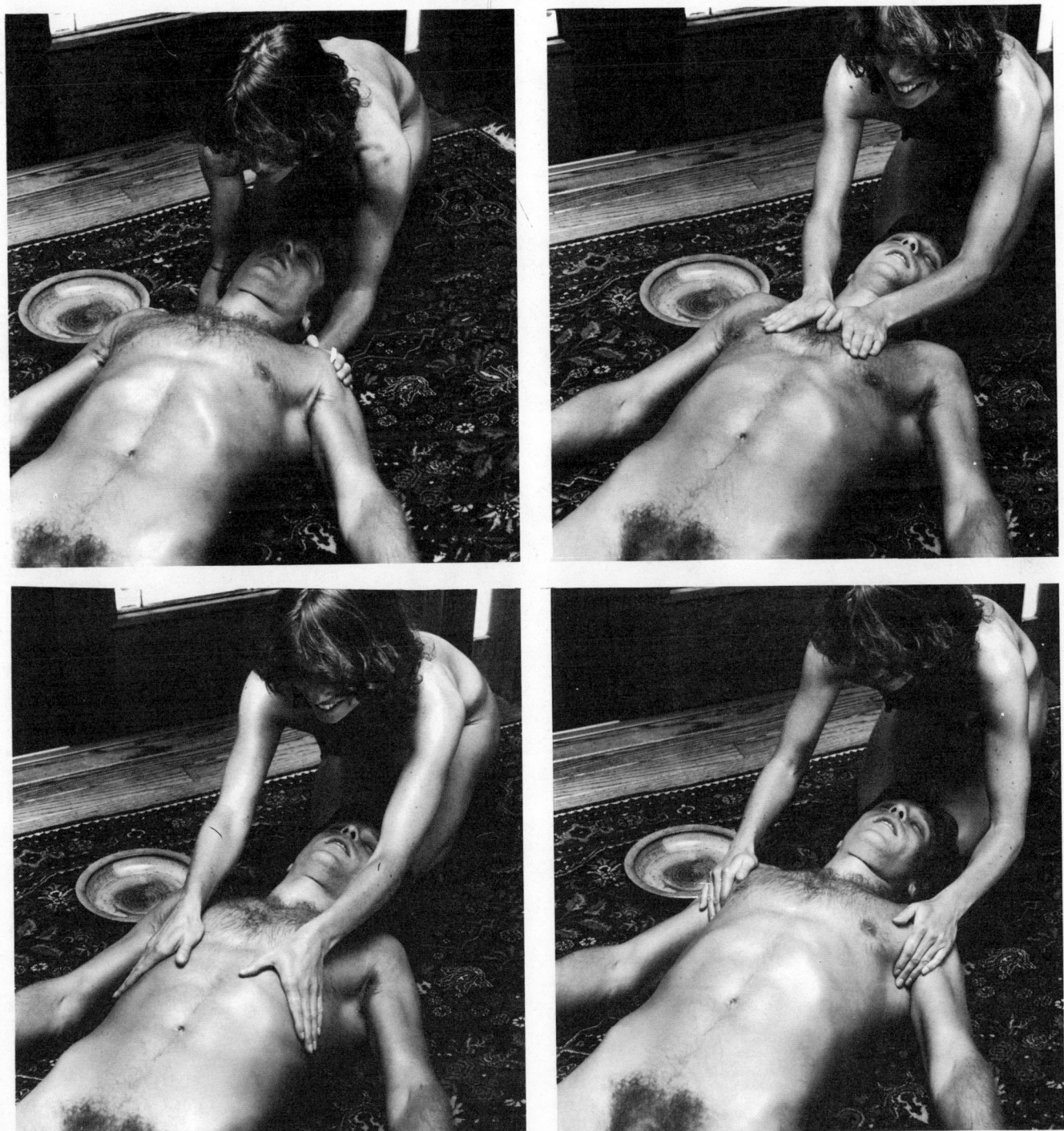

your partner's torso, and without leaning on that hand, make the move without breaking contact. Though you have a smaller area to work with while fan stroking from the waist, it's still possible to vary the size of your movements. Begin by pressing up just under the rib cage with the tips of your fingers. Do a few movements this way, and then begin to stop just a bit short of the rib cage. Again, your fingertips should mold to the shape of your part-

ner's sides on the return. Since you're working from both ends of the torso, this is the first of many movements that feel as though more than one person is massaging your partner—a delightful illusion and so easy to preserve.

The deceiving of the senses is one of the pleasures of the senses.
—SIR FRANCIS BACON, The Advancement of Learning

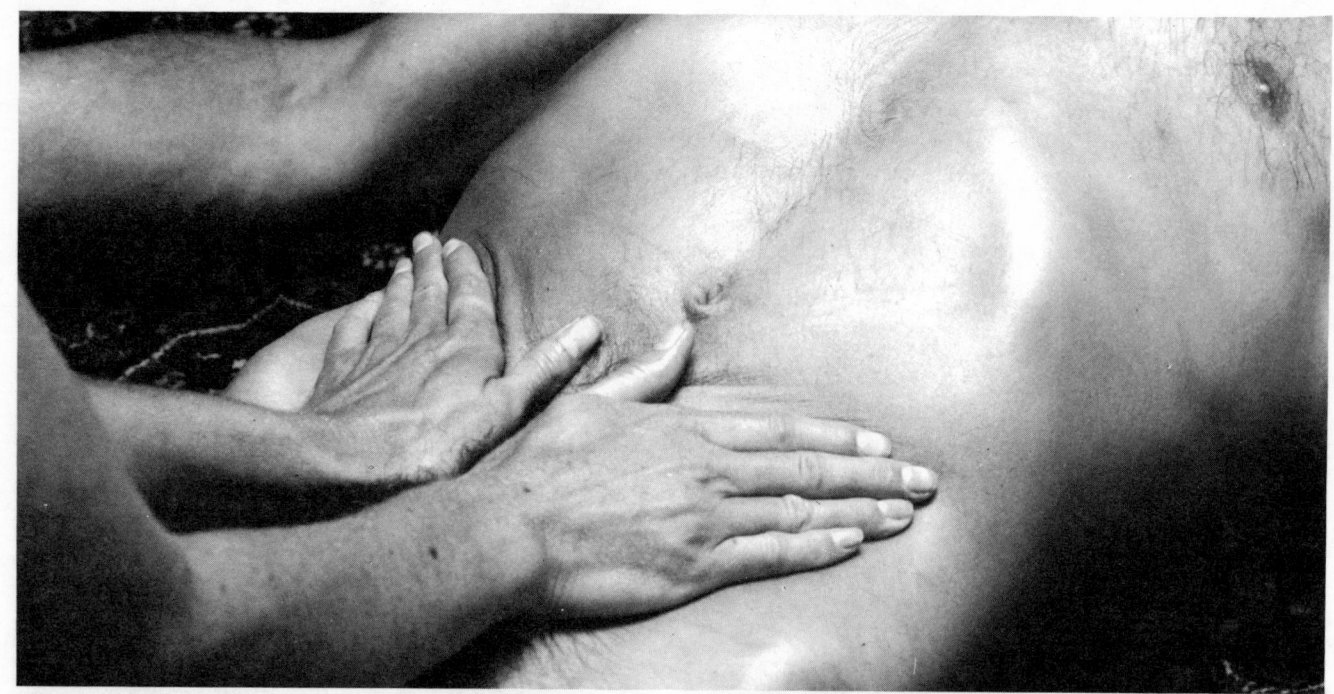

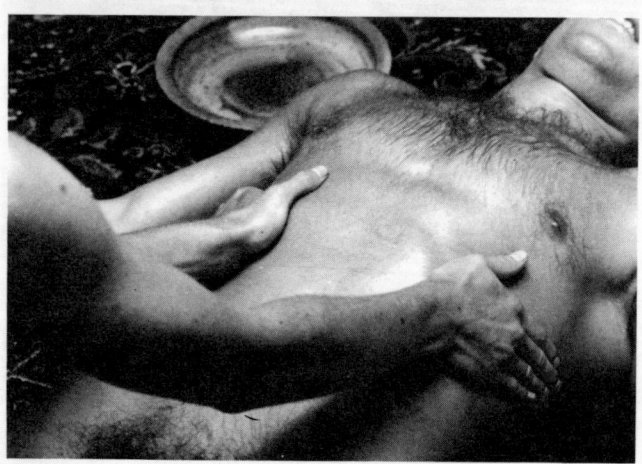

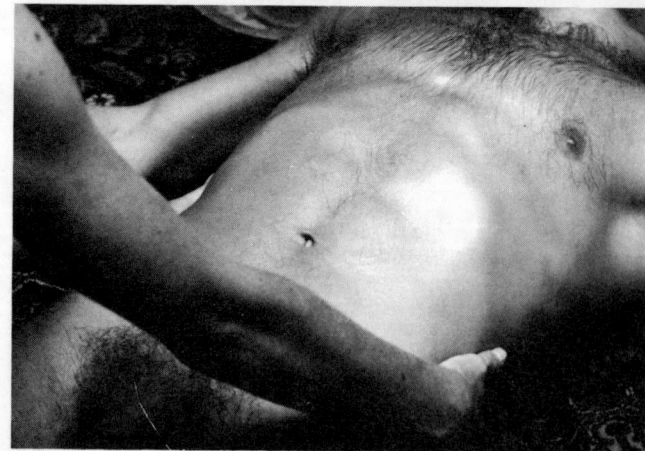

Kneading is probably the single most important movement in any massage. Again and again, wherever there is a broad or fleshy part of the body, you will return to it. On large, fleshy areas, like the sides of the abdomen, you can use the entire surface of your hand in a kneading motion that will follow the curves of your partner's body. Wherever it's possible to do so, without pinching your partner, try to lift and to squeeze folds of flesh gently as you knead.

The hands follow each other in a circular motion. If you favor the right hand, let the circle it makes intersect with the circle the left hand makes. Begin with the right hand by picking up a comfortable amount of flesh between the thumb and the four fingers (as shown). As you begin to release

this flesh, open the thumb and forefinger, and move into this open space with the left hand to pick up a fold of flesh in exactly the same way. As the hands move back and forth across various parts of the body, the one hand will always move into the open position created by the thumb and forefinger of the other. Again, remember to move your hands in a circular motion as you knead, not a jerky back-and-forth straight line.

If you're already involved in an exercise program, Fluid Release movements like this one make a tangible difference in the way you feel all day long. A good part of the intricate venous and lymphatic web that spreads across the abdomen can be drained with a gentle hand-over-hand squeezing motion. Squeezing the spongelike inner tissues of the abdomen creates a suction effect that drains wastes and then sucks nourishment back into the muscles. After this movement the blood vessels of the abdomen will actually expand elastically to a greater size than before the movement. Because squeezing serves to strengthen the abdominal muscles, it is an effective aid to digestion as well. Reach down with one hand at a time to pick up a fold of flesh. Squeeze gently, and keep your fingers together.

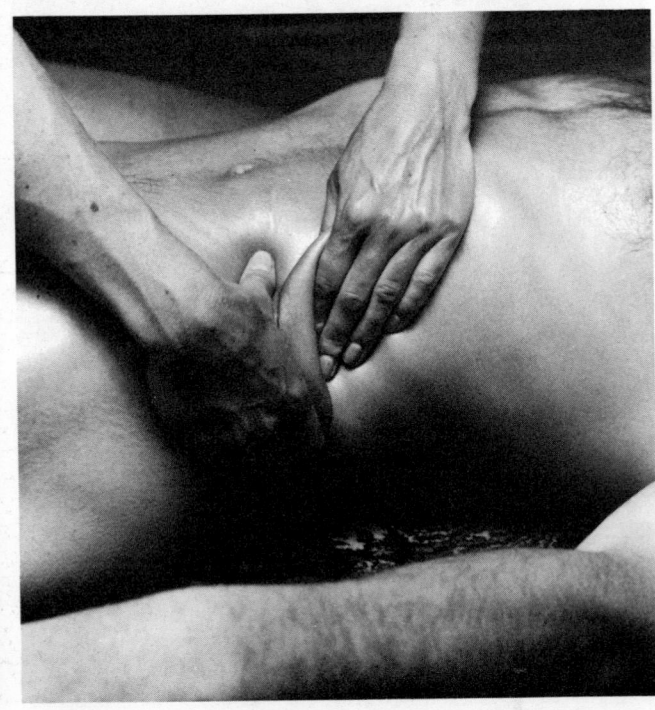
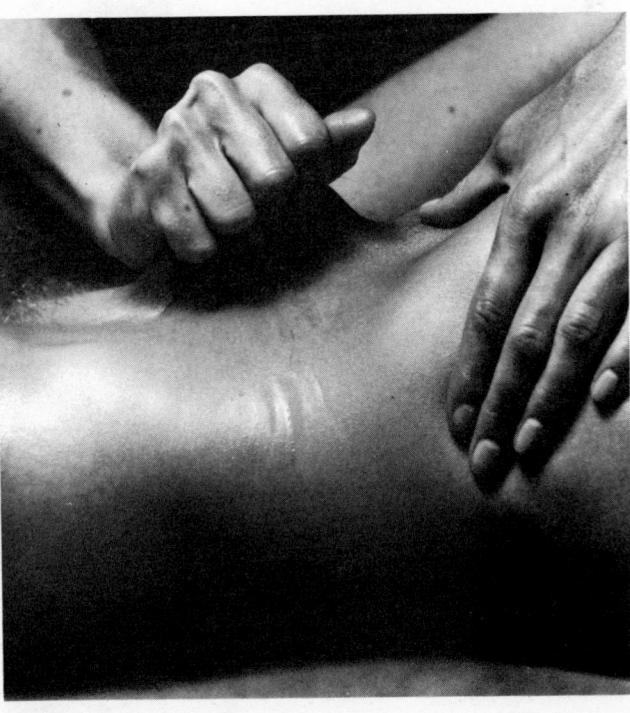

Hand-Over-Hand Compression—A Stroking and Kneading Combination Movement

Light Heel Thumping—A Percussion Movement

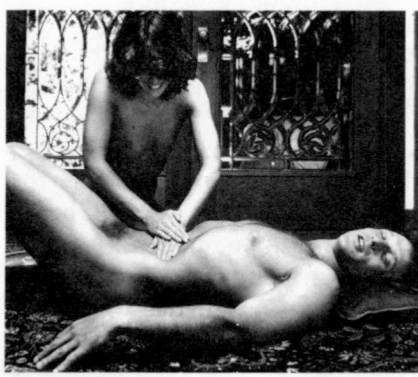

Compression movements allow you to apply pressure where muscles are tight while your hand, in direct contact with your partner, molds to whatever part of the body is being massaged. The circular movement of compression strokes is extremely soothing. Keeping your fingers tightly pressed together, simply place one hand over the other (as shown). Pressure with the top hand need be applied only when tightness is encountered. Even then the degree of pressure should never be so great as to cause the muscles to tighten. Mild, gentle pressure will have a far more satisfying result than intense force. The contact hand—that is, the hand actually touching your partner—acts as a kind of tension sensor. Whenever you feel tension in the muscles, press down on the contact hand with the anchor hand, and circle an extra half dozen times. Sometimes you can actually feel the tension begin to dissipate. More commonly your partner will feel the difference after the massage is over, perhaps even the next day. By focusing a compression movement on the tense muscle, you increase nutrition to the entire area and speed the waste disposal process. You also allow your partner to feel pleasure instead of tension for the duration of the movement.

Certainly one of the primary aims of any exercise program is lowering the pulse rate. By doing this, you not only strengthen the heart but significantly increase the capacity of the lungs. Light heel thumping will work beneath the rib cage directly on the lungs themselves to promote internal circulation. It will also loosen mucus and debris inside the lungs and, in general, clear the entire system.

The actual thumping, a light percussion effect, should be done with whichever hand you favor. The other hand presses against your partner's chest following the contours of the body (as in compression). Strike that hand with a loosely formed fist just above the heel (as shown). Begin slowly. Remember that a fast, erratic rhythm is far less effective than a slow, steady one. As you practice this movement, your speed will increase until you reach an ideal rate of about five per second. Muscle power, of course, is not important here. The hand in contact with your partner's body will cushion the blows and spread the effects throughout the lung cavity. Two minutes of light heel thumping will leave your partner feeling light and refreshed.

If you're working on a woman move around and above the breasts. The percussive effect, will reach within.

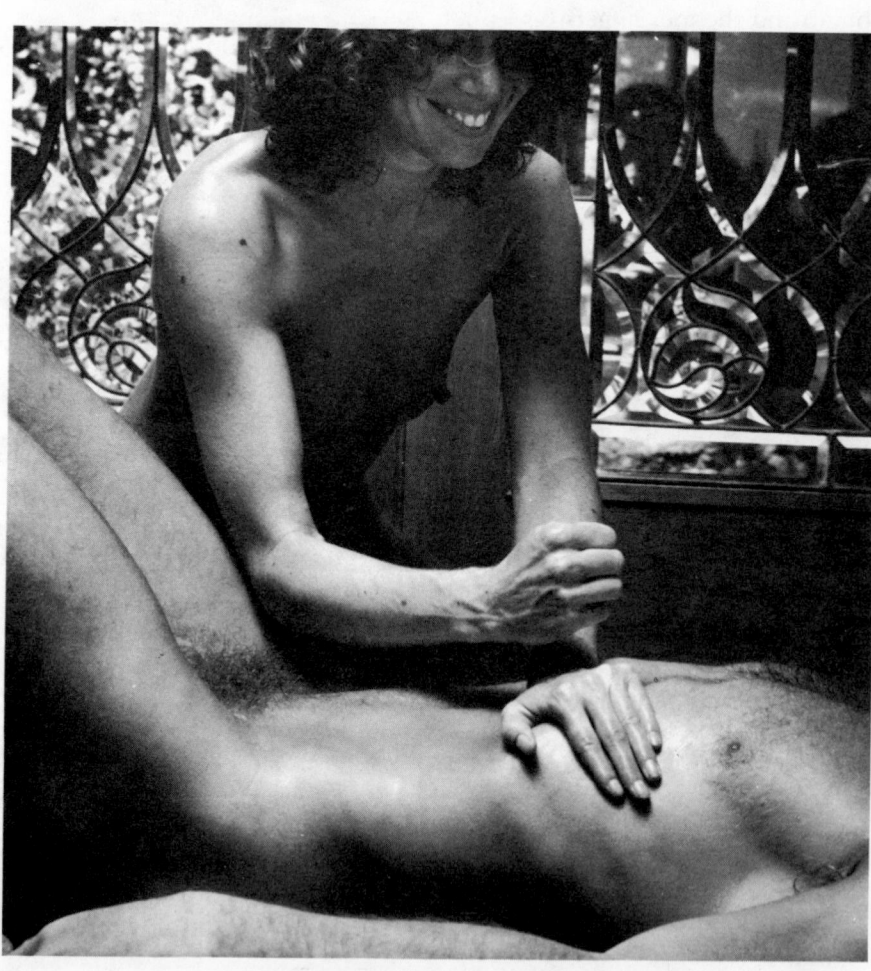

The Full Body Lift—A Passive Exercise

A popular stereotype of massage, fostered by certain health clubs, holds that masseurs are huge, dim-witted, muscle-bound types who thump on your body "to get out the stiffness." Thumpers are yet another manifestation of the "if it hurts, it must be good for you" philosophy that puritanically inclined Americans find so irresistible. For those who take the stereotype seriously, massage appears to be a grim ordeal requiring near superhuman strength and endurance.

The full body lift is one of those very rare massage movements in which strength actually

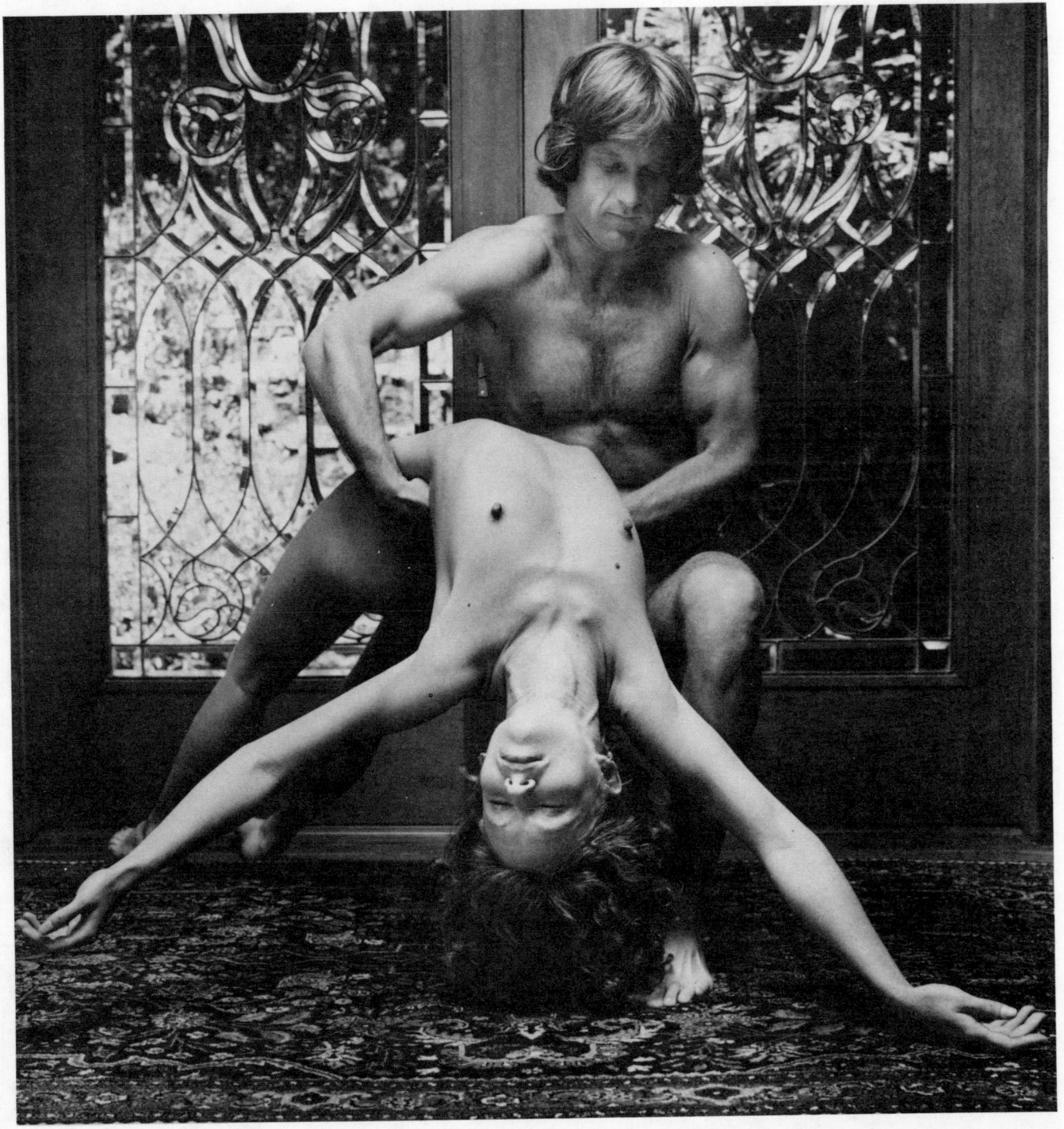

is a factor. Unless you're strong enough to manage it *easily*, it's best to settle for an abbreviated version of this movement, in which you simply pull up on the small of your partner's back while holding your hands. If you're going to try the complete lift, remember to raise one knee when lifting to steady yourself. Like any other massage movement, the lift should be smooth and fluid. One of the problems occasionally encountered here is that your partner sometimes unwittingly tries to help you by lifting her head or curling her toes inward. Sometimes it's a good idea to remind your partner, before you begin, not to help, but to let her body fall back.

Most of your partner's body will leave the ground when you lift her back. If you avoid the occasional temptation to jerk the back into position, your partner will stay relaxed when you reach the fully arched position. Like all stretching and pulling movements, you will eventually feel the usual point of tension, the point where your partner's muscles begin to tighten as you lift. (The height that is shown is just about as high as you want to go with the full body lift.) Never lift beyond this point. When you reach it, shake the back sideways three times and lower your partner slowly. When she's just a few inches above the ground, shake the body once again from side to side gently. This does great things for the lower back and will encourage the unique kind of trust that characterizes the massage experience.

Like hand-over-hand compression, this forearm movement allows you to vary the pressure as you work on different parts of the body. The forearm can cover large amounts of the body at once and feels massive to your partner. Begin at the shoulders, and work in slow circles. Be sure to cover all of your partner's torso. This movement feels very different from anything else you'll be

doing. If you skip a spot, your partner will definitely notice an omission. When you're at the very edge of the rib cage, you can lower your fist so that your knuckles make contact with your partner's side. On the flatter parts of the torso, it's best to keep your fist elevated (as shown) because lowering it on a flat surface will raise the wrist part of your forearm. When you reach the waist, reverse the direction of the movement up the center of the torso to the neck. Working up and back this way, cover the entire torso three times.

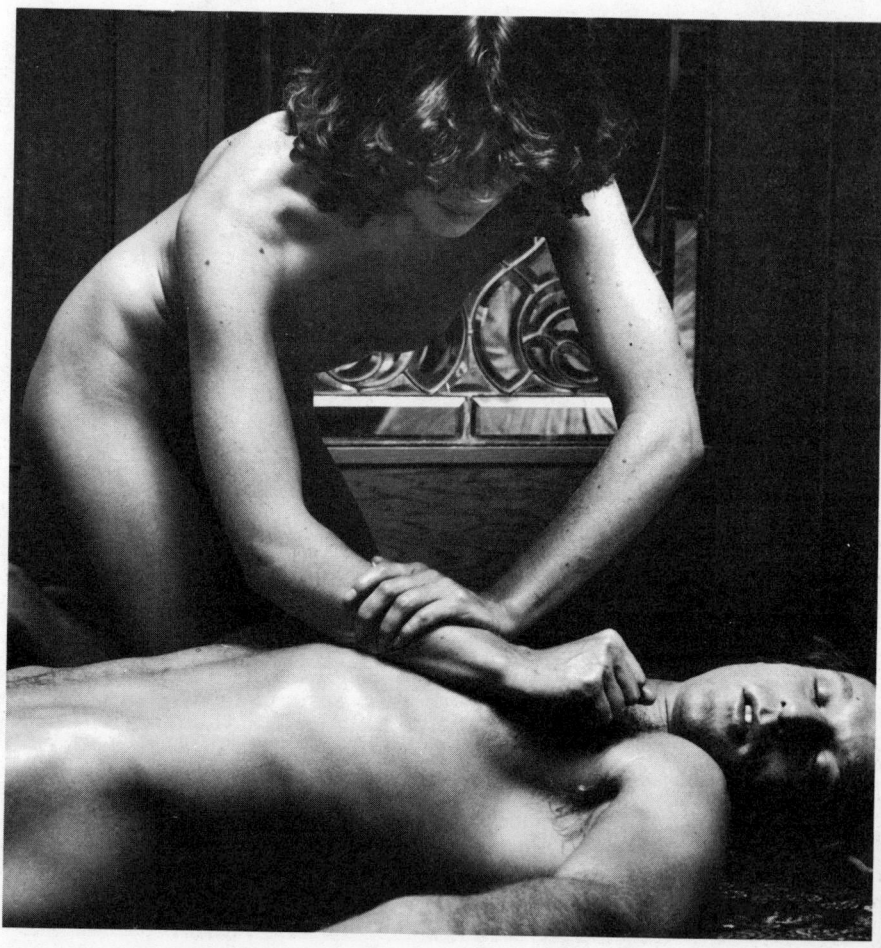

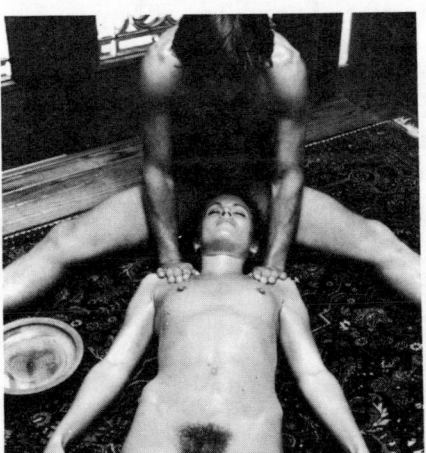

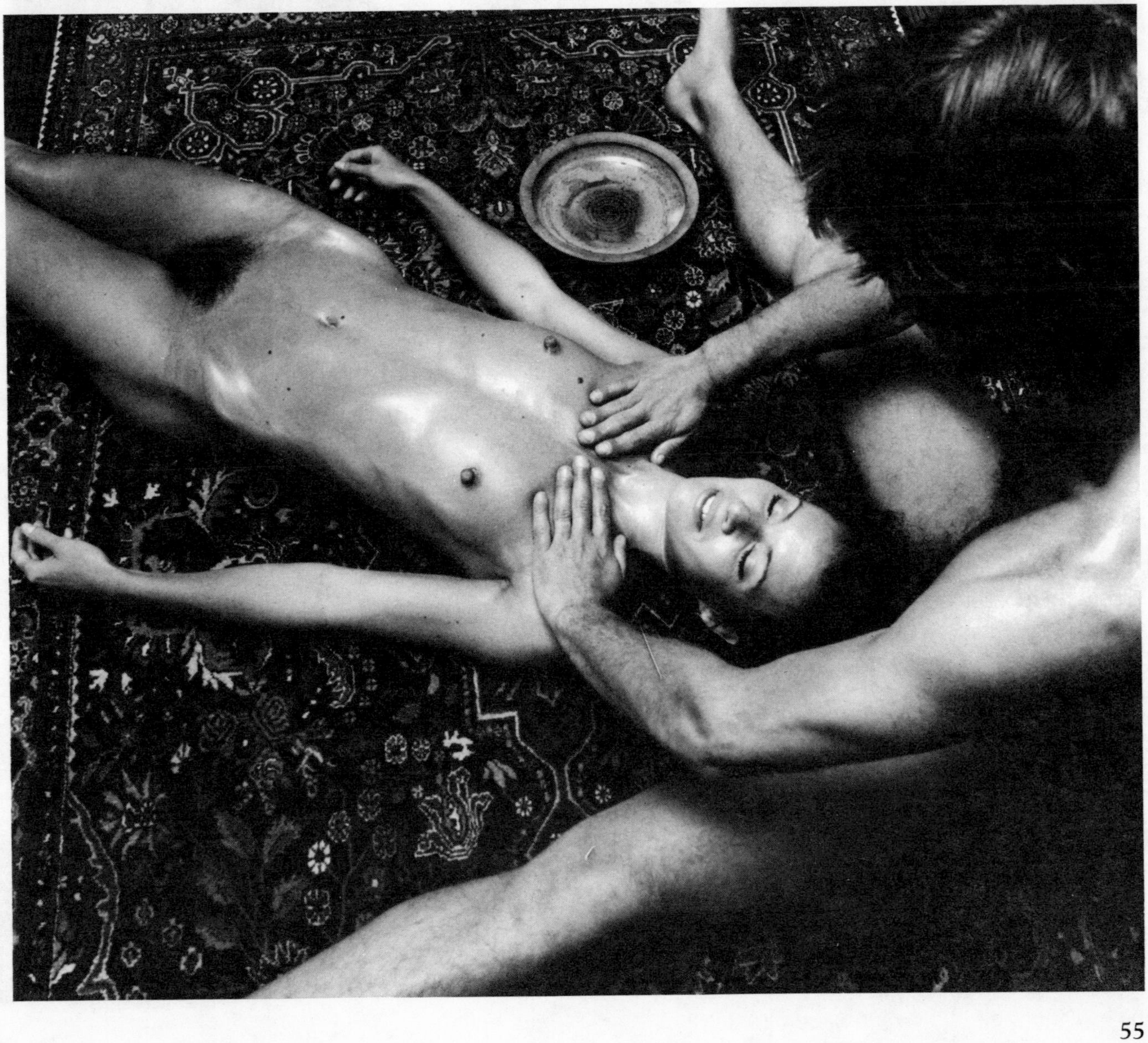

Kneel above your partner's head. This movement covers the entire front of the torso, both sides, and parts of the back in a single long sweeping motion. There is no deep stroking movement anywhere on the body that covers more skin. Since that is what massage is all about, everyone loves this movement. You'll want to repeat it at least ten times. Begin at the shoulders, making full contact from the base of the palm to the tips of your fingers. If

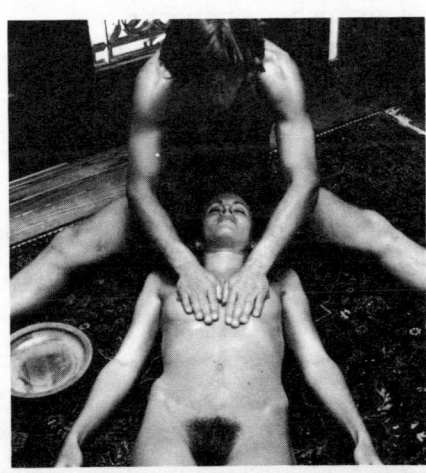

you remember to maintain this contact all through the movement and follow the sequence below, there's really no way you can go wrong. Be sure the entire torso is thoroughly oiled before you begin. Keep your fingers together, and arrange yourself in a comfortable position—either with your legs apart (as shown) or, if you prefer, with your legs crossed, kneeling, or sitting on the side of one thigh with your legs tucked under. Since the stroke covers such a large part of the body and depends on repetition for its full effect, you should be extra careful to get comfort-

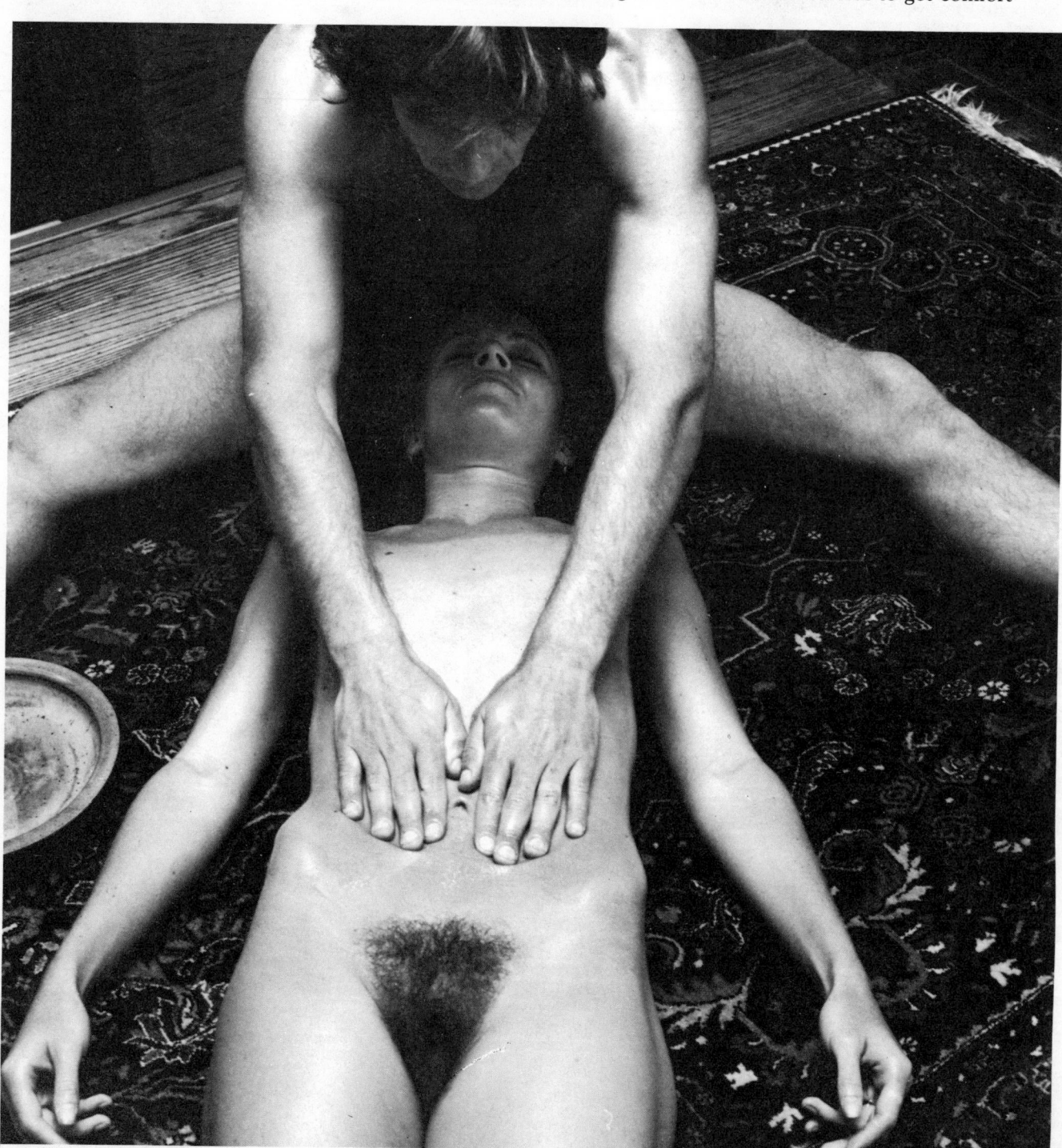

able before beginning so there's no chance you will have to break contact while changing position. Ideally you should press down as far as your partner's waist before starting up the sides of the abdo- men to the shoulder. If you're much shorter than your partner, it may be necessary for you to work from a kneeling position so that you can reach the waist more easily. On the return part of the movement from waist to shoulders you can, if you like, incorporate a lift. This simply involves sliding your hands under your partner's rib cage and lifting (as shown). In order to do that smoothly, you'll

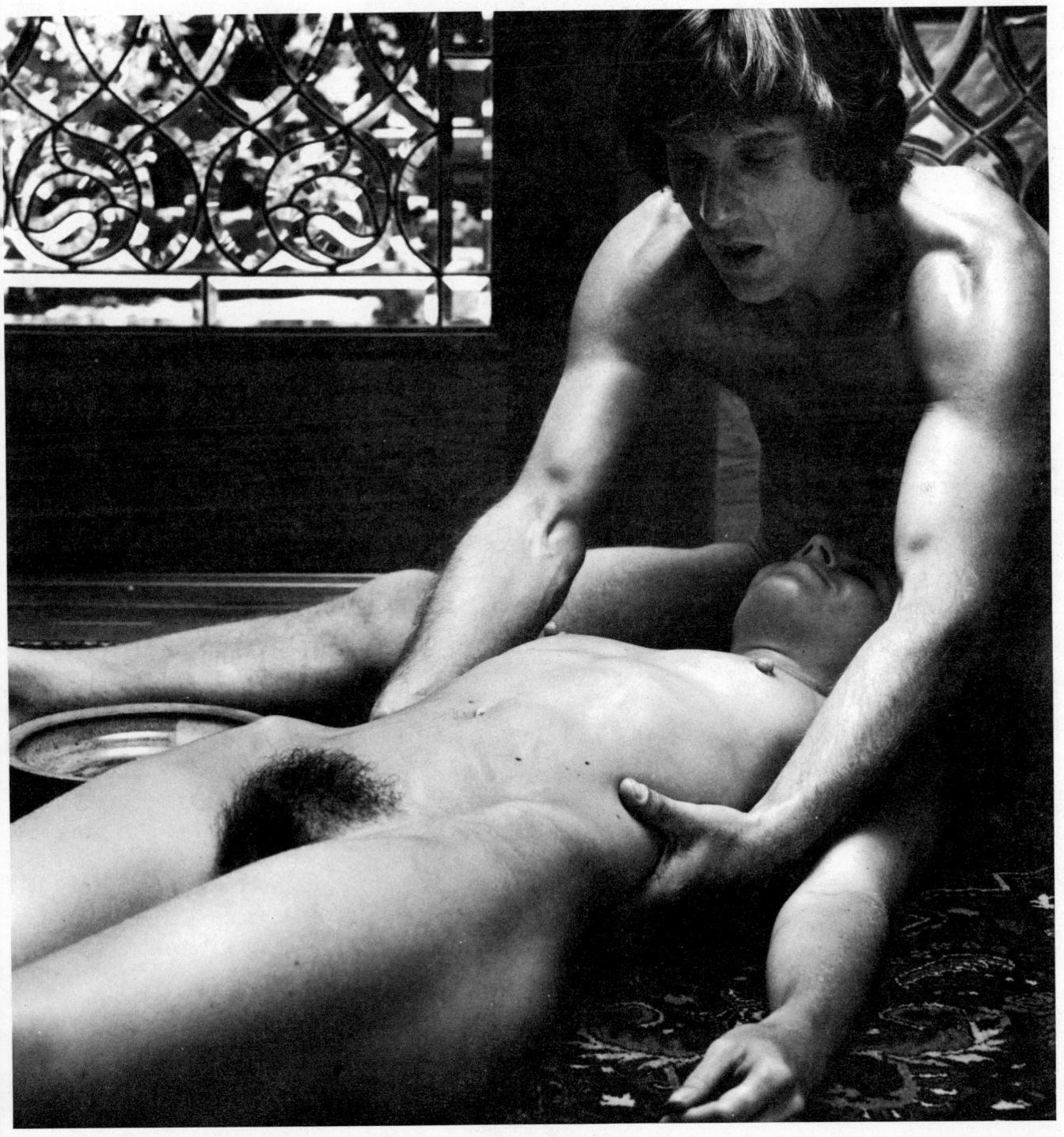

have to oil under the rib cage before you begin. This extra oiling can get a bit messy. Some people like to have their partners lying on a large beach towel, if the plan is to oil for the lift. Remember, too, that the lift requires strong arms and a steady hand. It's definitely an option, and under no circumstances should stroking the torso be aban-doned if you don't think you can handle this option. Your partner will still be quite thrilled if you content yourself with returning up the sides of the rib cage without lifting the back. Again, keep full-hand contact from the base of the palm to the tips of the fingers throughout this movement. On smaller surfaces like the shoulders you can simply bend your fingers so that your hands mold themselves to the shape of your partner's body.

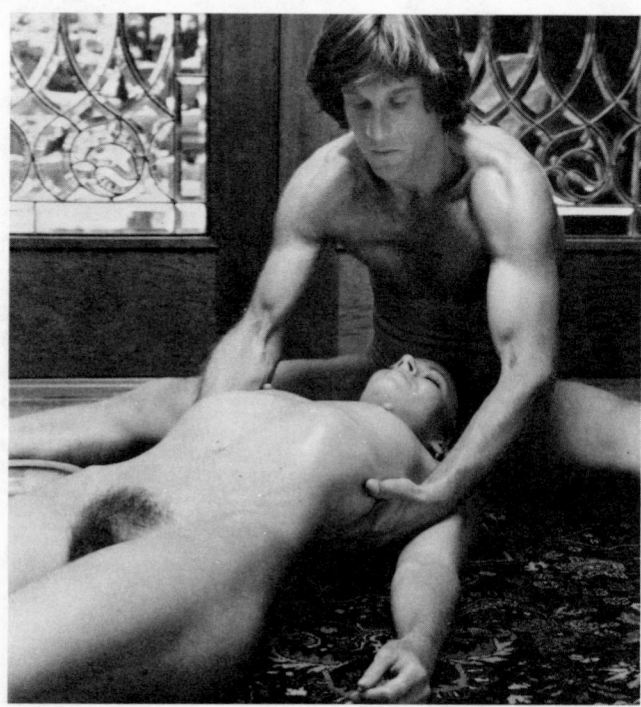
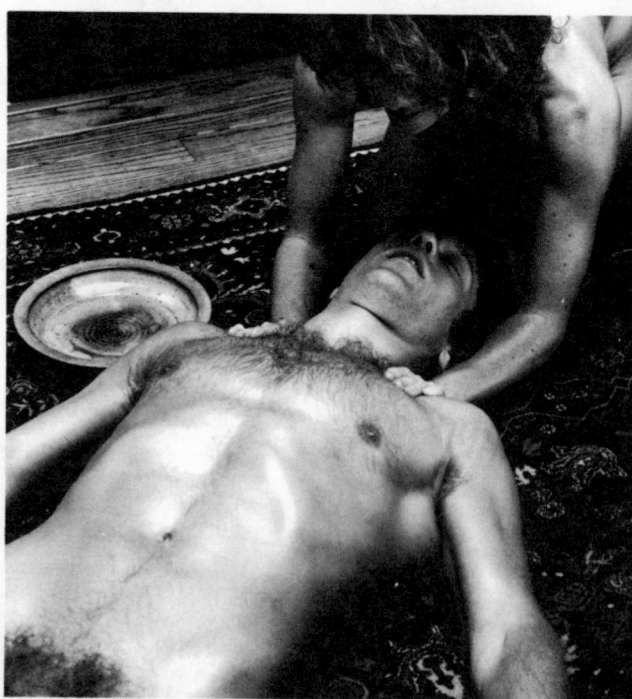

The Arms

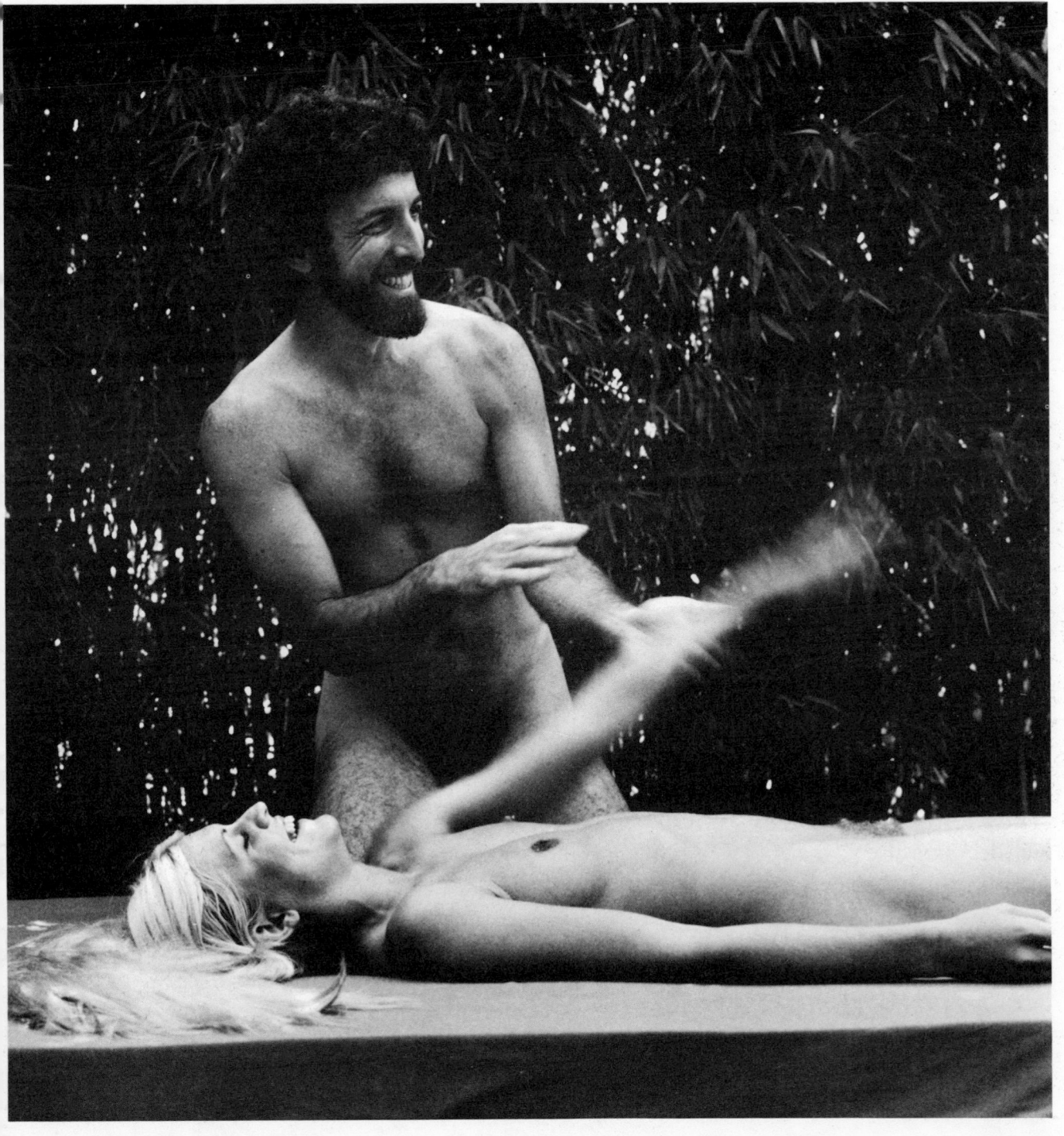

The Arms

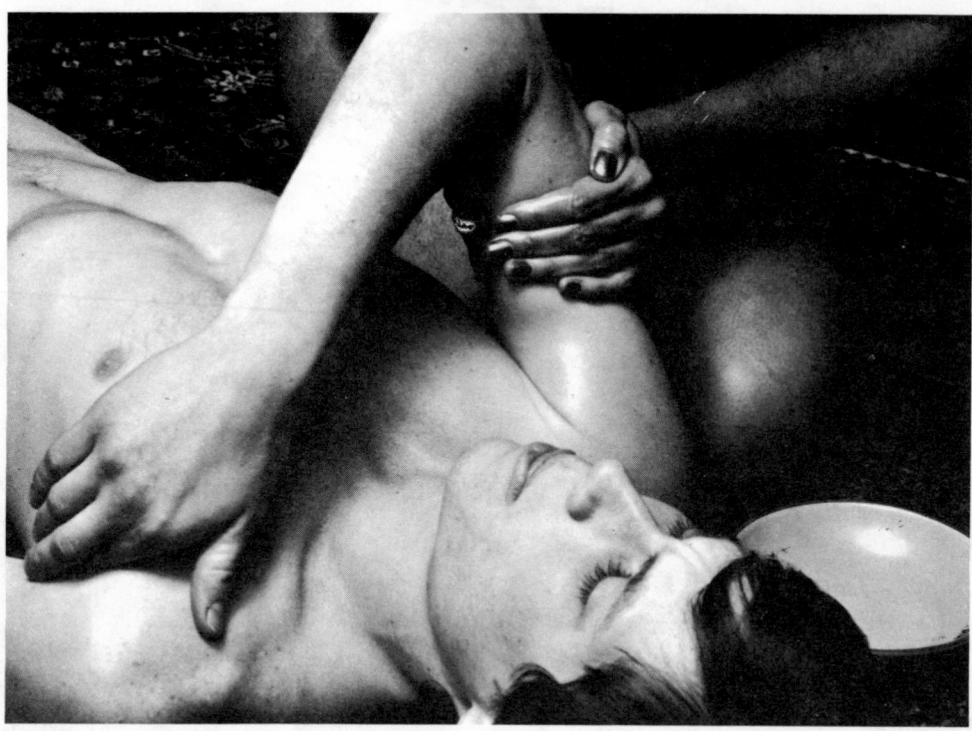

When people begin to exercise on a regular basis, almost every part of the body changes. One change of particular interest to masseurs is the way blood vessels within the muscles become more intricate. Networks of capillaries begin to develop within muscles to meet the increased demand for oxygen, to supply more nutrients, and to permit accelerated waste absorption. Like any physical change, this growth takes time. Usually weeks will go by before the body responds adequately, and meanwhile, exercise can become a real ordeal. While the muscles are being stretched into a new shape, they have trouble getting enough oxygen and blood-soluble nutrients. Wastes are backed up and begin to stagnate. The exercised limb feels sore and sluggish all day long. Many sophisticated exercise programs have come to regard constantly aching muscles as the inevitable price beginners must pay for developing their out-of-shape bodies. It's always a great pleasure to massage people who have stoically accepted this preposterous notion. Fluid Release techniques can be used to relieve almost all the painful aftereffects of exercise by pumping massive quantities of blood through the muscles without speeding up the heart. The kneading movements in this chapter will triple the blood supply to all of the arm's important muscle groups. They will also boost oxygen consumption in those muscles by 10 to 15 percent and promote more efficient fat combustion. Wastes are squeezed out of the tissues, and fatigue levels decline dramatically. Afterward, relaxation comes easily, and your partner can get through the day without being reminded with every movement of last night's exercise session.

Kneading the Lymph Nodes at the Top of the Arm

Arm Movement Series

Wringing the Arm—A Kneading Variation

Here is the perfect transition movement to take you from the torso to the arms. Each one of the four major lymph centers in the torso is located near the top of a limb. You can definitely enhance the Fluid Release effect by massaging the closest center before you begin work on a limb. This movement will complete your work on the torso and, at the same time, initiate massage of the arm. Use your fingertips to knead the thick muscles of the shoulder in a crescent right across your partner's armpit. Finish your kneading on top of the shoulder after clearing the important lymph center below one final time.

The series of four movements specifically designed to pump massive amounts of blood through the muscles of the upper arm include wringing, muscle pressing, thumb stroking, and thumb kneading. All these movements require that you develop a sensitivity to the size of your partner's arm. Large, thickly muscled arms will take a good bit more pressure than thin arms. But whether they are thick or thin, the same muscles are present and can be reached with these movements. The series of four movements, followed by a general circulation movement, constitutes a complete Fluid Release sequence for the upper arm muscles that are used in lifting.

If lifting with the arms is important to your partner for weight lifting, racket sports, dance, or gymnastics, these movements should be regarded as absolutely essential. Wringing is the first of the four movements. Grasp the muscles of the upper arm with both hands, and twist your hands in opposite directions. Move up and down the arm just a few inches at a time with this twisting motion. Be careful not to press hard on your partner's bones. Concentrate, instead, on the thickest parts of the arm. Remember to keep your fingers together as you twist.

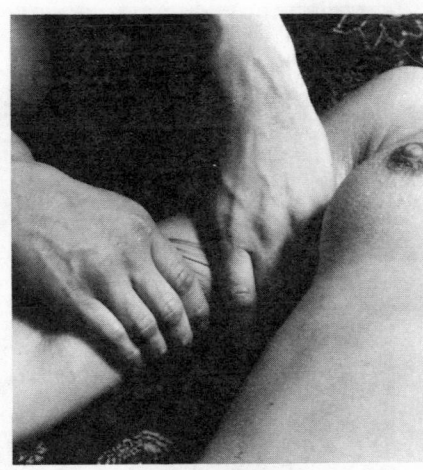

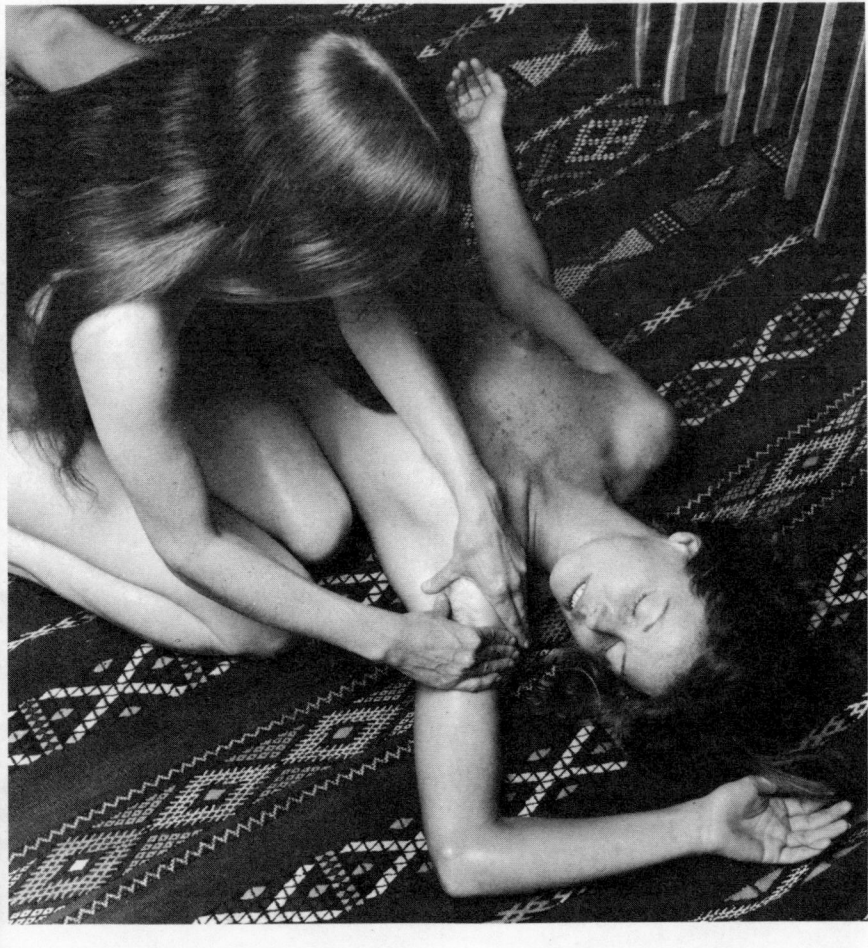

Muscle Pressing—A Kneading Variation

Thumb Stroking the Arms—A Kneading Variation

Kneading the Upper Arm

Extend the arm (as shown), and hold it in place with your free hand. Do this by spreading your partner's fingers so you can reach around through them to the back of the hand. Circle the muscles of the arm with the flat part of your hand, using as much of the hand as the arm will accept comfortably. This surface will vary a bit from person to person. On large, well-muscled arms you can use almost the entire surface of your hand, while children's arms will probably only accept your fingertips. Move up and down the arms in small, even circles.

During the kneading stroke the four fingers wrappd around the bottom of your partner's arm merely ride along while your thumbs do all the work. In thumb stroking, however, both sides of the hand are active in stroking down the arm. This is a pulling movement. Begin at the shoulder and work down the arm, pulling first with one hand and then with the other. Move in very small steps. Although your hands and thumbs are working on opposite sides of the arms, your movements should overlap. As you pull, press down with your thumb into the muscles of the arm. You can, if you like, vary your pulling speed. If you work fast, keep the pressures about the same.

Old-time masseurs used to work in rooms with ropes, straps, and pulleys hanging from the ceiling. Arms and legs were routinely trussed up and hoisted into vertical positions where they would hang motionless while the muscles and bones were manipulated. This quick hoisting technique is fine when you're working with sacks of potatoes, but it does tend to alienate human beings. There are two ways you can support your partner's arm while you knead; either will allow you to maximize contact and preserve the warmth that is part of every massage.

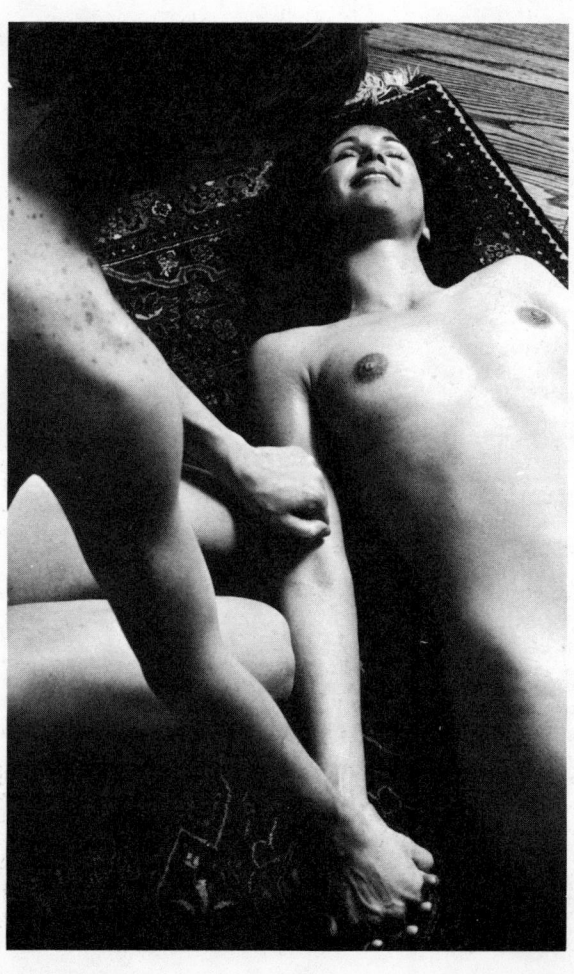

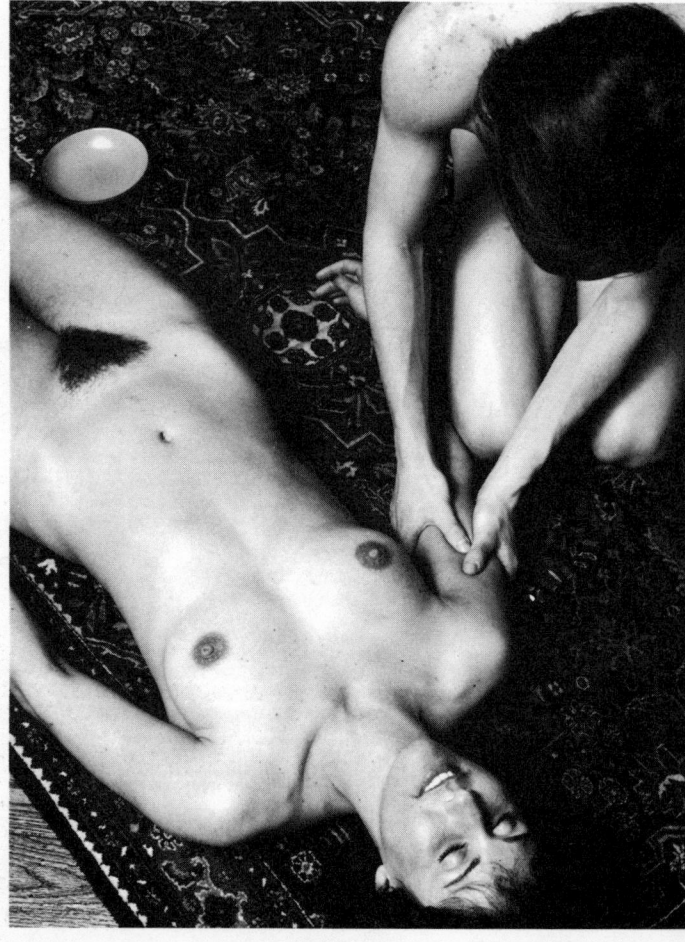

The easiest way to support the arm is to rest your partner's hand on your shoulder (palm down) and to tilt your head against it while you knead. You can hold the arm in place without much

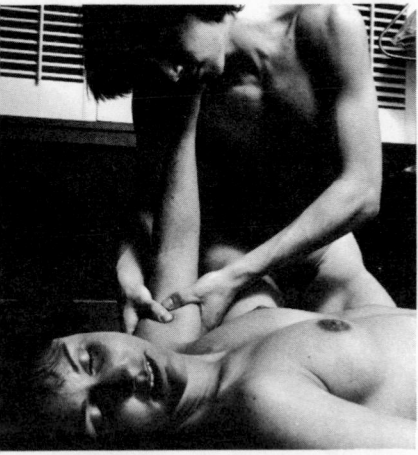

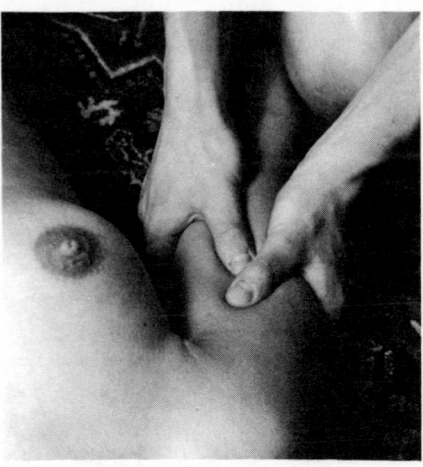

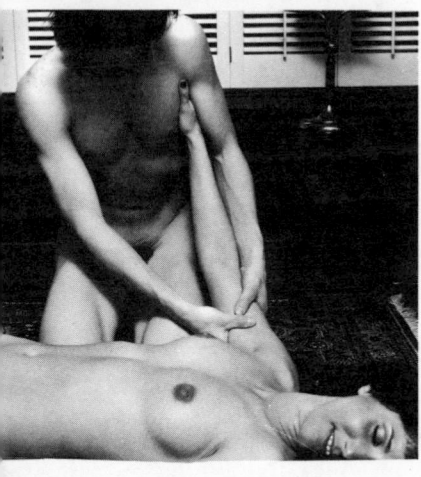

effort and with no help from your partner. Or, if you prefer, your partner's hand can be supported vise style between your arm and body (as shown). Be sure to keep the fingers together, if you choose this method, and fold the thumb around the front of your armpit. Once the arm is supported off the ground, you can reach underneath it with four fingers of each hand and press your thumbs into the thick muscle groups along the top.

Thumb kneading is one of the standard movements in massage, and you will use variatins of it on all the limbs. The emphasis is always on using the whole surface of the thumb from tip to ball as a broad, flat kneading instrument. Attempting to dig in with the tip of your thumb does not intensify the movement and may hurt your partner. The thumbs turn in smooth opposing circles. These circles will actually intersect, but since the thumb tips will always be at opposite ends of the circles, the thumbs complement each other perfectly (see diagram).

Like every kneading motion, these thumb strokes concentrate on the muscles. Here, on the upper arms, you'll be kneading the muscles that do most of the work when you lift things with your arms. The contour of these muscles is very easy to feel. Knead up and down the muscles, using moderate to hard pressure. As you feel the muscles decrease in size toward the middle of the upper arm, your pressure should decrease until contact just over the bone is almost superficial. Move up and down the thickly muscled parts of the upper arm from shoulder to elbow at least three times.

Joints are living hinges. Some of them work exactly the same way as door and cabinet hinges, while others operate like the familiar desk top penholder. But for certain of the body's more exotic joints, you will not find convenient models in any hardware store. At the joint between the thumb and hand two concave surfaces meet. The extraodinary ankle joints allow great flexibility while they support and balance the entire weight of the body.

One of the most troublesome and unnecessary constraints of aging is the way the joints begin to lose full mobility and impose limitations on the rest of the body. So many middle-aged people who suddenly become serious about fitness exercise the body within those limitations. Even after they have exercised for months, many of the limitations remain. How many runners could improve marathon times and enjoy running a whole lot more if they could somehow find a way to lengthen their strides or simply liberate the shoulders from a short, jerky arc that seems to work against the rest of the body all through a race? While the most well-intentioned exercise program may fail to compensate for reduced mobility in a joint, passive exercise movements can be used to restore a joint to full potential. Poorly toned ligaments and tendons that are attached to the bones where they meet at a

joint can certainly restrict movement. Passive exercise movements take the joint through its
full range of movement and
gently stretch the connective
tissues. The body's most flexible
joints—at the wrists, fingers,
elbows, shoulders, hips, knees,
ankles, and toes—all are lubricated by a thick liquid (called
synovial fluid) that absorbs heat
during movement. Passive exercise movements can be used to
stimulate production of this fluid,
to tone all the connective tissues,
and to develop full mobility in
joints all over the body. As in
every other massage movement,
your partner remains perfectly
still; you do all the work.

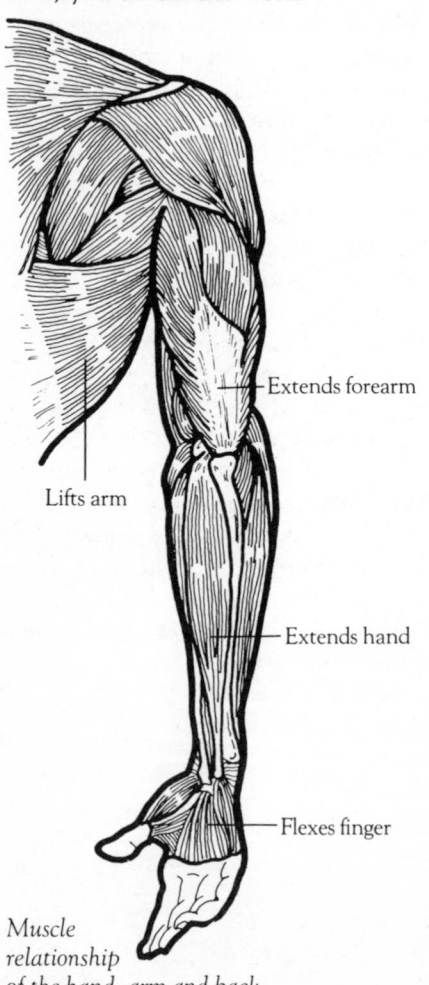

Lifts arm

Extends forearm

Extends hand

Flexes finger

*Muscle
relationship
of the hand, arm and back*

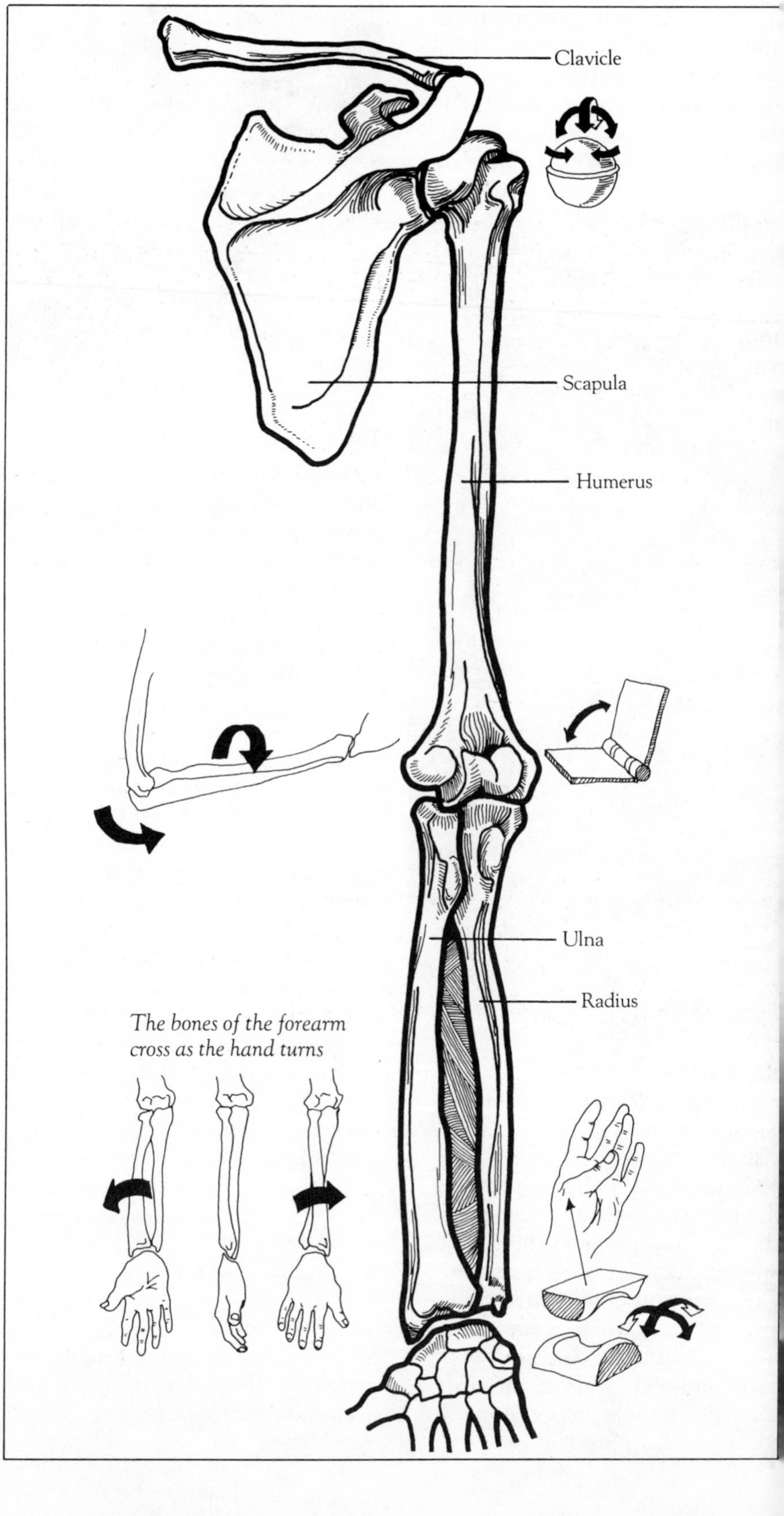

Clavicle

Scapula

Humerus

Ulna

Radius

*The bones of the forearm
cross as the hand turns*

his movement allows you to pull
n both arm joints as well as the
oint at the wrist. Grasp your
artner's hand handshake-style to
void any pressure above the
rist. Use your other hand to pull
own on the upper arm. This
osition distributes the pulling
ressure evenly over all three
oints and feels much smoother to
our partner than if you were to
mply pull the arm from the
rist. Pulling down on the arm,
se moderate pressure, and hold
or a silent count of twenty. You
an also use this movement to
xperiment with other effects on
he shoulder joint by pulling
vhen the arm is in different
ositions. The photo shows pull-
ng from the waist, but the same
and position will work when
our partner's arm is extended
traight out from the body or up
ver the head.

Hold the arm across the back of
the wrist just below your partner's
hand. This way the hand becomes a sort of natural handle or
stop that will prevent it from
sliding off the arm when you
turn. If your reach will allow it,
go ahead and anchor the stroke
on your partner's opposite shoulder (as shown). Press down with
your palm and fingers on the
shoulder while you pull the opposite arm. The anchoring will
prevent your partner from being
jerked around when you pull.
Turn the arm in a full circle right
next to your body. Circle three
times in each direction, pulling at
the wrist while you turn.

Flexing both arms at once is an
interesting variation on this
movement. Kneeling at your partner's head will allow you to lean
forward with the movement and
follow the arms. There's a wide
range of possible movement, but
don't try to overextend yourself.
Hold both of your partner's hands
just below the balls of the

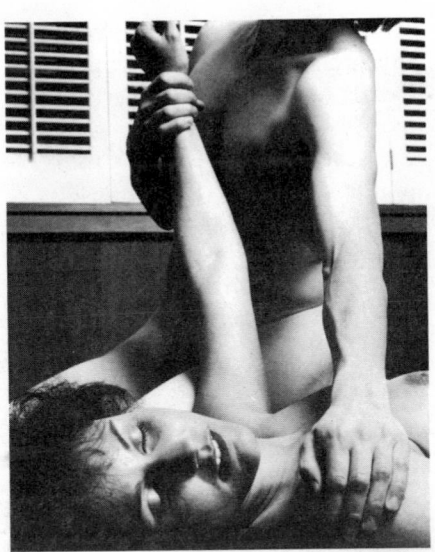

thumbs. Keep your pressures
smooth even as you turn the arms
in long sweeping motions.

One of the most exciting passive exercises for the shoulder
actually sends your partner's entire arm flying through the air.
Lift the arm by the forearm, and
guide it through a complete arc
from the waist to straight over
the head. Still holding the fore-

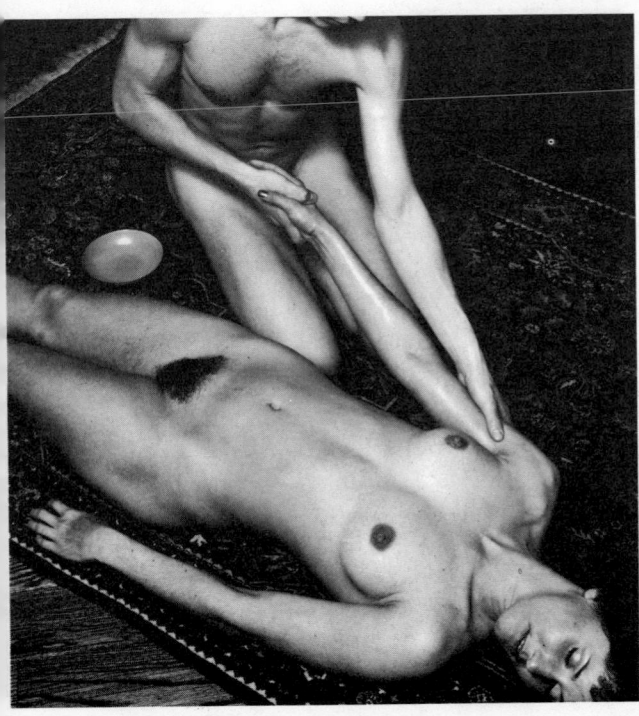

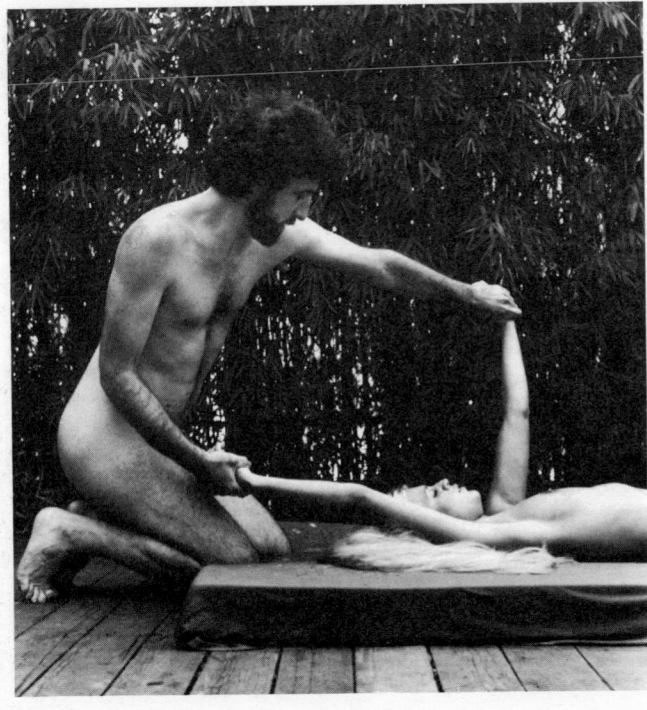

65

arm, go back and forth through this arc several times so you can clearly feel the point of resistance over the head. You don't want the arm to move beyond this point. By guiding the arm up to the point of resistance several times, you will learn exactly how far to go with this movement and give your partner the confidence to relax when the arm takes off. The movement involves lightly tossing the arm from one hand to another. Begin with a short throw, and gradually increase your speed and distance. Catch the arm at the forearm, and stay within the point of resistance you found when you tested the movement.

Lift your partner's arms just above the elbow, and let the hands rest on your shoulders. That way you can give full support to the whole arm throughout this movement. Lift straight up on the elbows (as shown), and the shoulders will rise along with the chest. Hold the arms up in position for a silent count of ten, and lower them slowly. Be sure to give as much support as possible to both arms as you lay them back down on your massage surface. This movement really does three things at once: It puts a welcome tension on the shoulder joint, it lifts the top of your partner's chest, and it stretches the massive back muscle that reaches from shoulder to shoulder. Much more on that one in the chapter on the back.

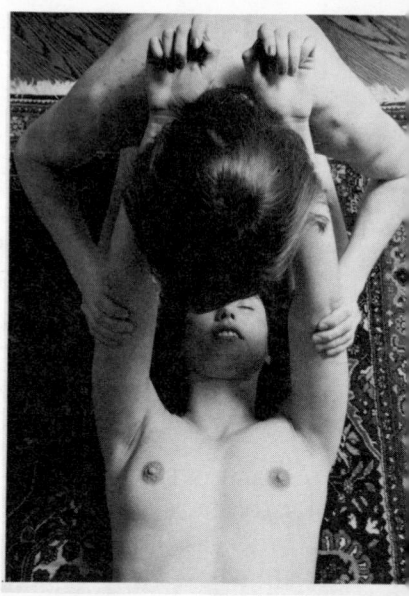

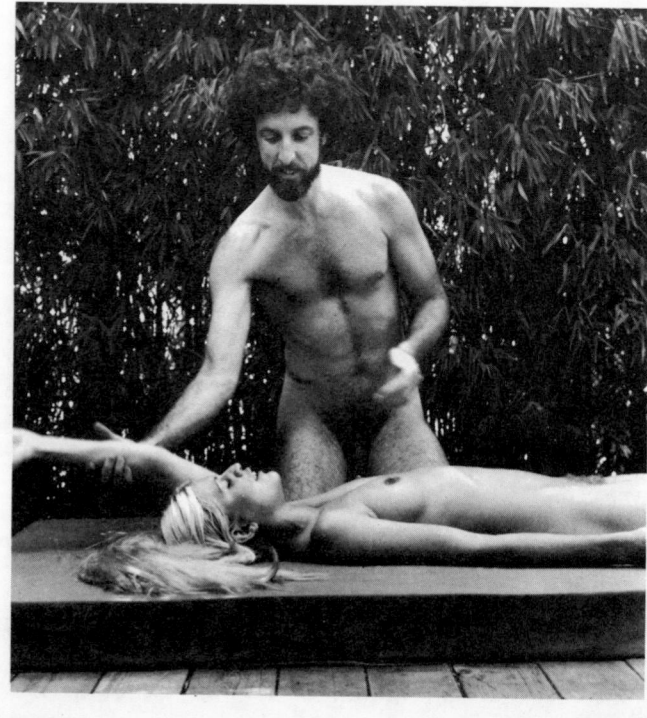

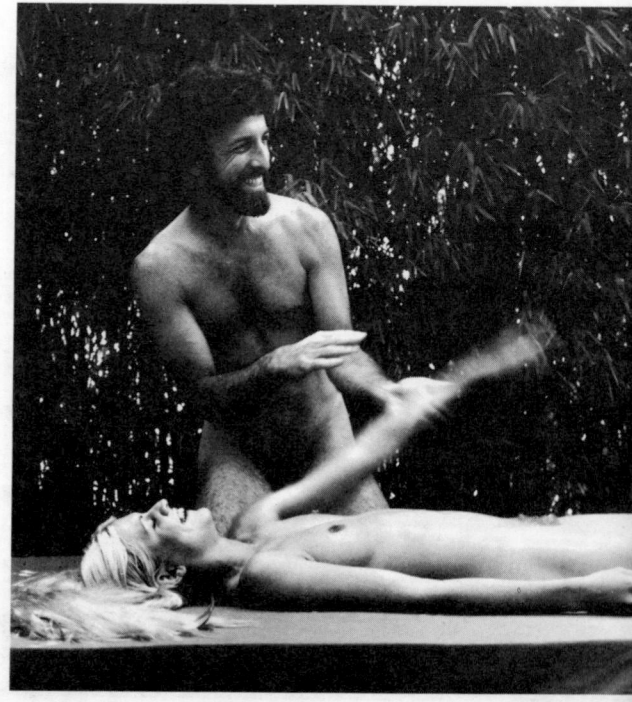

nchor the arm by pressing down
a it just above the elbow. A
eady grip on this point will
low you to confine all move-
ent to the forearm when you
rn it. The elbow is a basic
inge joint that permits an up-
d-down flexing motion of the
orearm. This straightforward ac-
on is, however, coupled with
ne of the most unusual bone
ovements in the entire body.
he two large bones of the
orearm actually cross over each
ther when the hand is turned
ver (see illustration). That cross-
ng takes place at both ends of
ne forearm; the elbow and the
rist. Passive exercise for the
lbow should combine movements
hat take place at the joint.
Depending on whether you grasp
our partner's wrist or hand,
ompletely different things will
appen when you turn the fore-
rm. If you grasp the wrist (as
hown), your partner's hand will
emain stationary. This, in turn,

keeps the forearm bones stationary and limits horizontal movement of the forearm. You can
make a small circle next to your
partner's side with the arm, but
for the most part, there isn't
much room to circle without
encountering substantial resistance. Most of the motion that's
possible is confined to a simple
up-and-back flexing movement.
But if you hold your hand over
your partner's fist instead of at the
wrist, a much wider range of
movement will appear. Keep your
anchor hand in place, but hold
the fist lightly as you turn the
forearm. This will permit the
hand, wrist, and entire forearm to
turn a full ninety degrees as you
rotate the arm. As the hand is
allowed to rotate, the forearm
will turn in a much wider arc
over your partner's torso and out
away from the body. The bones
cross over; your partner sighs;
everyone is happy.

If your partner complains of tingling or deadness in the hands,
look closely at the carrying angle
of the elbow. The carrying angle
is simply the angle formed between the elbow and the body
when the arms hang straight
down at the sides. While your
partner is still standing, before
the massage begins, you can see
this angle clearly. In men it's
usually about ten degrees; in
women, about fifteen degrees. If
the angle is substantially more,
it's likely that the most important
nerve to the hand may be overstretched at the elbow. Almost all
the important muscles of the
hand are supplied by the ulnar
nerve, which is wrapped around
the point of the elbow between
the bone and skin. Banging your
"funny bone," which sends shiv-
ers up and down the arm, really
means pinching the ulnar nerve.
For people with an exaggerated
carrying angle this can become a
nasty little habit. Folks who work
on their hands and knees, like
gardeners and carpenters, also do
a fair amount of elbow banging.
Either way, if you can persuade
your partner to take care not to
bang the elbow, there's a good
chance you can soothe a bruised
ulnar nerve and bring peace to
the hands.

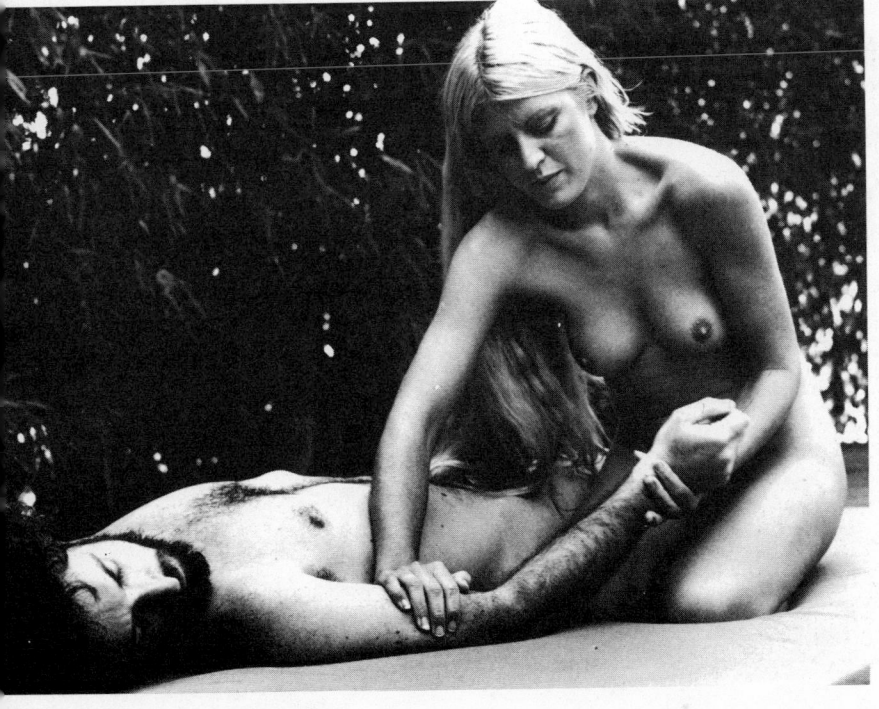

There are four ways to give elbow friction, and three of them are illustrated here. The fourth requires your partner to turn over so you can work from the other side of the body. If you're doing a full body massage and want to spend more time on the elbow, you can always return to it while you're massaging the back. Nobody wants to turn over more than once during a massage. Raising the arm over your partner's head gives you very good access to the elbow.

If you're ready to continue with movements in this position, go ahead and lift the arm. Give support with both hands above and below the elbow when you raise the arm. More typically, you'll reach the elbow on the way down to the forearm. If that's the case, the easiest approach is to bend the forearm across your partner's chest and to support the elbow with one hand. You can, if you like, reach across the body and massage the elbow of the opposite arm. If you choose to do that, be sure to include some general kneading movements up and down the arm so the friction stroke doesn't appear totally isolated.

The movement itself is simple. Press down and move the underlying tissues (not the skin). If you're specifically trying to soothe the ulnar nerve, work a bit faster than usual. Fast friction will quiet an irritated nerve, while slow friction awakens and stimulates drowsy parts of the body.

The veins unfill'd, our blood is cold and then
We pout upon the morning, are unapt
To give or to forgive; but when we have stuff'd
These pipes and their conveyances of our blood
With wine and feeding, we have suppler souls. . . .
—WILLIAM SHAKESPEARE, *Coriolanus*

Here is the massive circulation movement that masseurs use on all the limbs to move blood and lymph toward the heart. Wastes and impurities you've stirred up with kneading, friction, and other arm movements can be rapidly pressed through the larger blood vessels and metabolized. Toxins are flushed out, and at the same time, all the tissues from skin to bone are supplied with essential nutrients and oxygen. The entire Fluid Release sequence on every limb culminates with this sumptuous movement, which allows you to contact every raised surface of the arm in one uninterrupted sweep.

The idea is to make maximum contact while you press the blood toward the heart through the large surface veins of the arm. Press your fingers together, and hold your hands opposed to each other. On the right arm your left hand should begin on top; on the left arm it's the other way around. This allows

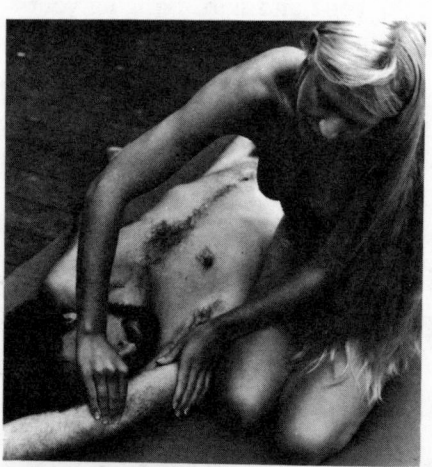

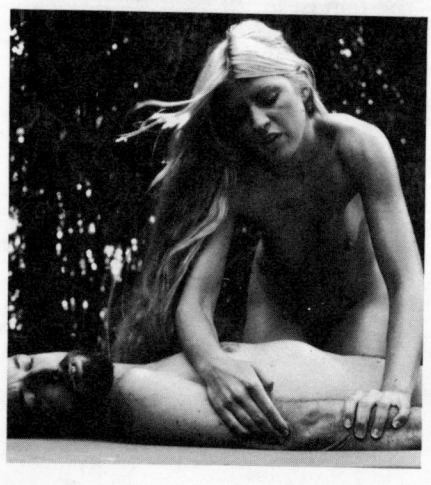

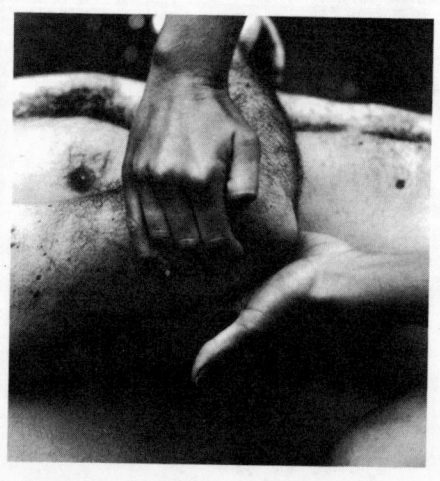

ou to extend the stroke up onto
e shoulder when you turn at
he top of the arm. Begin by
upping your hands over the back
f your partner's wrist. You want
onstant contact on both hands
om your fingertips to the base of
ur hand. Move up the arm with
oth hands, and allow your fin-
ers to shape themselves to the
hanging contours of your part-
er's arm. When you turn at the
houlder, your top hand should
lide right over the top of the

shoulder while the bottom hand
turns at the armpit. Make superficial contact with the sides of the
arms on your return to the wrist.
Turn again at the wrist, keeping
your hands flat and not breaking
contact with your partner's arm.
After you've practiced the turns
at opposite ends of the arm, you'll
get the whole movement flowing
up and down the arm so your
partner is no longer aware of

turns, hesitations, or changing
pressures. All those melt into
waves of sensation that flow up
and down the arm. Repeat the
full cycle at least ten times on
each arm.

There are also veins that run
along the side of the arm, and to
complement your circulation
movement, it's a good idea to
press them toward the heart.
Hold your hands with your fingertips pressed down and your
thumbs crossed over (as shown).
Push your hands toward each
other from opposite sides of the
arm as you press up toward the
shoulder. Begin at the elbow, and
work all the way to the shoulder.
Because of surface arteries that
move blood away from the heart,
it's not a good idea to use this
movement on the forearm.

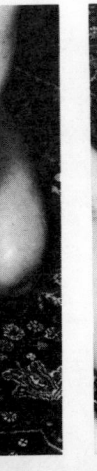
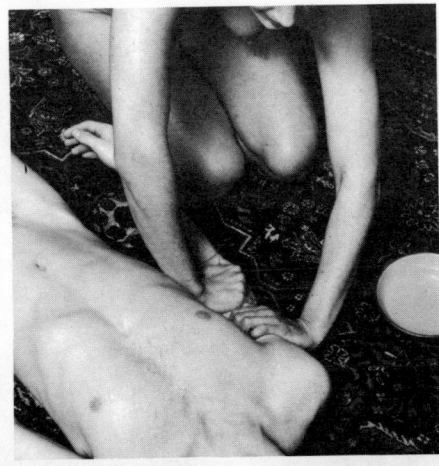
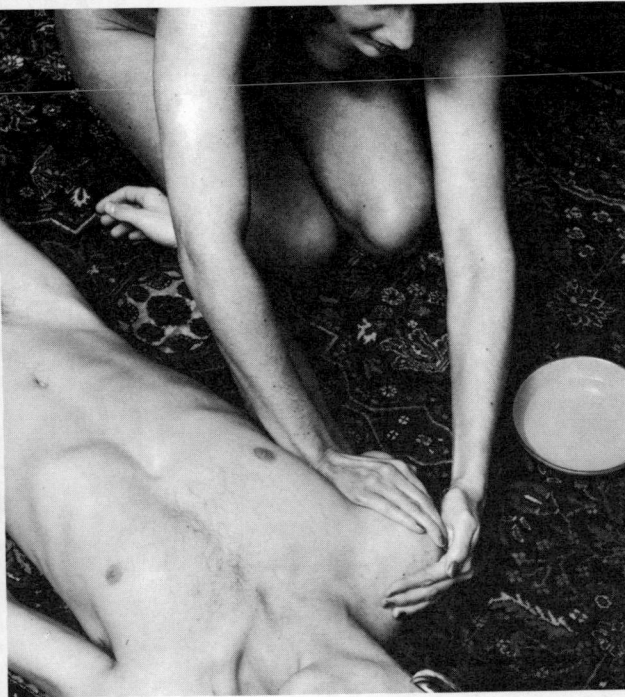
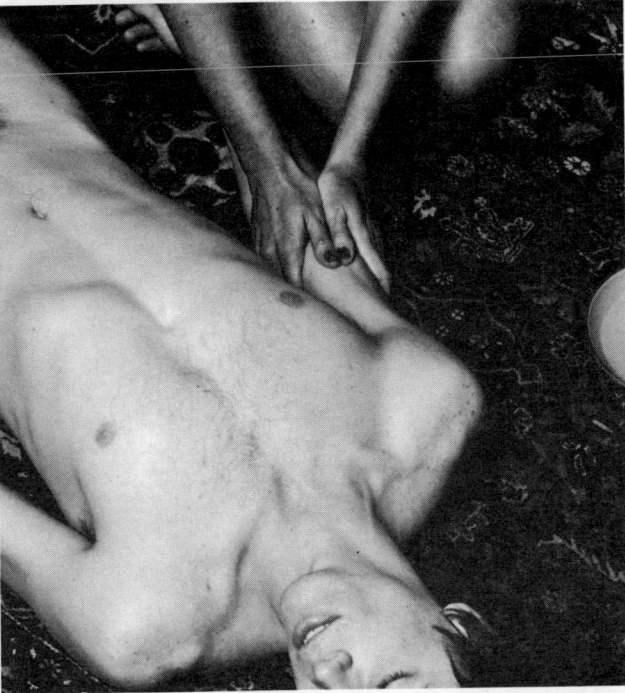

This long luxurious pressing movement covers the whole torso and half of the arm. Use it to end your work on the arms and at the same time to tie together the two parts of the body you've just massaged. Your hands cover a whole side of your partner's body from elbow to waist without breaking contact or changing position. Begin at the armpit with your thumbs together (as shown). Press out in opposite directions with your hands while your fin-

gertips follow every body contour. The top hand will go up to the elbow while the bottom hand descends to the waist. (If your reach is great enough, you can go on up to the wrist with your top hand, straightening the arm as you ascend.) The bottom hand has a bit more distance to travel, but generally the hands should always be equally distant from the armpit. Press up and back three times. Finish your arm massage by holding both hands perfectly still,

in full contact, at the two ends of this stroke. Hold that contact for a silent count of ten, and then release the hand at the waist. Keep your contact at the elbow until your bottom hand can join in a fingertip brushing movement up the forearm to the wrist, where you can begin massage of the hand.

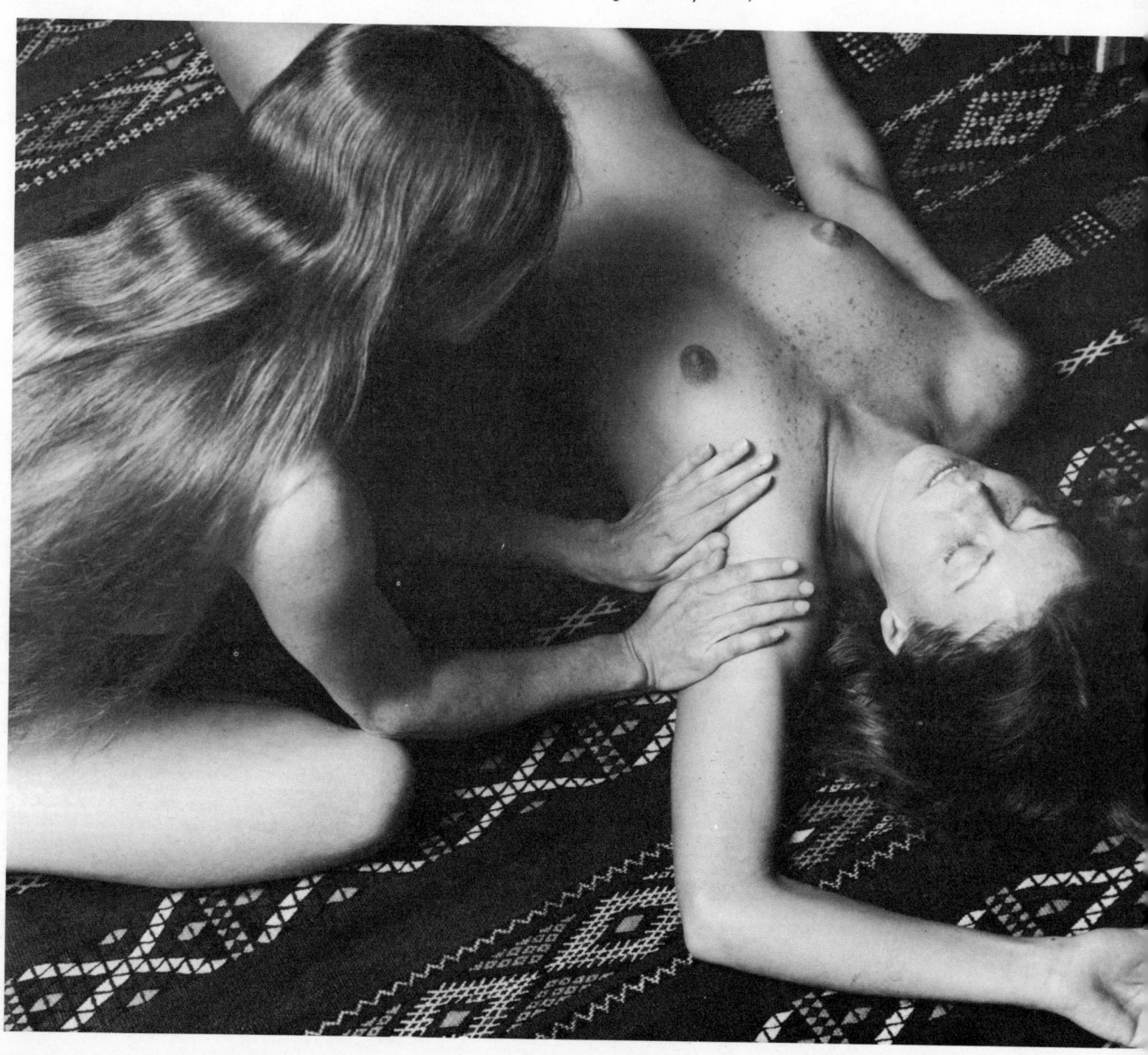

The Hands

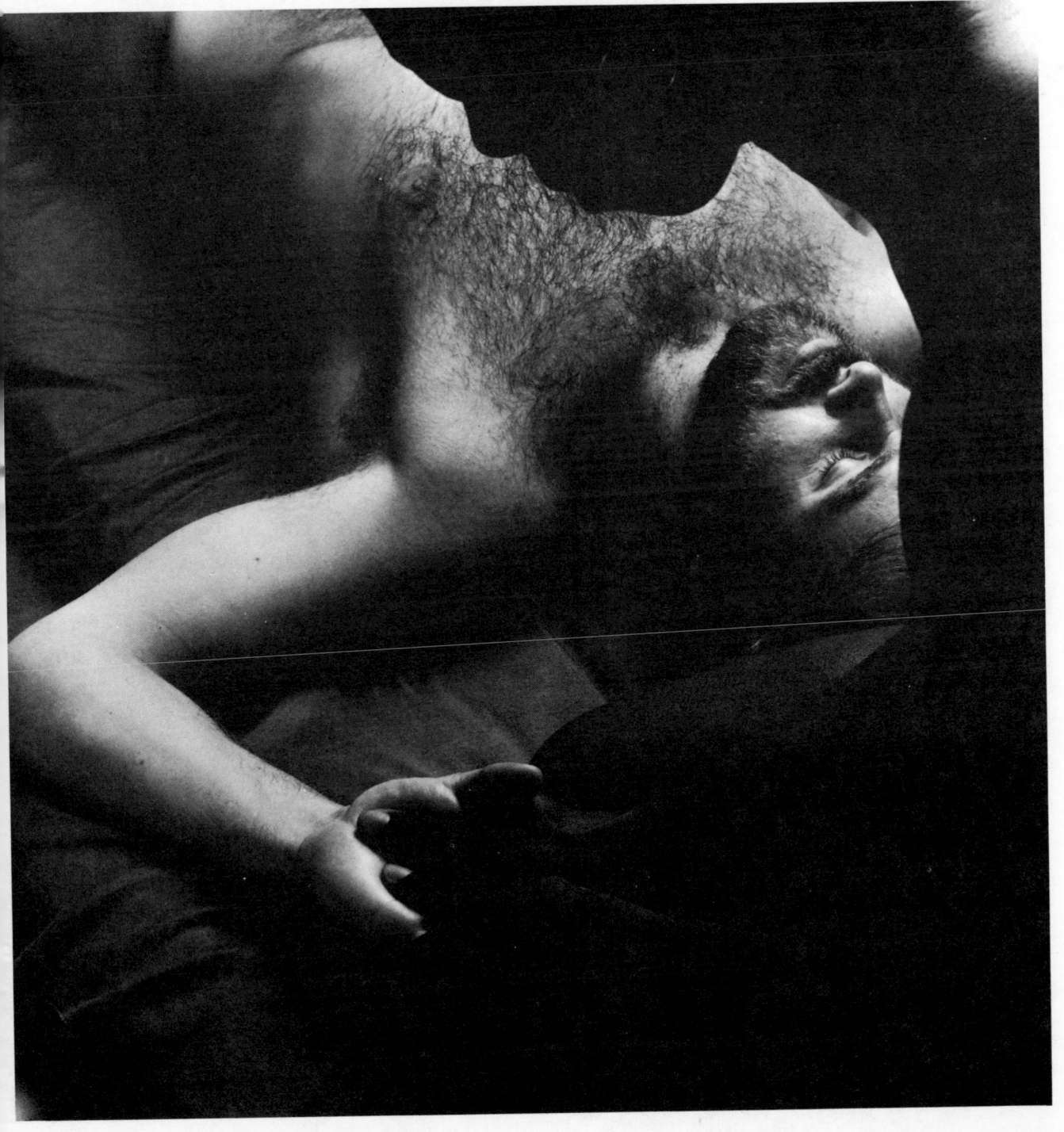

The Hands

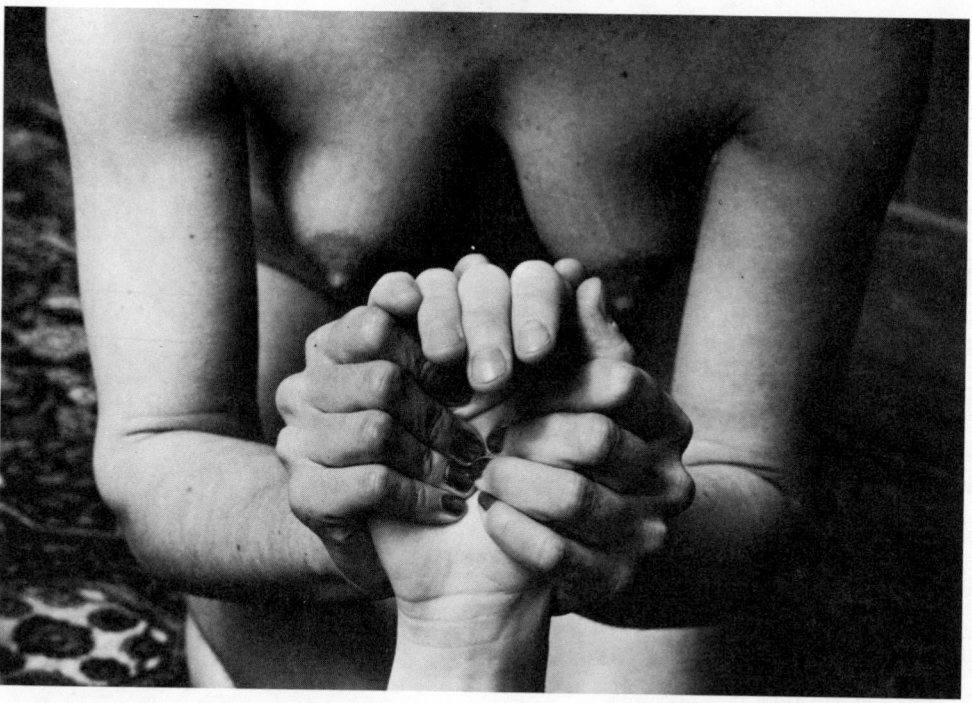

Hands are the only part of the body most adults will present naked to a stranger's touch. Since everyone is accustomed to being touched on his hands, it is a good place to begin massaging people who are afraid of massage. This irrational fear is shared by a great many people who would rather talk, worry, or watch than be touched. Marathoners who heroically carry on when body and mind say stop will often panic if somebody begins to massage their legs. I call this fear irrational because it's difficult to imagine anything more beneficial to a serious runner than regular leg massage. Even if you plan to work only on the legs, a few minutes spent massaging the hands first will serve to relax your partner and quiet his fears.

People are used to feeling things with their hands even when the immense tactile potential of the remaining 95 percent of the body is ignored.

Vacationers who eagerly strip to almost nothing on a 75 degree Fahrenheit beach will stubbornly remain fully clothed in a 75-degree living room. One of the real delights in massage is liberating the body from the suffocating influence of clothes, shoes, hats, gloves, and jewelry. Hand massage is an excellent way to begin this process simply because antitactile conditioning does not extend to this part of the body.

From the wrist to the fingertips, each hand has fifteen joints. All of them will respond to massage. Some masseurs will ignore the fingers because they are small and seem relatively insignificant. Is it really so much more important to dig into a thigh or the side of the back? If you like, the two of you can discuss this question and determine whether the thigh seems more important to your partner than a thumb or forefinger.

Hand massage begins on the palms. They are the fleshiest part of the hands, and the deepest strokes are possible here. If you start working on the hands just after completing the arms, your partner's hands will already be raised, and you can simply stroke down the arm and begin. But if you've decided to begin the entire massage on the hands, you may find your partner's arm straight down along the side of the body. Move the hand by moving the entire arm. Lift above and below the elbow, and put the arm down in the position you see in the photo.

Press up on the back of your partner's hand, and anchor the movement with four fingers from each hand. Bring your thumbs down over the top of your partner's hand (as shown). When you do this, be sure to reach around your partner's thumb so you can knead the entire palm right up to the root of the thumb. The kneading motion is exactly the

same as the one you used on the upper arm. On the palms you have to confine that motion to a limited space. Depending on the size of your partner's hands, it may not be possible to use the entire surface of your thumb when you knead. Make as much contact as is comfortably possible. The tips of your thumbs should follow each other in tiny circles across your partner's palm. When one thumb is up near the wrist, the other will be down toward the fingers. Keep your thumbs in contact with each other from tip to root. That way your rhythms will be smoother, and you will find it easier to direct pressures.

This movement allows you to exert much more pressure on the palm than simple thumb kneading. Lift your partner's hand and cushion it above your knee (as shown). That allows you to press down without hurting the bones on the other side. Anchor the whole hand at the wrist. All your contact should be right against the second knuckle of your fingers. Circle with this large flat area, pressing down hard. You may want to use just a bit more oil for this movement. Work around the whole surface of the palm up to the base of the fingers. Pay special attention to the fleshy ball of the thumb, the thickest part of the hand.

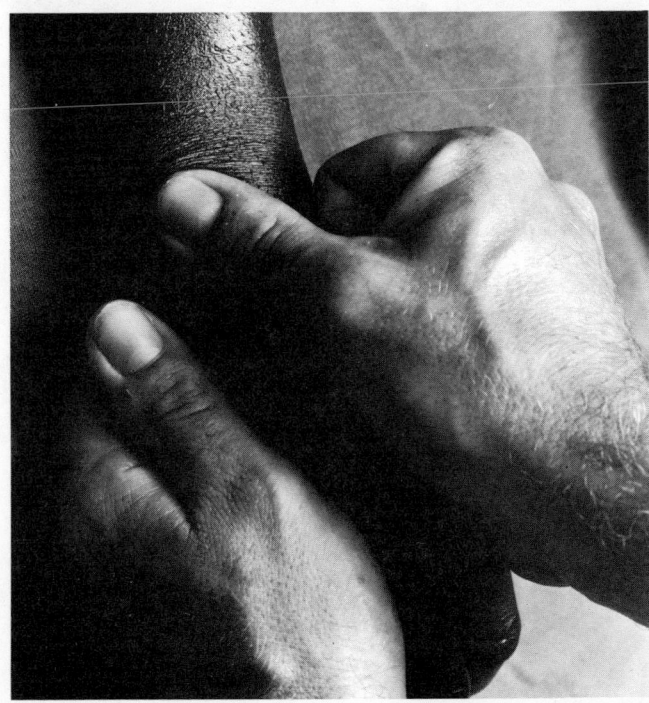
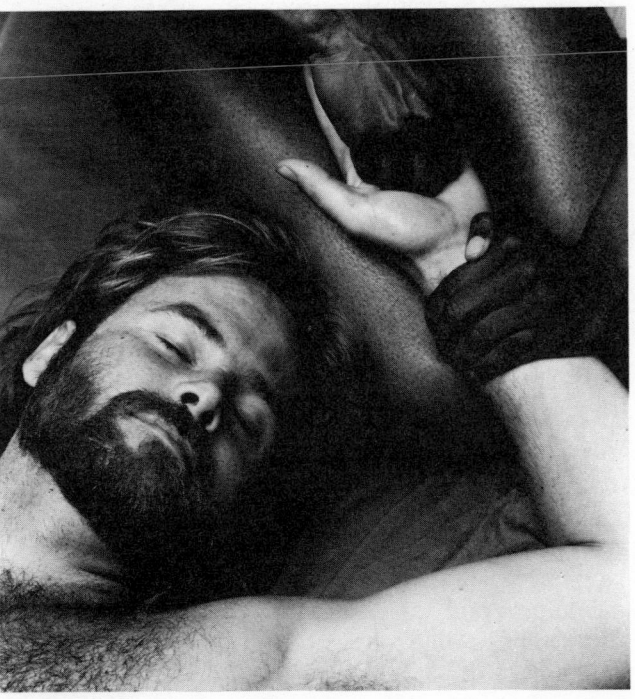

The joint at the wrist is one of the most complex joints anywhere in the body. At this point two bones in the forearm meet eight intricately arranged wrist bones. It is commonly assumed that pain in this joint merely indicates a sprained wrist. This is almost never the case. Wrist pain is usually caused by a fracture, a dislocation, or arthritis and calls for thorough medical investigation. Nevertheless, many skaters rationalize wildly after each fall no matter how serious. Is it possible that every accident is a learning experience which will never be repeated? One must certainly hope so if the wrist has been hurt. Successive falls after a painful wrist injury will manage only to confuse an X-ray technician. The wrist joint is complex but delicate and will not support the full weight of the body in high-speed crashes. Skating is one of the only sports in which you can badly injure yourself, yet continue playing. Masseurs must be ready to explain this to sloppy skaters who seek quick relief for intense wrist pain.

The top of the wrist is dominated by a massive ligament between the bones of the hand and arm. On the palm side of the wrist this ligament passes up onto the hand itself, leaving exposed the whole network of blood vessels that service the hand. Use your leg to support and flex your partner's hand (as shown), and this entire area will relax. The thumb kneading movement you use here is almost identical to the one you used on the back of the hand and the upper arm. Because you're kneading around a right-angle turn and space is limited, you won't be able to use the full flat surface of your thumbs all the time. Make as much contact as is comfortably possible, and avoid digging in with the tips of your thumbs. Begin at the wrist, and work across it from one side of the arm to the other. Light pressures are fine on the wrist, but as you work up onto the hand, you will want to increase them. Press down harder across the fleshy base of the palm, and finish by moving onto the palm itself.

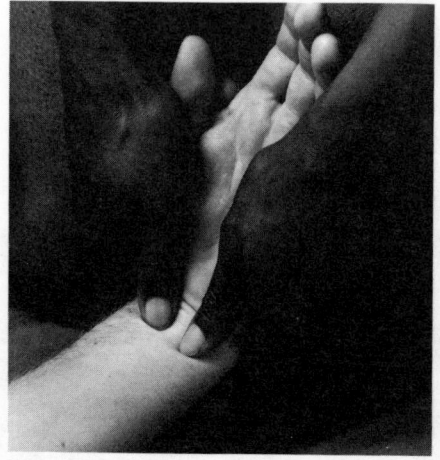

Two concave surfaces meet at the wrist and allow the hand to move straight up and down without permitting much deviation from side to side. This erratic pattern, so unlike the predictable ball joint at the shoulder, becomes apparent when you turn the hand. Flex your partner's elbow, and rest it on the massage surface. The movement is further anchored by supporting the forearm with your free hand (as shown). Take hold of your partner's hand around the back of the fingers, and bend it back until you feel resistance at the wrist. Keep the hand right at that point of resistance as you begin to turn the wrist. The whole hand will

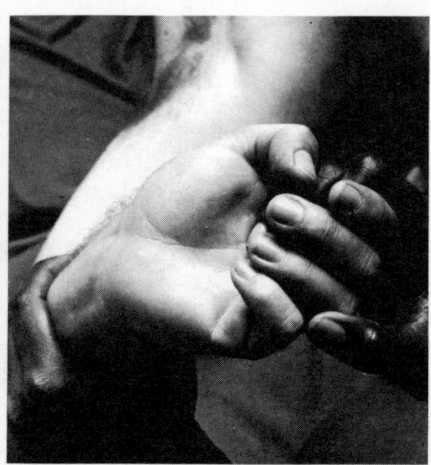

turn easily on the wrist joint as long as you don't try to press beyond the point of resistance. That point marks the comfortable limitation of both the wrist joint and the local muscles and tendons. Practiced daily as a passive exercise, this movement will eventually develop greater mobility in the wrist. After a while the point of resistance recedes, and the wrist will become much more supple than before. Practiced daily as a simple massage technique, this movement will allow your partner to feel and hear a major joint moving effortlessly. People for whom "elegance" means only the consumption of expensive goods have not had this experience.

The palm side of the hand is most easily massaged up near your partner's head. To massage the back of the hand, you need to move the whole arm so that it is parallel to your partner's body and the hand lies at the waist. Any other position will cause a tightening in the upper arm when the hand is rotated. This tightening is subtle, but then so are many of the effects in a full body massage. Remember to support the arm above and below the elbow when you lift it. Whenever you move a part of the body in massage, give as much support as possible. That way you do all the work and your partner is free to relax completely and enjoy the massage.

Almost all of the hand's twenty-eight bones form part of a highly mobile joint. The five bones that cross the back of the hand from the base of the fingers to the wrist are perhaps the least mobile. At the wrist end of these bones limited movement takes place when the thumb and fingers are brought together. If running is your only form of exercise, it's unlikely that finger grasping movements will get much use. This delightful stroke allows you to flex the least mobile joint on the hand by actually moving the large bones that cross the back of the hand. Since you're working with a joint that will permit some motion, a great deal of pressure is definitely not required. The idea is to position your hands correctly and simply to turn them in opposing circles.

Press up against the palm side of your partner's hand with your four fingertips. Press down on the top of the hand with the ball of each thumb. The tip of the thumb is not used in this movement. You should be exerting equal pressure with the fingertips and the balls of your thumbs. Once you feel comfortable with that position, you can begin to turn your hands in vertical circles. Always be sure that the hands are at opposite points in their circles. You may not feel much happening, but your partner will experience hard bones moving while the muscles remain completely relaxed. This is a very intimate movement because most people have never even considered surrendering control of their bones. Doing so usually makes your partner smile and brings the two of you much closer.

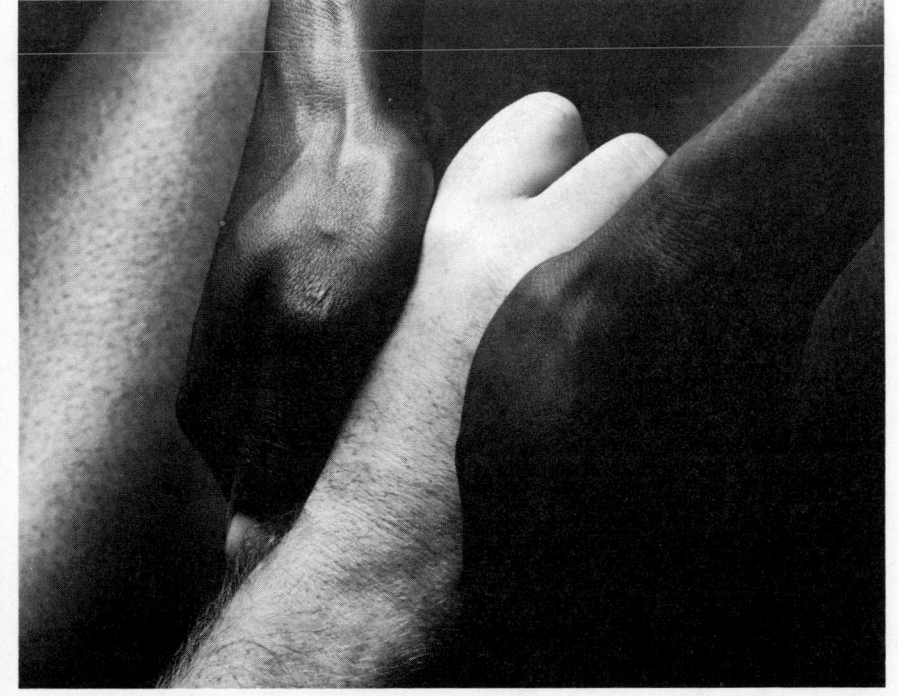

While massaging the arms and hands, you encounter thin muscular tissue that calls for long sweeping movements. A notable exception to this rule is the formidable carpal ligament that

If you cup the back of your partner's forearm with your palm, you will find that you can detect an interior quivering every time a finger is moved. Fingers are operated by a series of muscles that

begin at the elbow. Effective hand massage must deal with these muscles up on the arm and should also take into consideration their relationship to the hand and fingers. This movement

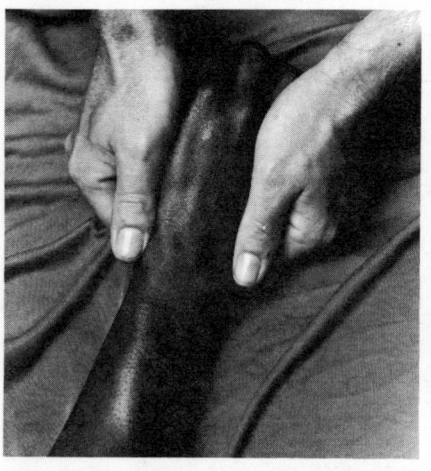 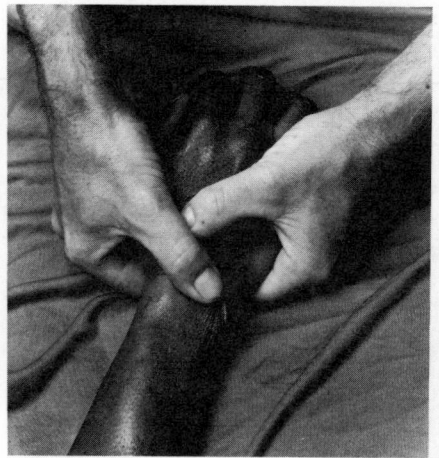 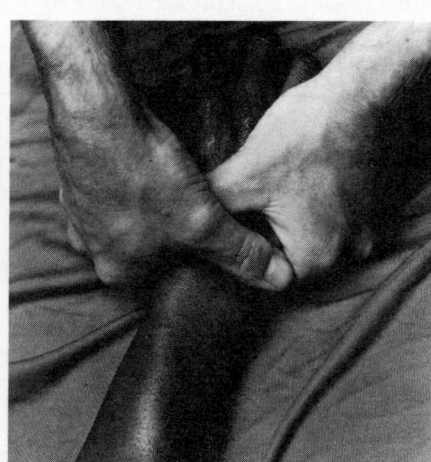

holds the bones of the hand and arm together. Massage it with a crisscross stroking motion, using both thumbs.

Begin with your thumbs in a parallel position crossed over the ligament (as shown). The movement is really nothing more than an unfolding of the thumbs toward your partner's wrist. There's usually just enough room for the thumbs to cross and uncross gracefully as you open and close the movement. Keep your four fingers flat and facing each other under your partner's hand. Glide slowly toward the outside of your partner's wrists, pressing down on the ligaments as you move. Use the full flat digit of your thumb to maximize contact. Stroke all the way to the sides of the wrists, and return three times.

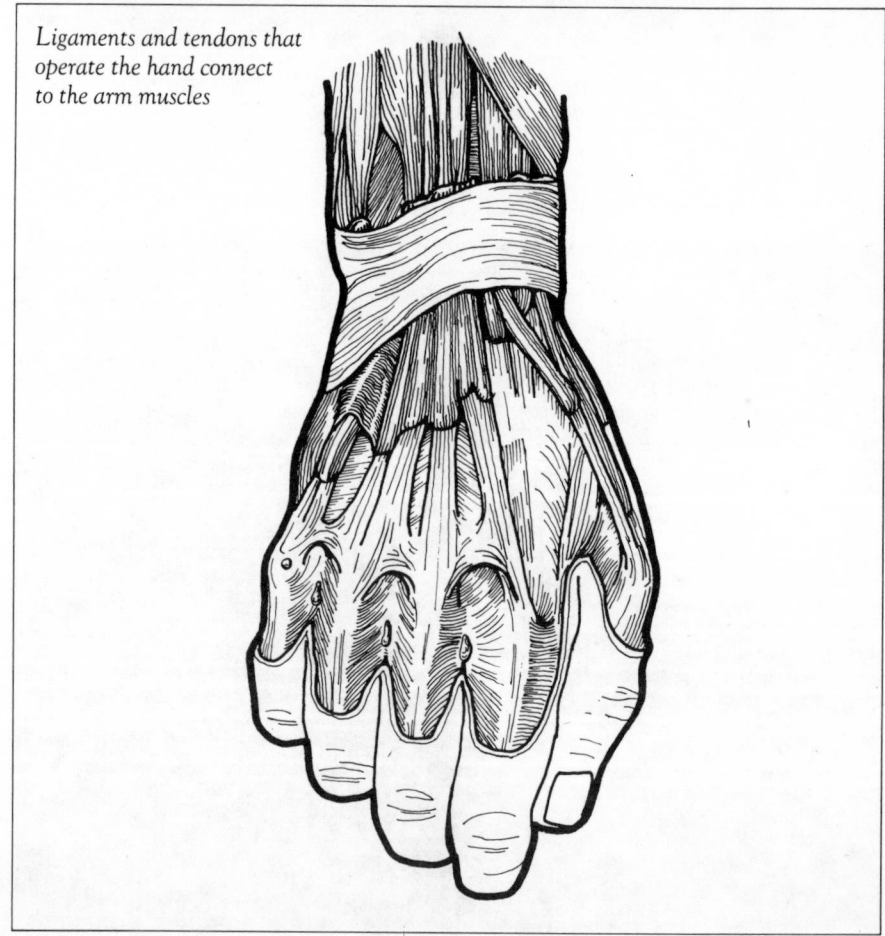

Ligaments and tendons that operate the hand connect to the arm muscles

allows you to integrate your work on the hand with the muscles that operate the fingers. Begin stroking about halfway up the arm, working toward the fingertips. Each hand cups the forearm to make contact all the way around from the thumb tip to the fingertips. Press down on the top of the arm with your thumbs, and be sure to keep them parallel all the way down to the fingertips. Keep your four fingers together under the arm, and use them to press up against the flesh while your hands travel toward the fingertips. Oil both sides of the arm and hand, and pull down toward the fingertips in short hand-over-hand motions. Your left hand will first glide down to

The extensor tendons that actually extend the fingers run right across the back of the hand and connect to the arm muscles at the wrist. They all can be reached with a simple thumb kneading motion to the back of the hand. Depending on the size of your partner's hand, you may not be able to bring your thumbs together full length (as shown). Even so, this movement works exactly the same way it did on the arm. Be sure to keep the thumbs moving in circles and remember that when one thumb tip is up, the other will be down.

Cover the entire surface of your partner's hand from the base of the fingers to the wrist. These are thin tendons that rest against the bones of the hand, so expect to press down lightly onto the bones when you massage them.

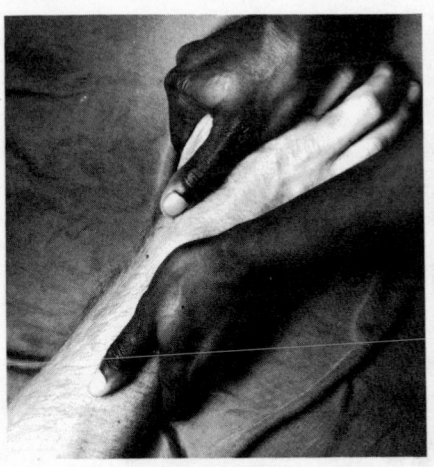
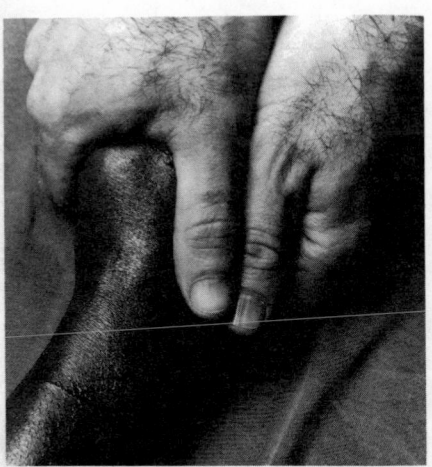
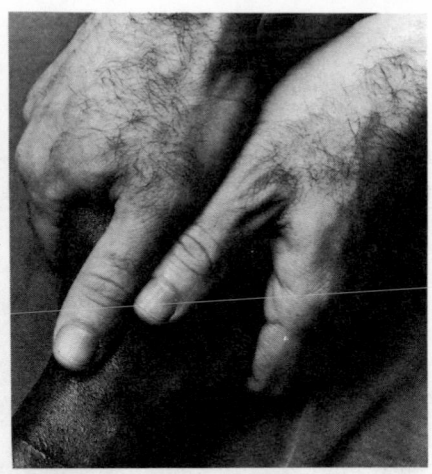
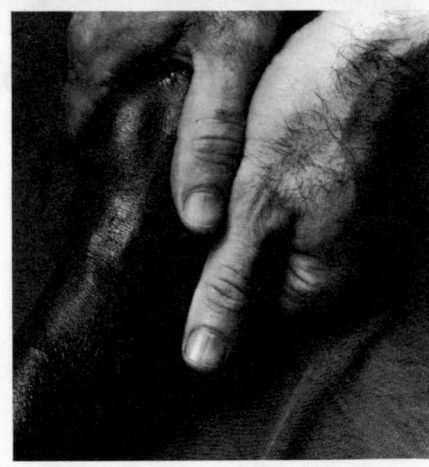

the wrist, then return to the beginning point as the right hand descends. Each time the hands descend they go a bit lower and return to a slightly lower point on the forearm. Final strokes begin almost at the wrist and extend all the way to the fingertips.

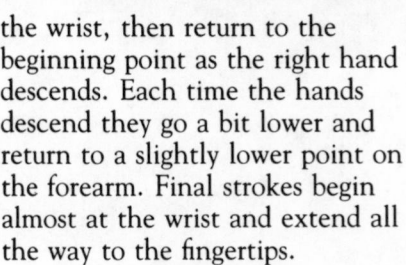

With the exception of the thumb, each finger is jointed three times. This movement will allow you to isolate each of these joints and to massage the area above it. Finger joints are covered with very thin tendons that extend the length of the finger. At the joints these tendons press right against the bone. Like other tendons that rub against bone, those in the fingers are enclosed in a protective sheath. If the sheath is poorly lubricated, an irritation commonly known as bursitis can develop. Finger massage will lubricate these tendon sheaths, passively exercise the joints, and spread good feelings out to the tips of your partner's fingers.

Begin your finger massage by pulling gently just above each joint on each of the fingers. On the first joint you simply grasp the whole finger all the way up to the knuckle and pull gently. On the second joint it's important to isolate the first joint so you don't

find yourself pulling both of them. Do this by folding your partner's finger between your third and fourth fingers (as shown). Press your fingers together to anchor the stroke. When you pull above the second knuckle, your anchor fingers will confine the effect to that knuckle. You can then go ahead and knead the top part of the finger by rubbing back and forth with your thumb and forefinger. Move your anchor fingers up above the second joint, and use the same movement on the top joint. Begin with the little finger, and work across to the thumb, pulling and kneading each finger at all three joints. Because the thumb is jointed only twice, you can anchor it with the thumb and forefinger of your free hand.

Finger stroking combines circulation with a general nerve stimulation on the sides of the fingers. Work toward the heart away from the tips of the fingers. Anchor your stroking movement on each finger by holding the fingertip with your thumb and forefinger. You can end this movement at the base of the fingers or by extending it down a bit farther and gliding around the knuckles. Return to the fingertips with a light superficial pressure. Do each finger three times.

If your partner has been experiencing stiffness in the fingers, you may want to follow these finger movements with extra kneading movements on the back of the hand and the forearm. The idea here is to invigorate the muscles that operate the fingers and stimulate the nerves throughout the area.

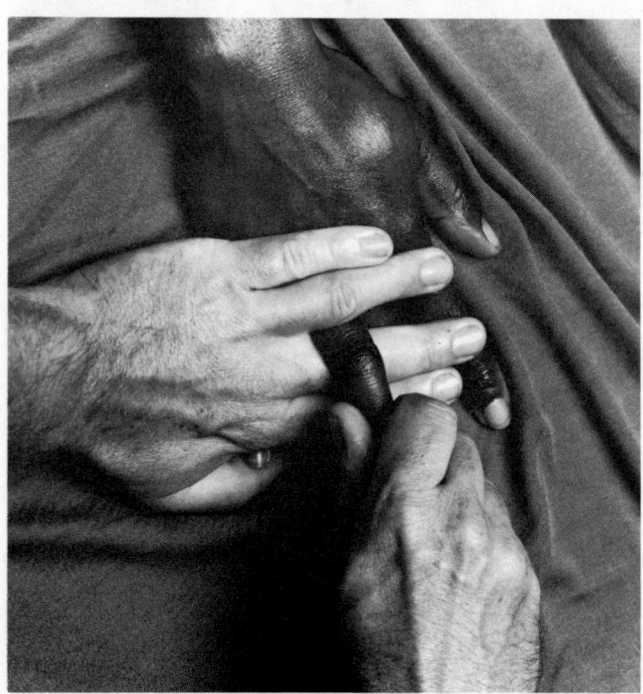

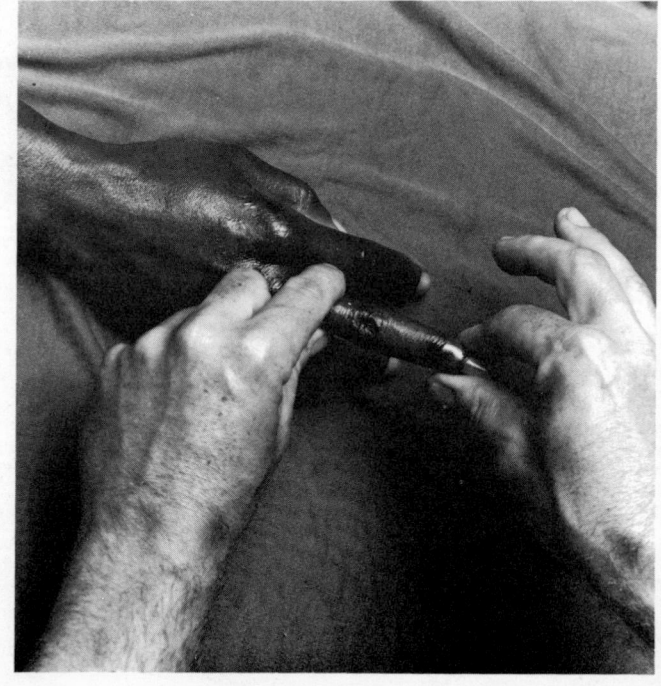

This is what happens when fifteen fingers intersect in an intelligent and deliberate fashion. Your little finger should wrap around the outside of your partner's little finger. If you begin there, you can

fingers straight back while they are spread apart. Press to the point of tension and relax slowly.

Normally one of the most tactile parts of the body, the hands become intensely sensitized after a few minutes of massage. Brushing enhances the sensitivity by allowing your partner to feel dozens of very light contact movements traveling toward the fingertips. You can start this movement up on the arms near the shoulders or just above the wrist. Either way, the brushing movement is an exception to several of the basic massage rules you've been following. Stroke here with your fingers slightly parted, and at the end of the movement break contact for a moment. More on that later.

There are a few ways to do the brushing movement. The important thing is to keep at least one set of fingertips moving toward the end point at all times. Both hands can work down the top of the arm from the shoulder, brushing in a hand-over-hand motion. A more interesting approach to the hands is to work from both sides at once. Slide one hand under your partner's, and begin

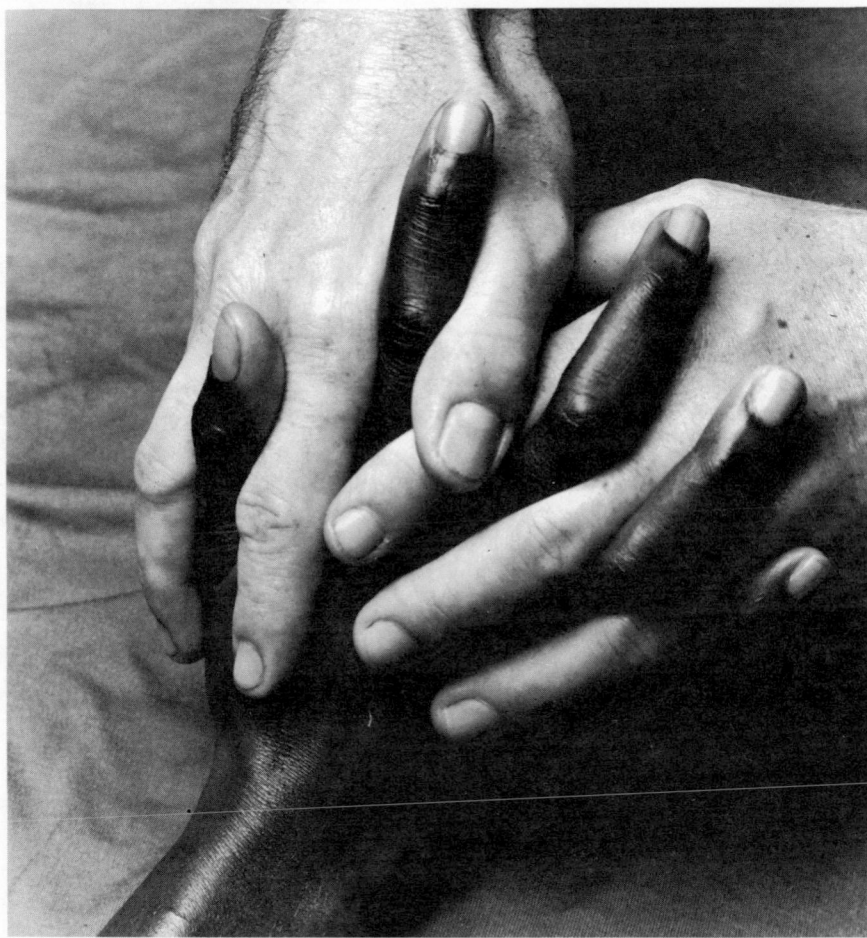

wrap all four fingers around your partner's fingers and tuck your thumb under. Now bring the thumb of your other hand around your partner's index finger, and press *your* index finger into the space between your partner's thumb and index finger.

Press all your contact fingers down as far as possible. Your partner's fingers should rest on the back of your hand. By rocking forward with your hands, you can flex all of your partner's

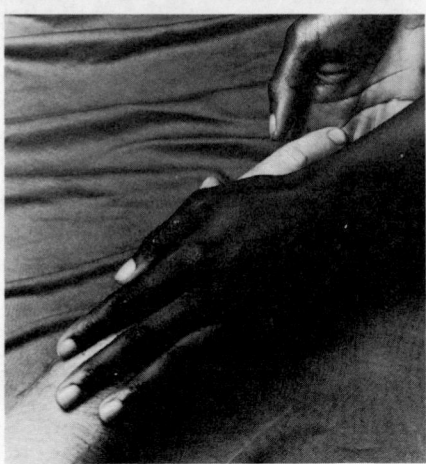 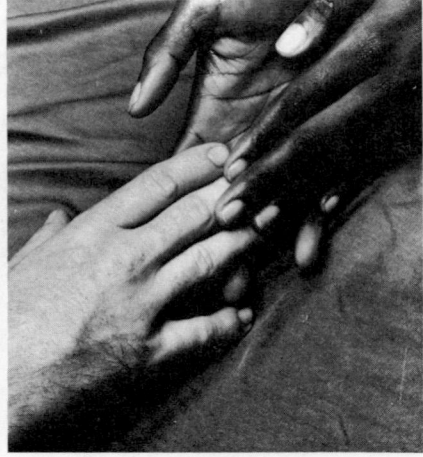

brushing down slowly on the top of your partner's arm near the elbow. As you reach the palm with your top hand, your fingers will line up on both sides of your partner's hand. Move both your hands together out toward your partner's fingertips. Break contact first with your top hand and then very slowly, finger by finger, with your bottom hand. Finally, you will just be touching each other with a single fingertip. This is one of the most powerful mo-

ments in massage. The extravagant tactile delight your partner has been enjoying all over the body focuses here on one fingertip. Make it last.

After a part of the body has been massaged, it feels revitalized. Energy appears out of nowhere, and the whole body seems less sluggish and more powerful than before. That's because it actually is (see Introduction). Energized feelings begin as soon as you start massaging; your very first contact is always a transfer of energy from one part of the body to another. The instant you break contact with your partner's fingertip, you should touch the face in prepara-

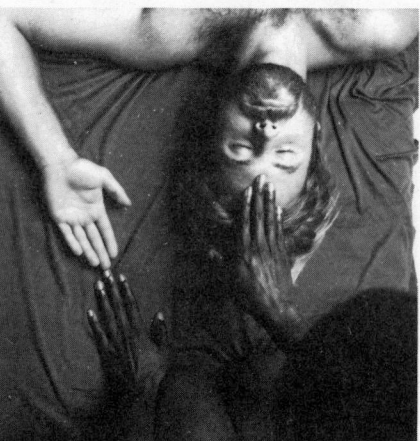

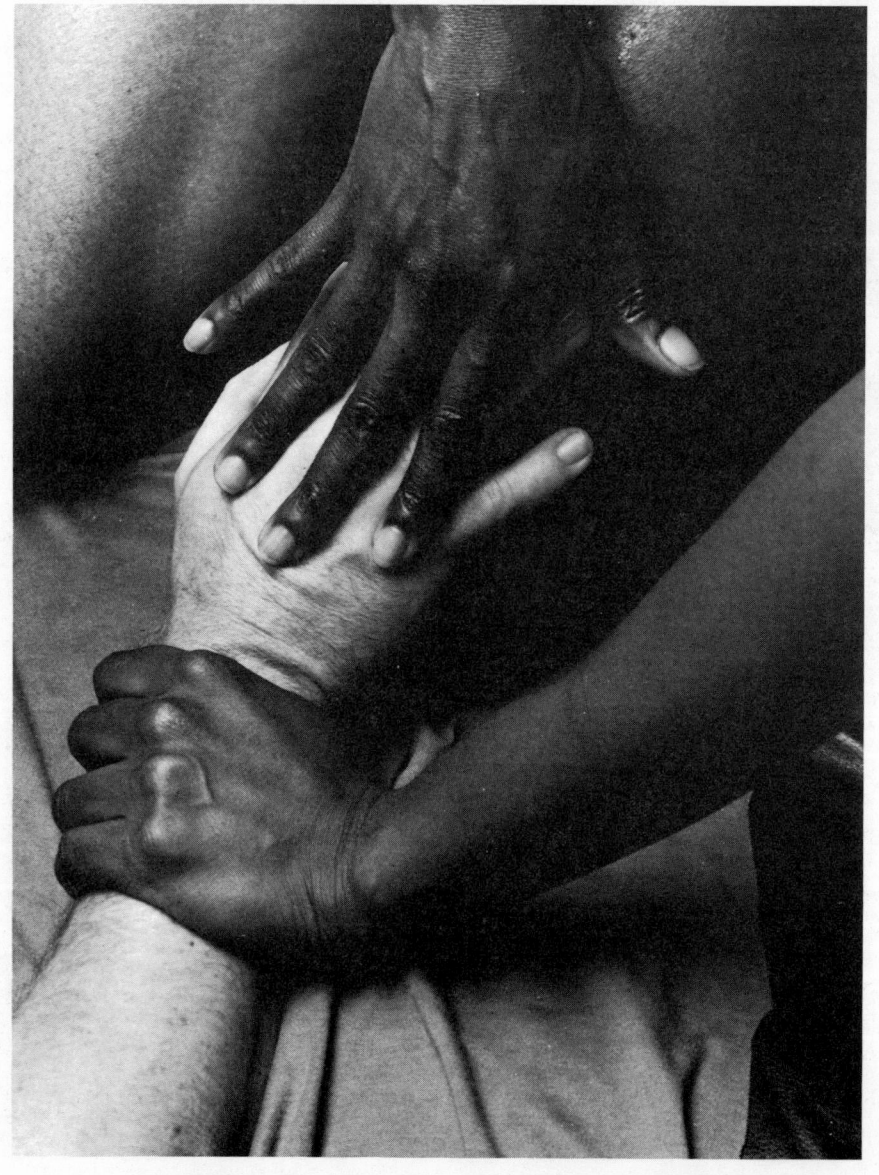

tion for your work there. Brushing sequences coupled with an energy transfer can be used throughout the massage as you move from one part of the body to another.

The Head and Face

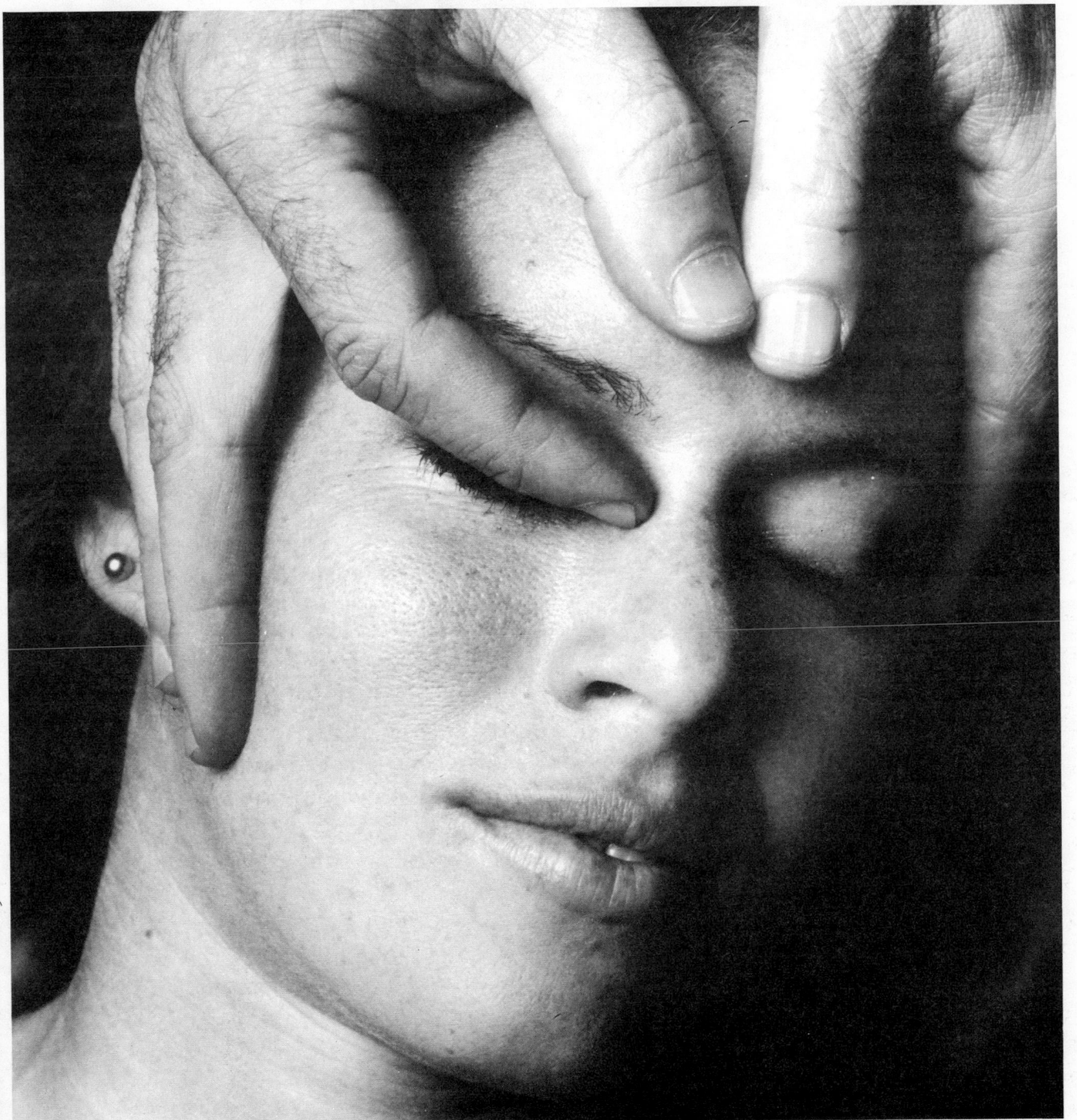

The Head and Face

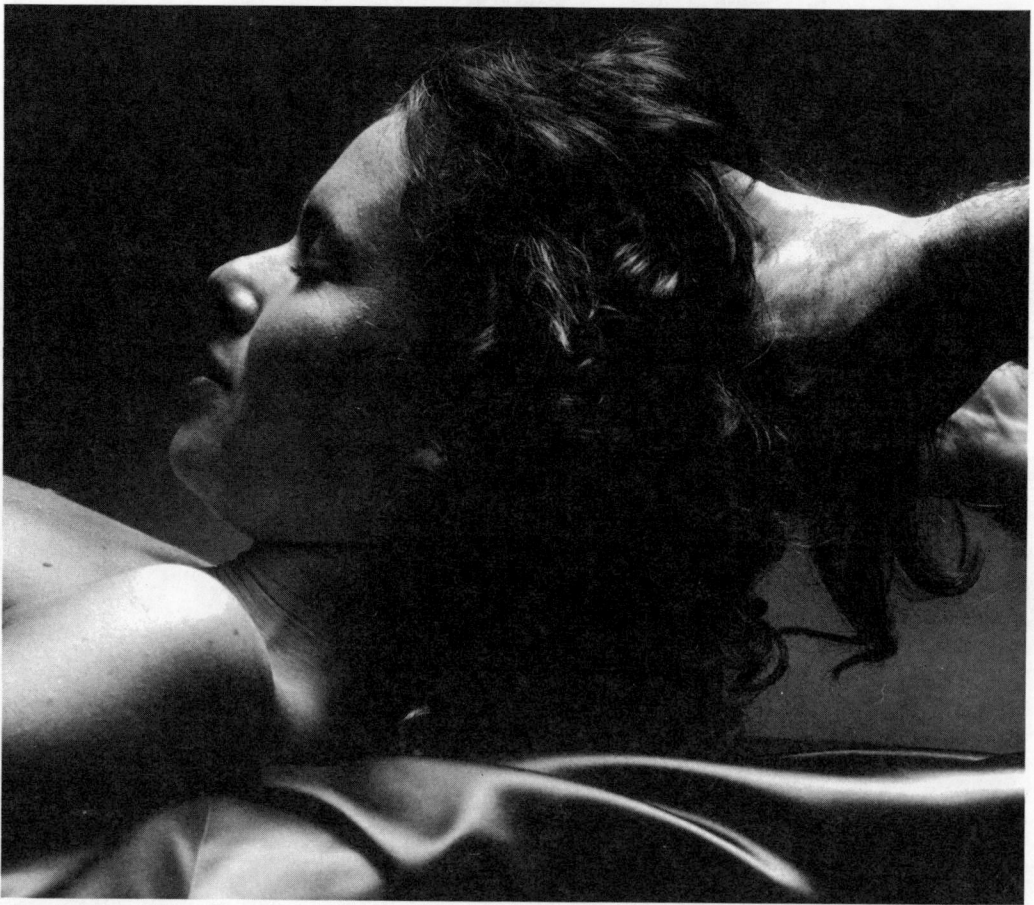

The head offers direct nerve paths to the brain at the temples, through the eyes and ears, and at the base of the skull. By using these unique paths to reach the brain, masseurs can create the most profound sorts of mood changes. But the most dramatic change of all will occur when you work on your partner's face.

Because the face is routinely exposed to the elements, it is always one of the first parts of the body to age. Fortunately, there are movements you can use to help restore the skin's resiliency and improve subcutaneous muscle tone. The specific technique for this kind of massage leaves people feeling tremendously refreshed and actually looking younger. For this reason the secrets of this technique, called a facial, have for the past few lifetimes been the closely guarded, almost exclusive property of beauty parlors. There the emphasis is more often on consumption than technique and a great deal of time is spent spreading the nectar of rare flowers and bees around worry and frown lines. Even so, the nervous thrill of being dabbed by fabulously expensive jellies and creams falls far short of the exquisite peace that facial massage performed with three cents' worth of safflower oil can bring.

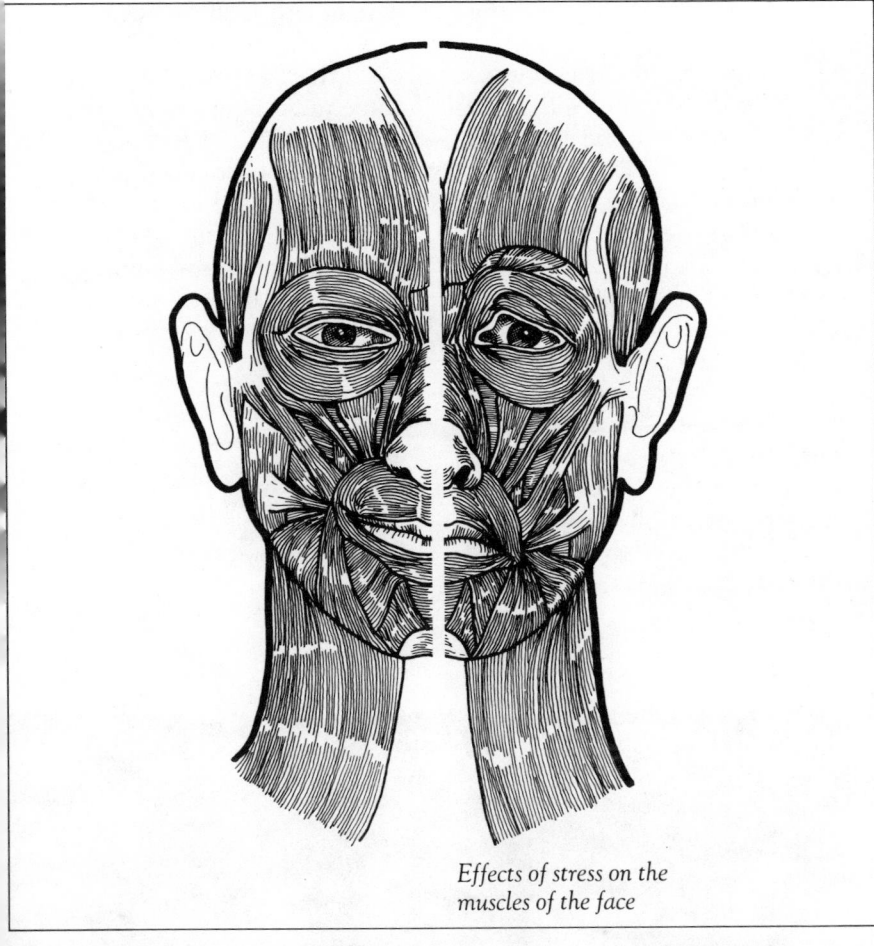

Effects of stress on the muscles of the face

Look in thy glass, and tell the face thou viewest
Now is the time that face should form another;
Whose fresh repair if now thou not renewest,
Thou dost beguile the world, unbless some mother.
—WILLIAM SHAKESPEARE, Sonnet III

A great many people become intensely preoccupied with facial treatments as soon as the first wrinkles appear around the eyes and mouth. Most of these treatments insist on steaming, creaming, powdering, and oiling the skin to smooth out and finally to erase the marks of aging. The reason that none of them works is that wrinkles are caused not by trouble in the skin itself, but rather by a general weakening of the underlying muscular tissue. Unless you're very serious about yoga, massage is the only way to reach and strengthen these mus-

cles. Most modern exercise programs dismiss the face as a bony, unchangeable part of the body. It's not.

Tiny muscles, not bones, shape the expression; like muscles anywhere else in the body, they will respond to massage. Along with broad general movements like nerve compression and circulation, facial massage involves a series of very fine strokes that affect precise parts of the face. Some of these areas are so tiny that they must be kneaded with a single finger. This does not mean they are any less important to your partner's sense of well-being than massive back movements that require half an arm. A facial begins with a series of movements which are specifically intended to benefit the muscles of expression. Six strokes form the core of a facial massage which you can then vary according to your partner's taste. If you're working with one person over a long period of time, you may want to change the facial slightly each time. One of the most tempting areas for exploration is an herbal steam treatment.

No way you can get away from it—layered hot towels steeped in fragrant herbs feel absolutely wonderful when they are pressed against your face. You can concentrate on massaging a single part of the body during an herbal steam facial to pamper your partner totally, or incorporate it into a full body massage. Since the facial has been transformed into an expensive beauty treatment, available only to the customers of certain exclusive salons, very few men have experienced it. Nevertheless, you will find that they rapidly learn to appreciate it.

Speculation on the precise effects herbs have on human beings has filled many volumes. This might be a good time for you to open one of them, or if you don't have that kind of time, simply choose herbs that your partner enjoys. It's not terribly unreasonable to suppose that people can smell or taste the herbs that are best for them. Like everything else on this planet, herbs were put here for a reason.

Ordinary spice rack herbs, like thyme, sage, and lemon peel, can be used to scent your hot towels. Once you find a few favorites, it's easy enough to grow your own the year round in a window box or flower pot. All you'll need to prepare for an herbal steam facial is a large pot (preferably enamel or stainless steel), a stove, and a half dozen or so small smooth towels. Fill the pot with enough water to cover the towels completely. Sprinkle in a half teaspoon of the herb your partner has selected, and begin to heat the water. You can tell when the towels are warm enough simply by touching them. When they're pleasantly warm, they are ready for your partner's face. Each towel

remains doubled throughout the facial and should be unrolled slowly from the forehead down. In two or three minutes the towel will begin to cool, and it should then be replaced. Repeat this process three or four times, and be sure that the time your partner's face is exposed without a towel is very brief. You can, if you like, vary this procedure by unfolding the cooled towel to the bottom half of the face and then draping the new hot towel across your partner's forehead. That way constant contact is maintained, and you can unroll the new hot towel just as soon as the old one is removed.

The mouth is surrounded by a ring of tiny muscles. Once you've oiled the face, you can massage these muscles by circling the mouth with the tip of your index or middle finger. Press down moderately hard, and work around the mouth in tiny circles. Stay just above and below the lips.

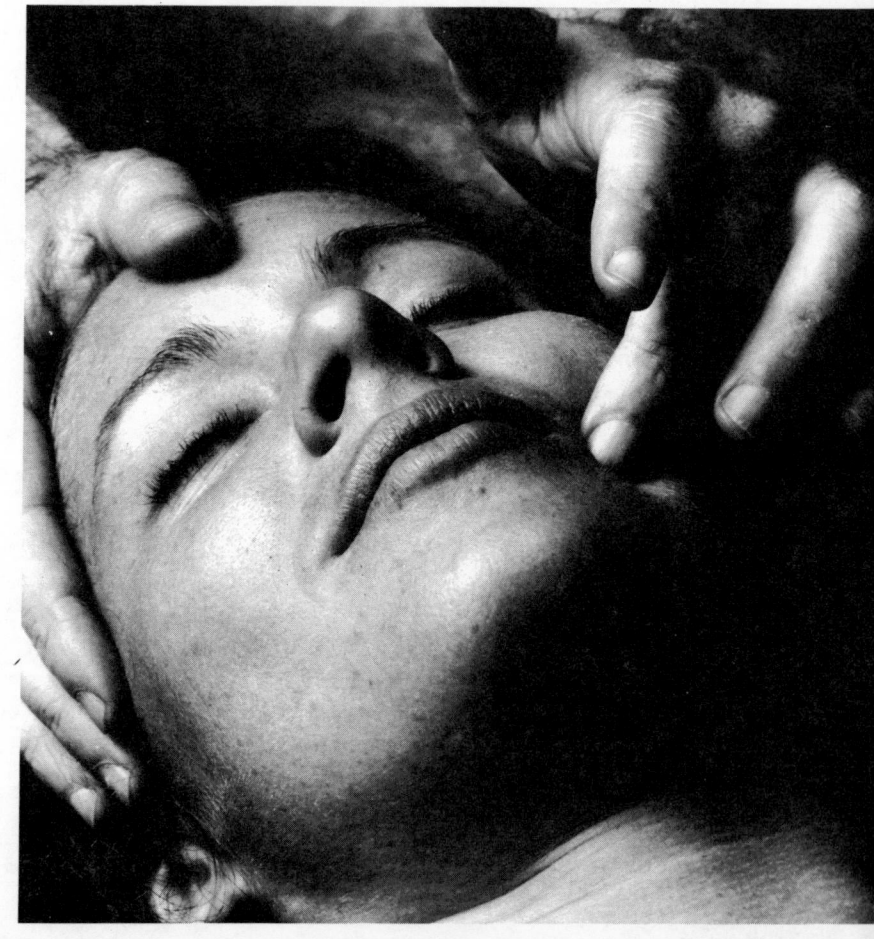

Wrinkles and Crow's-feet

Kneading the Face

Single-Finger Contact Movements

Smooth out wrinkles by tightening the skin around them before you begin massaging. Your aim here is to reach the underlying muscles; loose folds of skin will only interfere. At the corner of the eye you can tighten the skin between the forefinger and thumb (as shown) before you begin friction movements with the fingertips of your other hand. When the skin is tightened like this, it's a good idea to limit your friction movements to a rapid back-and-forth movement. Circling will tug against the skin. You can also move around the face with this arrangement, tightening the skin with one hand and applying friction with the other.

Even on the forehead and in the depressions around the nose, it's possible to pick up tiny folds of flesh with your fingertips as you knead. Squeeze gently as you pick them up. In the corners around your partner's eyes, you will find yourself kneading with just the thumb and forefinger. Begin at the third eye, and descend over one side of the face with both hands. Turn at the cheek, and knead up the other side of the face. If you knead slowly back and forth—from the eye to the temple, from the nose to the cheekbone—you will cover most of the muscles and nerves of your partner's face. People always enjoy having their expressions manipulated and changed, and almost everyone has spent some time complaining about the way he looks. Remember that while you knead around the lips, and watch your partner's normal expression melt as lips and cheeks twist into bizarre and unrecognizable shapes.

Above all, massage is contact. No contact, no matter how insignificant it seems, will go unappreciated. On your partner's face, there are crevices on the sides of the nose, around the mouth, and even inside the ear that are too tiny to reach with anything larger than a single finger. This contact, once you decide to make it, should move in the same rhythm that all your stroking has followed. Stroke back and forth or in tiny circles. Avoid random, jerky movements that will leave your partner feeling poked or probed rather than massaged.

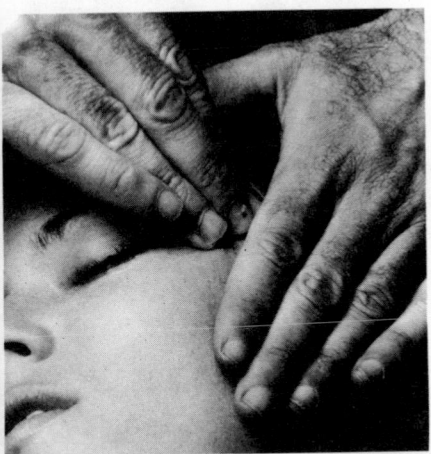

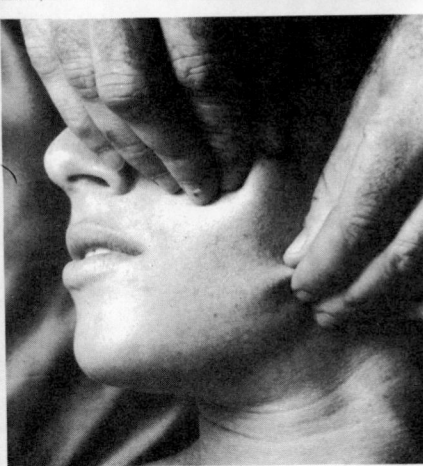

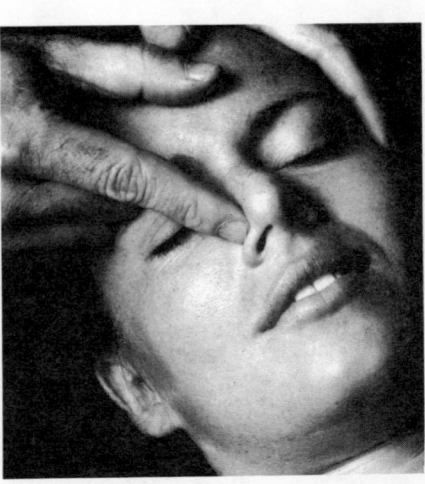

Pick up a fold of flesh, and roll it gently between your fingers. The hands work on opposite sides of the face, beginning at the forehead and working down to the mouth. To keep your pressures even, be sure not to release your grasp with one hand until the other begins its grasp.

As with every other part of the body, you can drain wastes and increase circulation to the muscles of the face. Once you've worked individually with the lower facial muscles, it's always a good idea to stimulate the whole mass. This simple movement allows you to reach the entire face below the temples: Anchor your thumbs at the center of your partner's forehead, and press down to the chin with your fingertips. When you reach the chin, begin moving back up toward the temple. As one hand begins to move up, the other descends. You may want to stop along the way with either hand to circle on the cheeks or along the sides of your partner's mouth.

The face registers every emotional change, no matter how subtle, and all these changes involve the exceptionally sensitive muscles of expression. Precisely because they are so sensitive, these muscles are

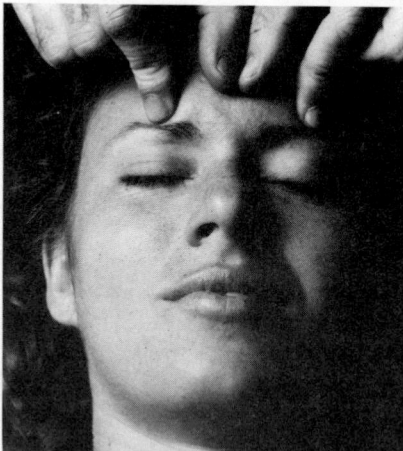

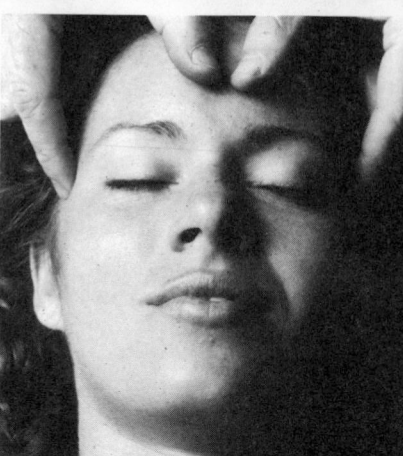

very often the first part of the body to pick up and register tension. If your partner has experienced a great deal of anxiety, the muscles of expression are likely to be permanently fatigued.

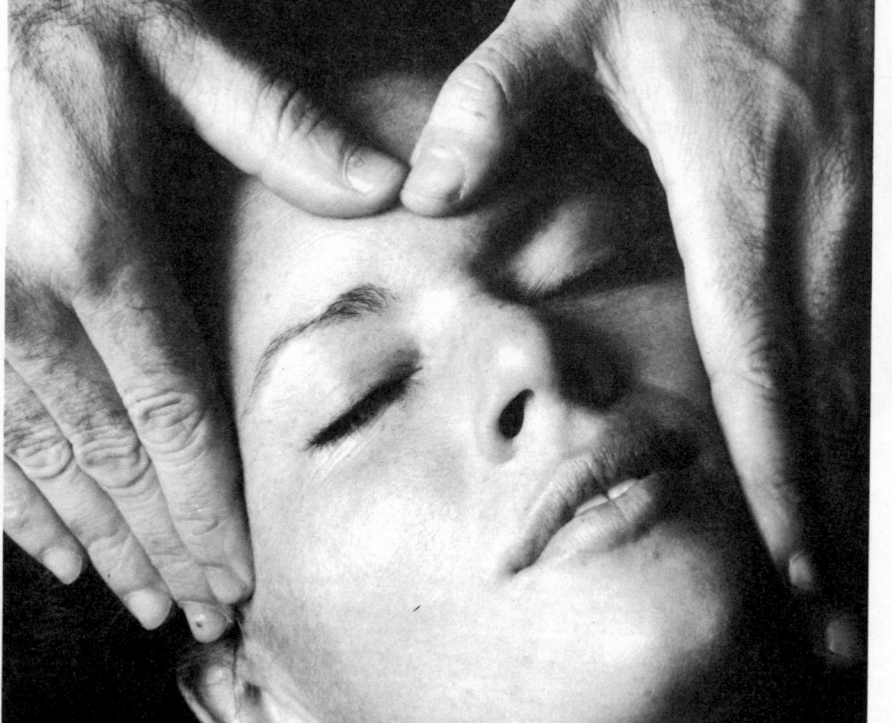

This fatigue is translated rapidly into a frozen expression and a smile that seems difficult and forced. Begin massaging the muscles of expression by soothing the nerves that supply them.

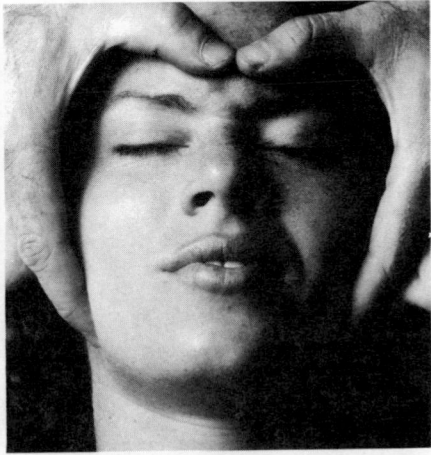

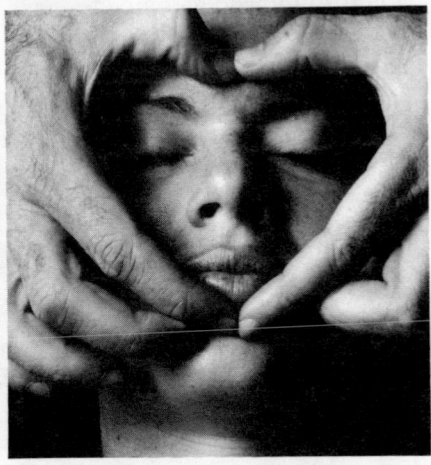

Throughout a massage your eyes should follow your hands. Here, on the face, you will have a chance to watch the wonderfully subtle changes that take place while you work.

This movement begins on the sinuses above the eyes (source of many headaches), moves to the temples, continues down the nerve branches on the side of the face, and ends just below the lower lip. It soothes the facial

nerves so effectively that you sometimes see your partner's face begin to change during the movement. Lips that were tightly pressed together begin to open, and the brow relaxes while you massage.

Like many of the eye movements that will follow, this stroke begins with both of your thumbs anchored to the center of your partner's forehead. They should stay at that spot throughout the movement unless the size of your partner's face in relation to your hands makes this impossible. If you find that you have to move your thumbs to stretch down to the lips, let the thumbs glide out toward the temples, and be sure to return to your original position as soon as it is comfortably possible.

Your contact point all the way down the face is with the fleshy ball of your index finger. Stroke from the forehead to the temples (as shown). Coming down the side of the face, turn when you reach the jaw, and press in to the point just below your partner's lips. Press this point, and return to your starting position on the forehead. On your return you need make only superficial contact up the sides of your partner's face.

Eyestrain, overeating, blocked sinuses, and muscle tension can cause headaches. More commonly, though, ordinary headaches are an exotic manifestation of the body's most intimate problem: brain pain. The brain, like the heart, is protected on all sides and completely hidden by bone. Even though you can't reach it directly with massage, no part of the body is more responsive to movements that work through referred pain centers. In this case the referred pain center, simply the spot where your head hurts, may indicate congestion on the surface of the brain. The brain coverings are supplied with a fine network of veins, arteries, and very delicate nerve endings. In stressful situations these blood vessels contract and blood pressure may rise. Tension is usually transmitted directly to the surface of the face either through the eyes or through other nerve channels.

Everyone has noticed the temporary relief that occurs when an aching temple is rubbed. This rubbing, an instinctive response to pain throughout the animal kingdom, gives masseurs a most important clue to dealing with headaches. Headache massage always begins with direct pressure on the referred pain centers and then seeks to lower blood pressure throughout the body. Severe headaches will sometimes miraculously disappear after only thirty seconds of pressure over the temples and forehead.

Try to get some feedback from your partner before you begin to work on a headache. To determine exactly where the pain is, have your partner touch the spot rather than attempt to describe it. Your first and last movement in dealing with a headache should always be thirty seconds of direct pressure on this spot. Very often headache pain is concentrated on the forehead just above the eyes or at the temples.

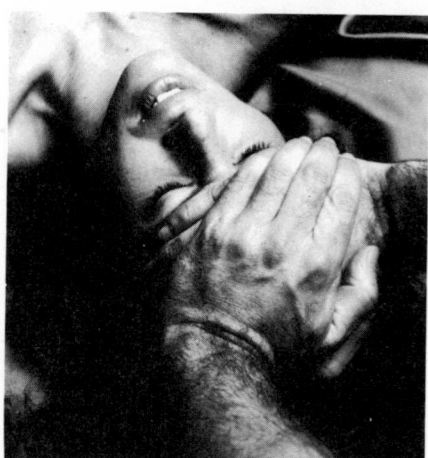

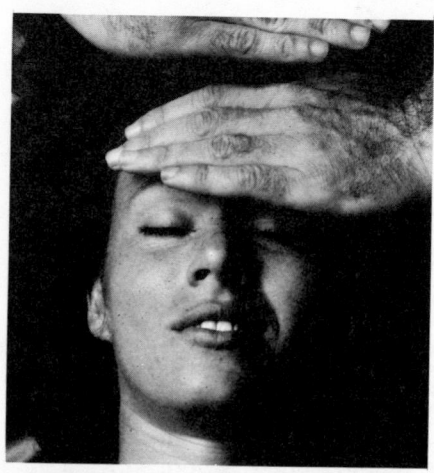

The Forehead: The formidable compression sequence for the forehead (see page 91) is an excellent way to begin dealing with pain in that area. Contact is even from your fingertips to the base of the palm. Be careful not to arch your hand, and leave a contact gap in the center. Your hands should overlap. Press down moderately hard for a silent count of thirty, and release the pressure slowly. Break your contact by flattening out your hands so that just the center of your bottom hand touches the center of your partner's forehead. Release that final contact very slowly and go on to the next movement.

The Temples: Depending on the size of your partner's head, you'll want to use either your fingertips or the heels of your hands to concentrate pressure on the temples. There are movements in this chapter to illustrate both techniques. If the area around the temples seems too large for your fingertips, don't hesitate to go in with the heels of your hands while you bend your fingers around the skull and press down to the point where your fingertips meet.

The Eyes: Because they are so delicate, direct pressure to the eyes should always be anchored just above them on the bony shield (see "Eyes," page 88). Press down slowly with your middle fingers until you make a very light contact with the center of the eyelid. Once you've established eyelid contact, move on to a more complete eye compression movement. You can use one of the fingertip compression movements in the eye section, or simply press down on the eyes with the soft tissues at the base of your palms. Sit below your partner's head when you do this, and anchor your fingers on the forehead and scalp.

After treating the specific problem areas, headache massage can go on to include a complete head massage or even a full body massage. This is a particularly important consideration during head massage since stress is almost always a factor in headaches.

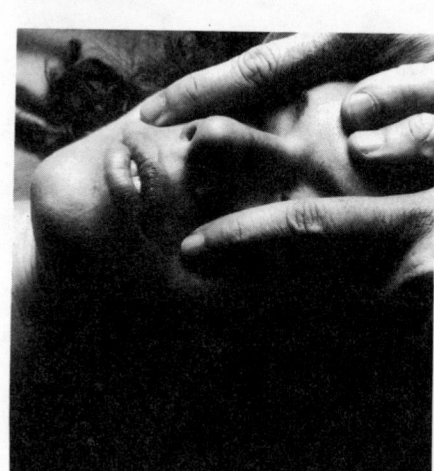

. . . I began thinking mechanistically enough to accept migraine for what it was: something with which I would be living, the way some people live with diabetes.
—JOAN DIDION, The White Album

How many people have resigned themselves to accept regular bouts of excruciating migraine pain? The cause of these terrible headaches is not fully understood. When aspirin and painkillers fail, migraine sufferers are often advised that their ordeal is nothing more than a purely imaginary, neurotic indulgence. They are left alone to suffer the terrific assaults that come every few days, even scorned because they suffer. Unfortunately, though, the pain is quite real. Nobody understands this better than a migraine victim who goes temporarily blind while driving in rush-hour traffic.

Massage was the standard medical approach to migraine at the end of the nineteenth century, and there are many documented cures in the medical literature of that time. Now that modern medicine has found ways to fiddle with chemical levels inside the brain, it's tempting to regard these cures as anachronistic and quaint. Migraine sufferers who are already on a first-name basis with the druggist cannot afford the luxury of this temptation. If merely rubbing the surface of the body seems like a superficial approach to something as intense as

a migraine, I must point out that I have seen migraine headaches disappear with a first massage and never return. I have also seen migraines diminish in force and finally vanish completely after daily massage practiced routinely for one month. That sort of limited massage takes about twenty minutes each day. Migraines can last for ten hours.

Follow the entire routine suggested for general headache problems, and pay specific attention to knotted muscles around the shoulders and upper back. You may want to include other parts of the back, like the muscles along the spine, in your deep kneading sequences. Occasional feedback from your partner will help you decide where to concentrate your efforts. Repeat each movement on the back at least fifty times. If you're dealing with a migraine, first massage the back and shoulders, and then go on to the head and face. On the face, work over the areas where the pain usually occurs, repeating your movements at least fifty times. Keep your pressures steady and even. When conversation is necessary for feedback on painful spots, try to keep it brief. Since migraines are not fully understood, it's difficult to explain why massage sometimes works. Perhaps it's merely a case of relaxing knotted muscles along the nerve paths in the neck, shoulders, and back. Or it may be that twenty minutes of pleasure each day, twenty minutes of gentle physical contact with another human being, is enough to exorcise the migraine demon.

Hand-over-hand movements, like this can be used throughout the full body massage. Never break contact with your partner. When one hand is up, the other is down; even if the contact hand is perfectly still for a moment, your partner does not feel abandoned. Forehead movements come off the forehead onto the bridge of the nose, maintaining a superficial contact. Break contact with one hand at the tip of the nose while the other hand continues to stroke down on the forehead. Maintain full contact from temple to temple, and begin stroking just below the hairline. Work through

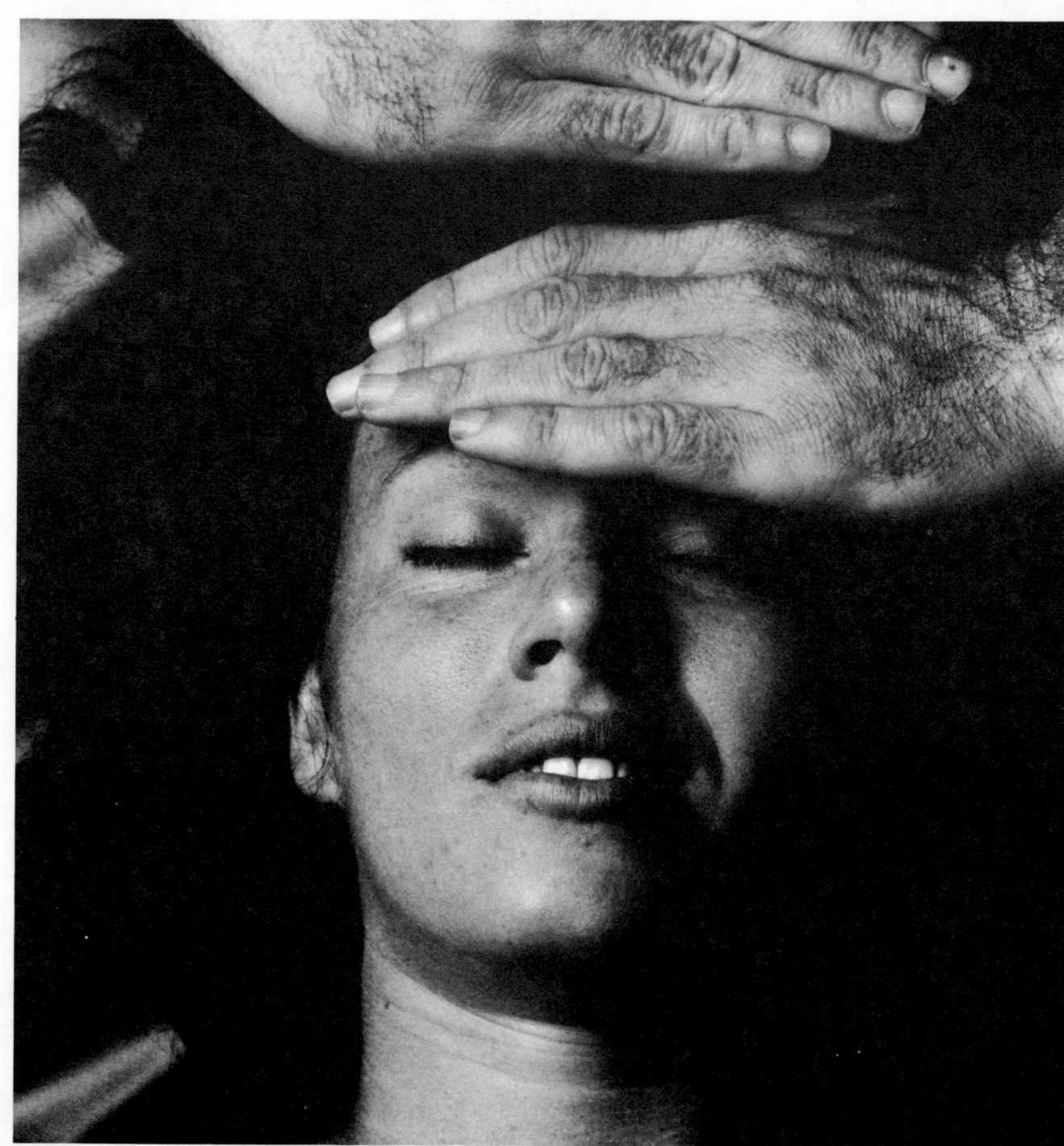

the complete hand-over-hand cycle from the forehead to the tip of the nose ten times. Then go on to your next movement.

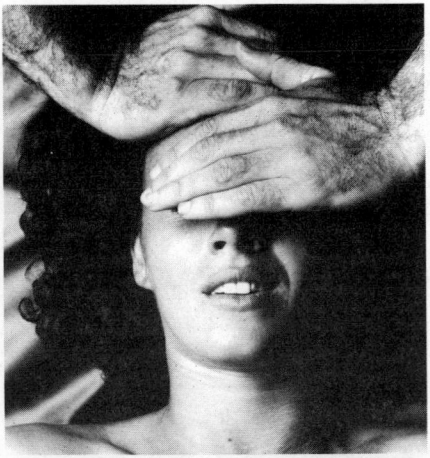

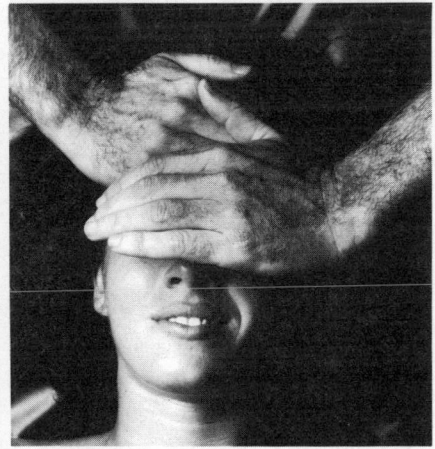

The forehead is the only hairless part of the body where you can massage right over the brain. Although the brain itself is hidden beneath the skull, nerves that connect to it directly emerge above the eyebrows and crisscross over the entire forehead. These surface-to-brain nerve connections are among the shortest you will find anywhere in the body. They are absolutely crucial whenever you want to relax your partner because the moment you soothe these nerves blood vessels throughout the head dilate. When this happens, your partner may experience the most remarkable mood changes. Anxieties dissolve and are replaced by calm and peaceful feelings. Such miraculous disposition changes merely serve to prove how much consciousness is dependent on the condition of your body.

Forehead nerve compression works best as a sequence of four movements that travel back and forth across this exquisitely sensitive part of the face. The nerves are just beneath the skin, and this sequence allows you to vary your pressures while your partner's mind is focused on four different compression sensations which will spread from the center of the forehead to the temples.

Begin by pressing both your hands, one on top of the other (as shown), on the middle of the forehead. Center your fingers so they line up with each other; that way you can equalize the pressure

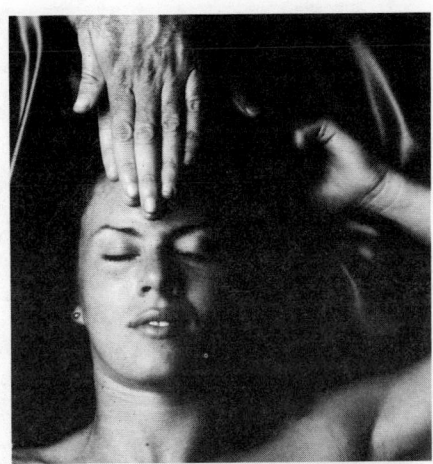

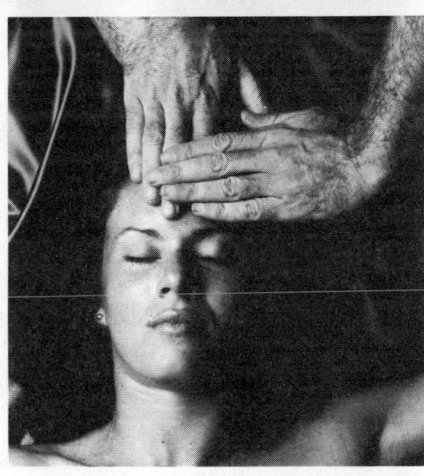

on your contact (lower) hand with your upper hand. Raise both thumbs slightly, but be sure that pressure is distributed equally between the four contact fingers. Contact. Press down on your fingers to the top of the forehead. Working this close to the brain, you can focus all of your partner's attention on the center of the forehead. Press down slowly for a silent count of thirty, release slowly, turn your top hand, and go into the second part of the sequence.

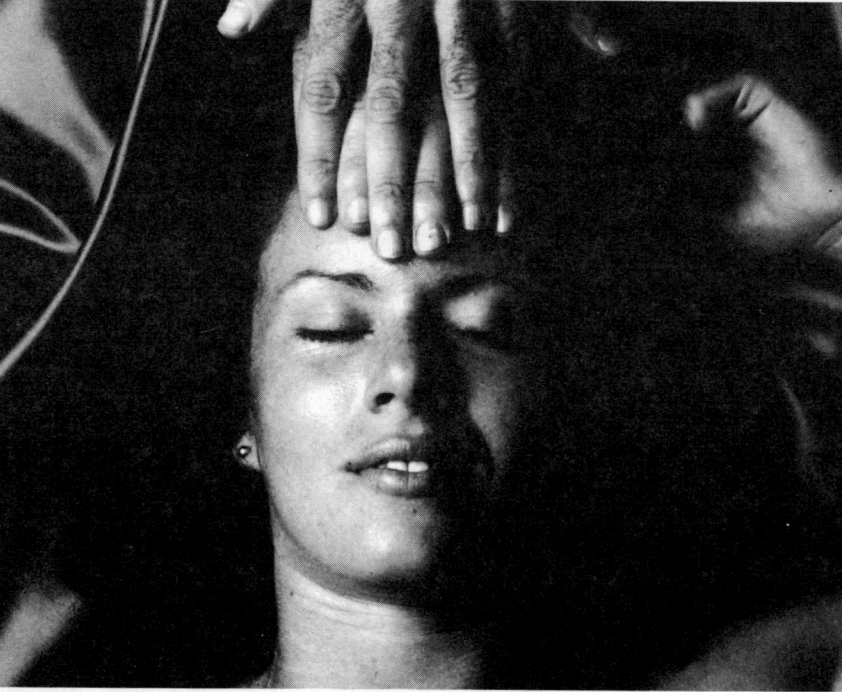

Turn your top hand at right angles to your contact hand without breaking contact with your partner. The difference here is subtle—more pressure on the middle finger of the contact hand, a sense of covering half of the forehead without touching it. Some people can feel this hand covering the forehead even though there is no actual contact. You need only glance at your partner's face to see it reaching for the hand that isn't quite there. Press down again for a silent count of thirty, release slowly, and go on to the third part of the sequence—a ten-finger forehead compression.

Weave the fingers on both your hands together (as shown). You'll be able to cover most of the forehead with your fingertips. Equalize the pressures. You might try bending your hands over the top of the skull while you maintain contact. Again, you can feel your partner reaching for your fingers wordlessly. There is a definite sense of the whole body focused at the forehead, precisely at the point of contact. Without breaking contact, turn your hands and go into the final part of the sequence, the lavish full-hand nerve compression. Your contact hand should maintain pressure from the fingertips to the heel. Use the top hand to help balance and equalize this pressure. Maintain full contact and maximum pressure for thirty seconds. This magnificent movement contacts all the nerves of the forehead and temples in one voluptuous sweep. People will yield to it; they will give in. No human being can resist it.

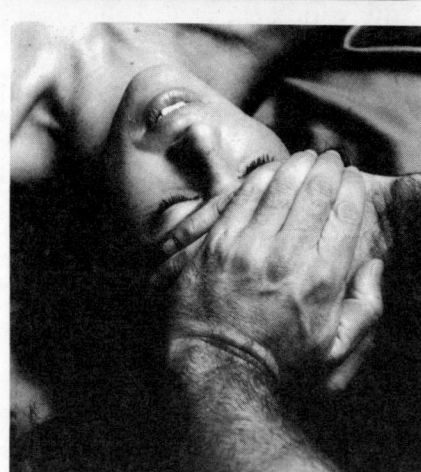

The skin of the eyelid is the thinnest anywhere on the body, and the eyes beneath connect directly to the brain. Eyes are brain windows. That's always interesting to meditate on when

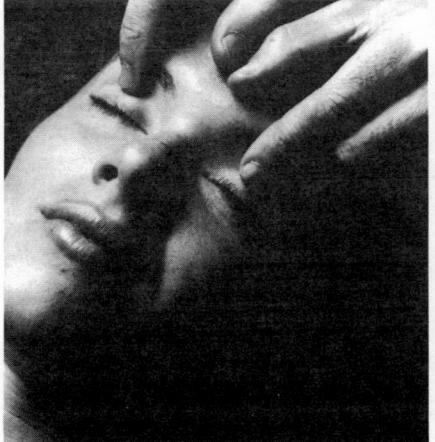

you work on this part of the body. Eyelid skin is so thin that any slight contact, even the most delicate pressure you can manage, will register. Begin contacting your partner's eyelids with a single finger from each hand. Everyone has spent plenty of time rubbing his eyes, but very few people are accustomed to the strange gossamer sensation of someone else doing this for them. Single-finger contact establishes this connection and allows your

partner to get used to being touched on the eyes before you go on to more involved movements. It also allows you to circle gently on specific parts of the eyelids.

To avoid putting too much

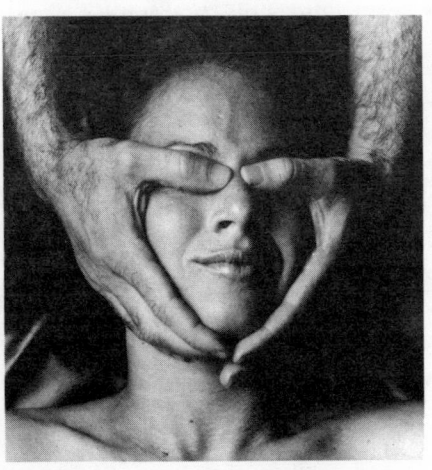

pressure on the eyes, anchor your hands on the bony ridge just above the eye socket. Do this by making a fist and resting your knuckles on the ridge. You can then extend your index or middle fingers out over your partner's eyes. Lower your fingers together or one at a time. Sometimes the mere weight of that single finger is pressure enough on the eye. Use the soft ball of your finger. Maintain contact for a silent count of twenty, and release

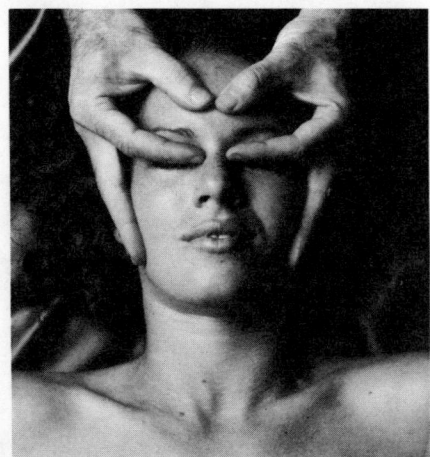

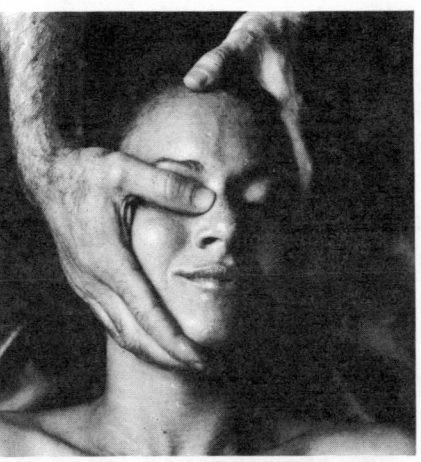

slowly. Don't move your hands until both index fingers are clear of your partner's eyes.

Another, more thorough way to press the eyes is by using the whole surface of your thumb. You can compress the entire eye this way without putting a great deal of pressure on any one part of it. If you're working on a headache that seems to involve pain behind one of the eyes, try concentrating pressure on the problem eye while you anchor your other hand above. The anchor hand can press flat against the forehead horizontally or press against the forehead and temples (as shown). The entire surface of your thumb-contact hand should cup your partner's cheek and chin, pressing gently. Anchor the tip of each thumb (as they contact the eye) against your partner's nose to avoid pressing down too hard on the eyes.

There are a number of interesting things you can do with the eyes by using the bones above and below to anchor your fingers. Some of them are illustrated here, and you can, of course, invent a few of your own.

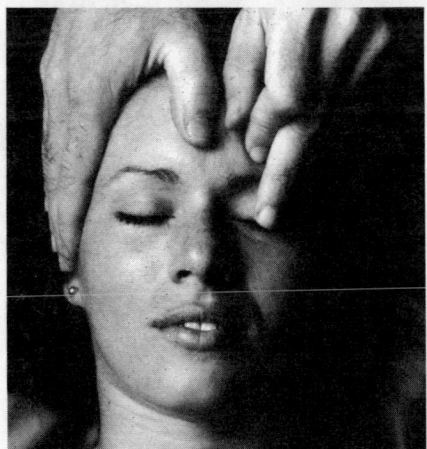

If your partner has been pursuing pleasures, he will be happy to discover here a pleasure most people have never even considered. Executed correctly, stroking the eyes can be one of the most exquisitely intimate moments in massage. You can actually put the four fingers of your hand down on the top of your partner's eye. Anchor your thumbs over the center of your partner's forehead, and press down gently to the inside corner of the eye with your little finger. Bring the finger over toward the outside corner of the eye, pressing half against the eye and half against the eye socket. As your little finger moves away from the inner corner of the eye, bring the second finger down to

that spot. Repeat this process, gliding toward the outside corner of the eye, until all four fingers are down. When you reach the outside corner of the eye with all your fingers, keep the thumbs in place on the forehead, circle with your fingers on the temples a few times, and return to the beginning of the movement. You can work along the top and bottom of the eye exactly the same way. There's a soft feeling along the eye and a hard, bony sensation just against the socket. The balls of your fingers should glide along between these two surfaces.

Just beyond the corner of your partner's eye you will find a shallow depression surrounded by a bony ridge. All your temple movements should work inside this depression. Anchor your thumbs at the center of the forehead (as shown). Temple movements should be soft and full. Even though you're working on a relatively small area, you can reach it with the fleshy parts of the three middle fingers. There are many different movements you can do here, but none of them should involve digging in with your fingertips.

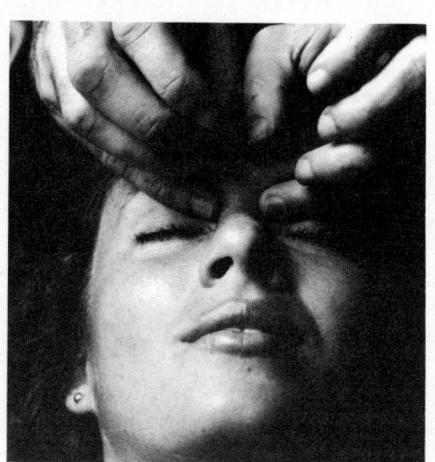

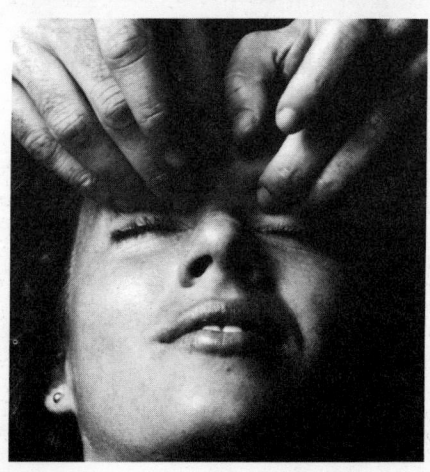

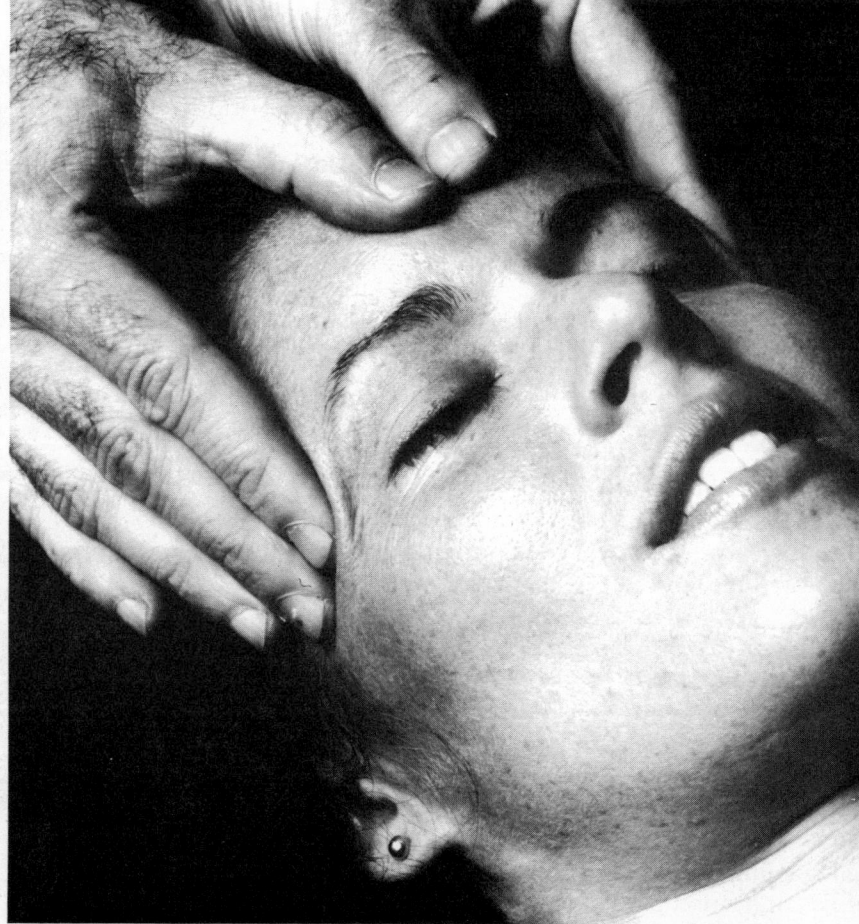

Circle the temples with your three middle fingers, keeping both thumbs steady on the center of your partner's forehead. Begin by moving both hands in the same direction, working within the bony ridge. There are several interesting ways to vary this movement without breaking contact or even interrupting the circling motion. You can circle with both hands in the same direction, but while one hand is at twelve o'clock, the other will be at six o'clock. You can also circle in different directions with each hand. You may want to blend all three techniques, but whatever approach you choose, be sure to keep your rhythm and pressure smooth and even. Generally six complete circles of each variation are about right. This movement is so popular that you may want to continue with it for a while. Nobody ever complains if you do.

To isolate the effects of forehead kneading, press down with four fingers of one hand on one side of the forehead. Anchor this contact hand with your thumb up on your partner's scalp. Pressures should be light to moderate because the aim here is merely to steady the skin and underlying tissues while you knead the opposite side of the forehead. If the skin on your partner's forehead is tight, press over to the kneading side with your contact hand. This will create some slack and make the kneading a bit easier.

This is one of the most delicate kneading movements anywhere on the body. There isn't enough flesh on the forehead to use your thumb, which you must keep

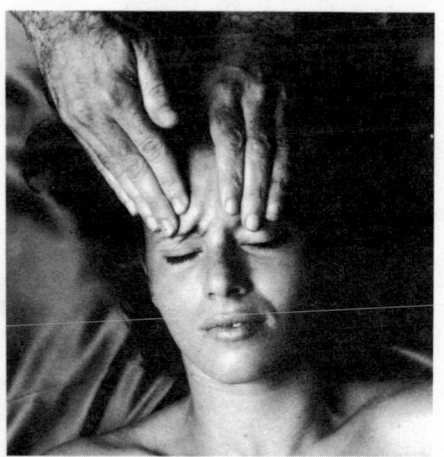

pressed against your other fingers. Working in very small circles, press the forehead skin into folds ahead of your fingers (as shown). Work back and forth across the forehead until you've covered half of it up to the contact hand several times. Then switch hands, and knead the other half.

Face circulation is divided into movements that work above and below the eyes. They are fairly vigorous, so it's best to avoid pressures that will jerk tissues away from the eyes. These movements will aid circulation throughout the face and speed the return of venous blood to the heart.

On the Forehead: Begin with both hands at the top of the scalp, and holding your fingers together, press down with one hand (as shown). Keep moving down until the heel of your hand reaches your partner's eyebrow. (That's the position you see in the photo.) When you reach this position, be sure no part of your hand touches your partner's face

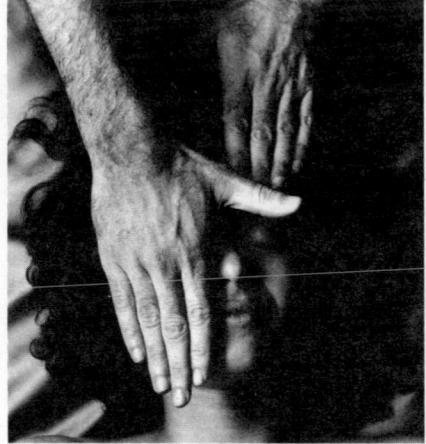

below the eyebrow. Your only contact in this movement is on the forehead itself. This is easy to do since the eyebrow is higher than the face below. It's always better to alternate your hand movements than to bring both hands down together in a scrubbing motion. When the heel of one hand reaches your partner's eyebrow, lift that hand, and as you return to your starting position, the other hand can begin to descend.

On the Cheeks: On the forehead you pressed down toward your fingertips to avoid pulling on the eyebrows. Here, on the cheeks, the circulation movement is reversed; you'll be pulling away from your fingertips. Press four fingers of each hand across your partner's face at a slight angle so as to avoid the eye socket. The longest fingertips should rest against the side of your partner's nose. Pull away from the nose, maintaining contact with all your fingers right to the edge of your partner's face. Here again it's best to alternate the movements, pulling first with one hand and then the other. This is one of those movements where you may want to experiment with different speeds, but even if you're moving very fast, be sure to keep the motion itself smooth and even. Never come down sharply on your partner's cheekbone.

Throughout this book you will find naked people massaging other naked people simply because this sort of thing has been going on for thousands of years. Nevertheless, your partner may come to a massage fiercely in love with a pair of earrings and utterly determined not to part with them. Worse yet, you may have gone this far into the massage without even noticing the earrings. Either way, do not interrupt the entire massage to get rid of an earring. No other piece of clothing or jewelry requires more effort to discard. All jewelry will usually come off easily at the beginning of the massage or not at all. Unless your partner is wearing extravagant earrings that cascade onto the neck, you can work around the earlobes and sacrifice less than two square inches of a full body massage.

Nobody comes away from a full body massage without a bit of oil in the hair. There are worse things you can put on your hair than a few drops of vegetable oil. Even so, be sure to move your partner's hair back before you begin stroking the ears. Begin with four fingers just above the hairline, and hold your thumb out (as shown). Press down around the ear without bending it back. Light contact is fine. This movement follows the contour of the ear and, below it, the jawbone. The lower fingers make contact with the neck, but most of your pressure is concentrated on the face above. When your thumb touches the top of the ear, stop and come back up again.

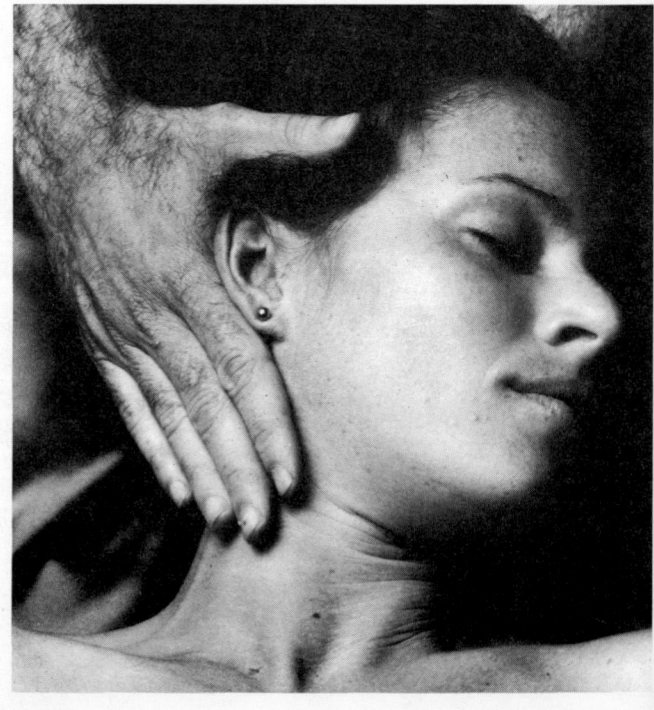

Closing your eyes during a massage serves to intensify the tactile sense. When you gently press your smallest finger into your partner's ear, the tactile sense is further enhanced. There are a number of other interesting things you can do with your hands while the ear is being entered. Press down lightly with your thumbs over your partner's eyes and squeeze the cheeks with your middle three fingers (see photo). Or you may prefer to make steady, silent contact with your partner's temples. Whatever you decide on, be sure your partner has something to feel when everything becomes suddenly silent.

Squeeze one ear at a time. Hold your partner's head when you squeeze to be sure it remains perfectly still. Since you must steady the head, why not incorporate a simple temple press with the thumb of your anchor hand? Squeeze the ear gently between your thumb and forefinger. Move up and down the soft outer tissues. Take your time with this movement. Very few people have ever had anyone show this much interest in their ears.

Inside the brain everything you have done so far has been noted. Unless your partner meditates, it's unlikely that the brain has ever had this much "waking rest." You could call massage an active meditation because waves of induced pleasure connect your partner's mind and body. What is more relevant to living in the here and now than the experience of your own body? The same nerves that torture people with worries and anxiety can bring peace and tranquillity to the brain.

Stroking down the sides of the neck along with vigorous scalp massage will pull blood away from the center of the skull and relieve congestion. That leaves the brain free of internal physical pressures which can be distracting. Inside the free brain, body massage is felt. That feeling has no name and cannot be described. Only the mind can know it.

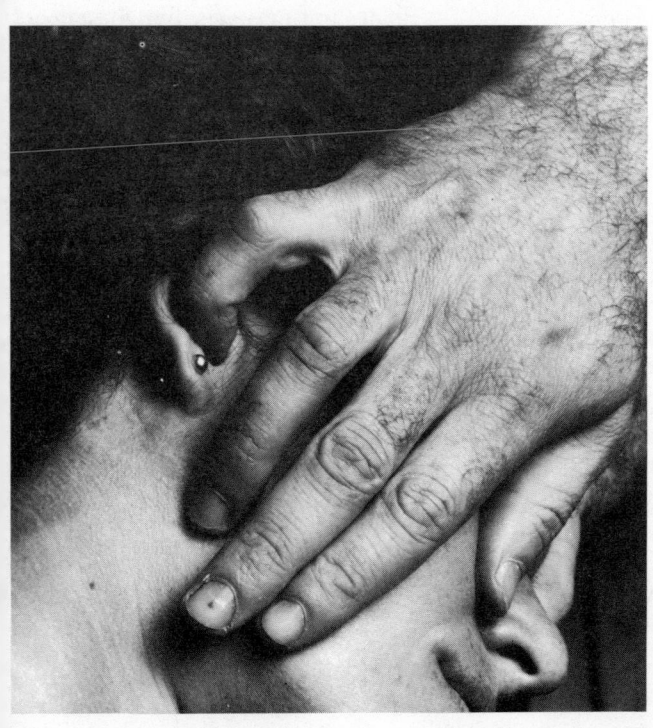
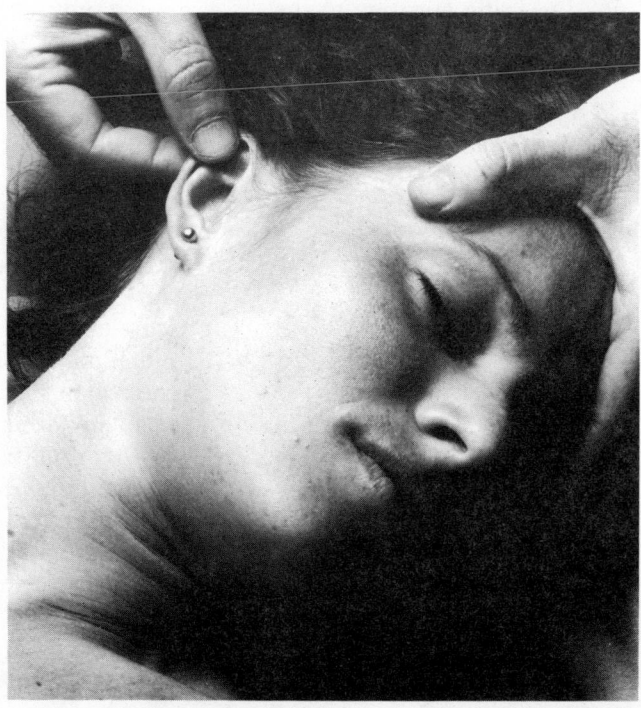

When your friends discover the effectiveness of massage throughout the body, they may ask you to work on hair and scalp problems. It seems evident that a treatment powerful enough to deal with back pains, headaches, and sprains should be able to dispatch dandruff quickly. People with itchy scalp, pattern baldness, eczema, brittle hair, and falling hair seek in massage a quick solution to their problem. With all these folks it's always instructive to begin by reviewing the ingredients of their shampoo, conditioner, or (especially) dandruff preparation. This can be an extremely sobering experience. Would you willingly rub coal tar into your hair? What about resorcinol, quinine, or arsenic? Many people with hair and scalp problems are paying for the privilege of dumping chemicals on their hair that would destroy the living-room rug.

Once this poisonous assault on the scalp ceases, massage can be used to bring nutrition to the tissues within. Remember that hair, once grown, is not a living tissue. Scalp massage aims to reach beneath the hair and skin via friction and kneading movements.

When your partner's face begins to register the physical effects of stress, the scalp, which is the unseen top of the face, will tighten along with the tissues below. Normally you can reach up and move your own scalp quite easily. But if you reach up and the scalp feels very tight, like the stretched head of a drum, subcutaneous hair follicles are definitely undernourished.

Every year balding hair lovers spend lots of money on chemicals that are supposed to "feed the roots" of their hair. The implication here is that human hair has roots like the roots of a tree and can be fertilized from above. Fortunately, for those of us who live in damp climates, this is not true. Hair roots are internal structures that receive nutrition from within the body. Nevertheless, popular baldness remedies come with explicit instructions directing the buyer vigorously to massage some evil-smelling miracle ointment into the scalp. These ointments do manage to leave existing bald spots looking waxed and shiny. This calls attention to the problem, thereby causing more stress, scalp tightening, hair loss, and ointment purchasing.

Hair lovers would do better to skip the ointment and concentrate, instead, on the vigorous scalp massage. You can bring nutrition to hair roots and relax the scalp exactly the way you relax any other part of the body, by soothing the underlying muscles and nerves while you promote circulation throughout the entire area. This is one of the few situations in which self-massage has any real value.

After twenty-four years of lecturing on massage at Harvard University, the late Hartvig Nissen wrote in his book *Practical Massage and Corrective Exercises*:

. . . there is no doubt that the circular kneading of the scalp will produce new growth of hair. In fact, I have seen several excellent proofs thereof. One, a lady of 65 years, who had worn a wig for more than twenty years; she began after my advice to give herself scalp massage twice every day for about ten or fifteen minutes each time, and when I saw the lady again after a couple of years, she had a good crop of hair all over her head. The simple reason is that the massage will bring nourishment to the roots of the hair and thereby awaken Nature to new life.

If ten minutes of kneading your own scalp seems tiring, you might want to invest in an electric vibrator (see page 185). These wonderful little machines were not around when Nissen was practicing massage, but the effects of stress on the scalp muscles were certainly apparent to him. If your partner is massaged regularly, he may find it no longer necessary to reach for the vibrator every morning. As in dealing with any other stress-related problem, it's best to boost nutrition to the problem area and then to relax the whole body.

You can tell a lot about people by ubbing their scalps. A tight scalp definitely a sign of tension lsewhere in the body, and you'll ant to remember this fact when ou work on the spine and the erves of the back. The scalp as n indicator of tension elsewhere n the body is one of many silent ues you'll be dealing with as you nassage your partner. I call them ilent because you should resist he temptation to share this information with your partner until fter the massage is over. People ome to a massage not to be eminded of how tense they are, ut rather, to relax and forget bout all their problems.

Cup the top of your partner's head with the full surface of one hand. You may want to anchor the head at the very back of the skull while you do this movement. Press down, making even contact from your fingertips to the heel of your hand. Maintain this even contact throughout the friction movement. As you move your hand back and forth, the scalp will move with it. Each scalp you massage will allow different amounts of movement. Feel the limits of movement that your partner's scalp will comfortably permit and do not attempt to press beyond. Friction movements on the scalp can easily change from a straight back-and-forth motion to a light circular one. Work from the front hairline all the way back to where your partner's head meets the massage surface. You can, if you like, lift the head with one hand and continue scalp friction down the back of the crown to the neck.

Unless your partner is completely bald, there's no reason to oil the scalp. Hair tangles easily, and it may not be possible for you to keep your fingers tightly closed while you knead. Even so, scalp kneading feels wonderful, and your partner won't want to miss it. Work over the entire scalp at least three times in small circles. Your hands will slide a bit over your partner's hair, but it really doesn't matter. You can compensate for the slippery contact by using more pressure on the scalp.

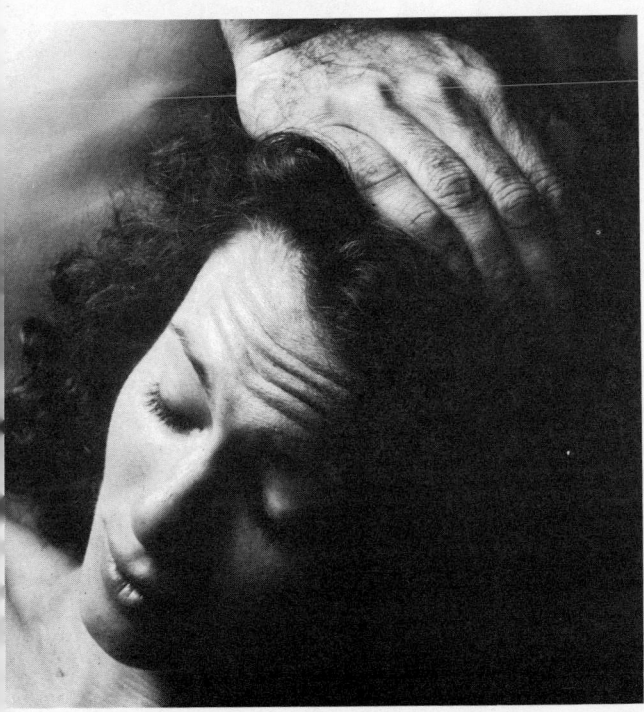 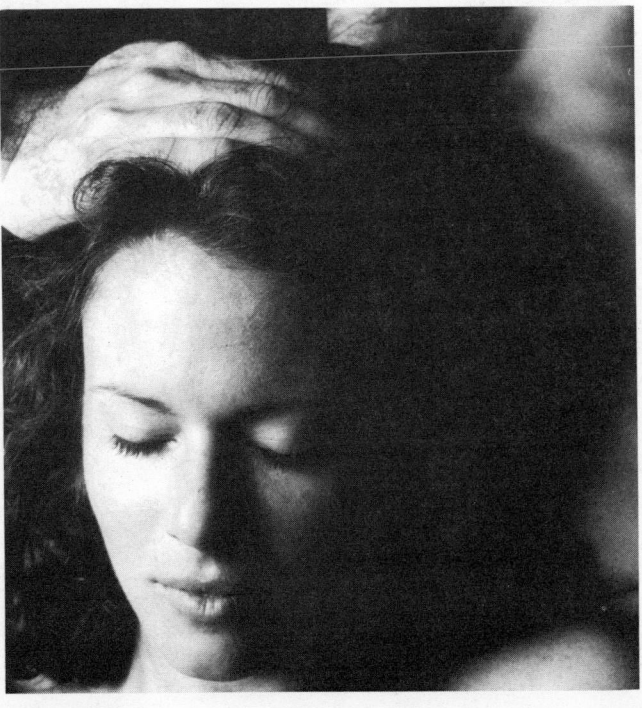

A complete head, face, and neck massage will take you in a sweeping half circle from the top of your partner's head all the way around to the side of the torso. For movements like this one, where it's easiest to reach up toward the face, sit alongside your partner's arm, facing the chin. If you decide to begin massage on the head, this is a good way to transfer sensation from the face down onto the torso. From there you can either go on to the arms or work on the torso itself. This single voluptuous movement allows your partner to experience a kind of miniature head-and-shoulders massage. Sensations range from a delicate light show at the eyes to firm pressure over the large muscles at the top of the shoulders.

In a six-part series of easy turns you cover the eyes, face, temples, neck, top of the back, and shoulders.

1. Begin by pressing the soft heel of your hands against both eyes. Your thumbs should be perfectly parallel and touch at the center of your partner's forehead. Light to moderate pressure over the eyes is usually just right. This is definitely one of those movements in which some feedback from your partner the first few times through will help you understand what pressures work best. Hold your pressure on the eyes for a silent count of ten.

2. Slide your hands to the side so that your thumbs rest over your partner's temples (as shown). You can, at this point, put pressure on the temples, but be sure to maintain contact from the bottom of your palms to the top of your partner's face.

3. Move your hands straight down, caressing the cheeks.

When your fingertips are near the top of your partner's mouth, turn your hands and press forward to the back of the neck. Contact on the neck should be with all four fingers while your thumb remains

raised (as shown).

4 and 5. Stroke down the back of the neck, and turn at the shoulders. Reach around the shoulders as far as you can without catching the massage surface.

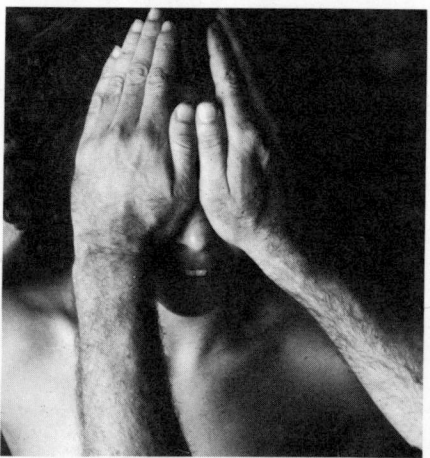
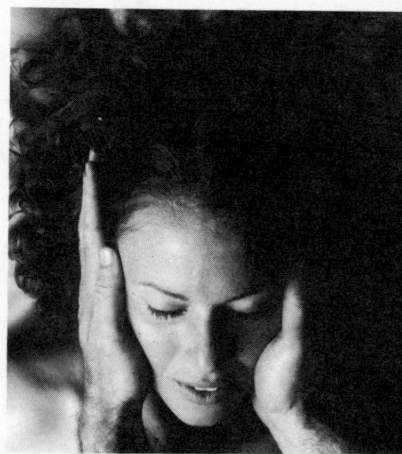

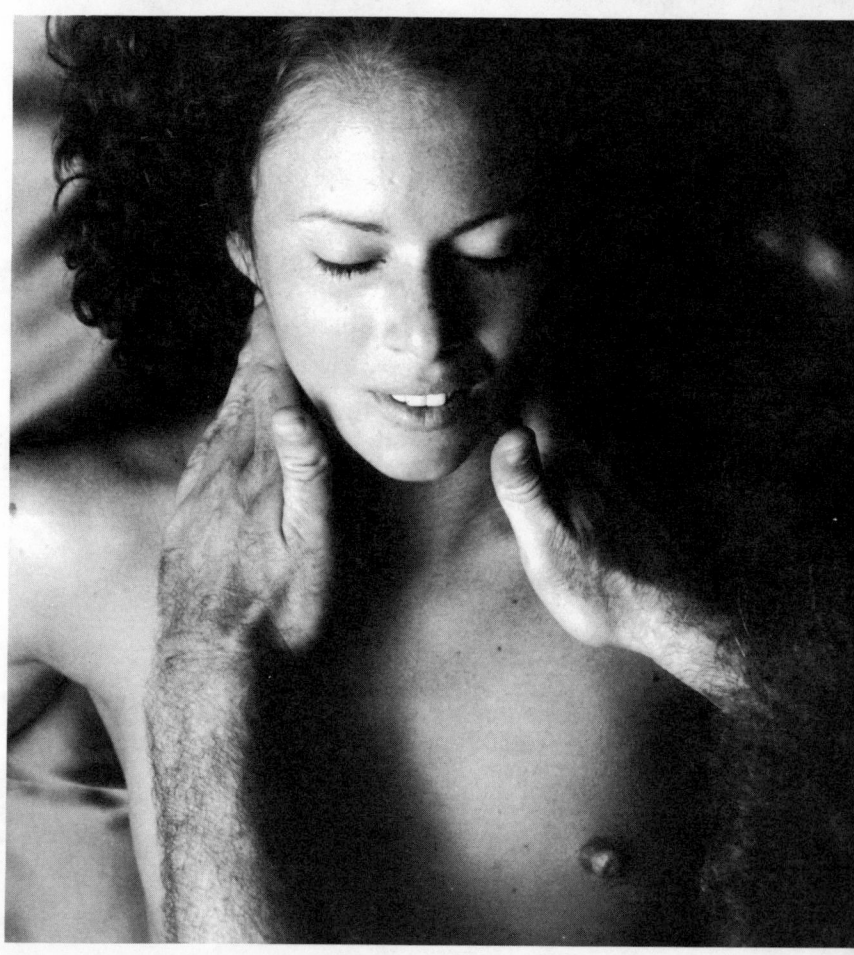

As you move away from your partner's neck, you can lower your thumb. Glide over the shoulder bones. Just after these bones you will feel the thick muscles at the top of the arm

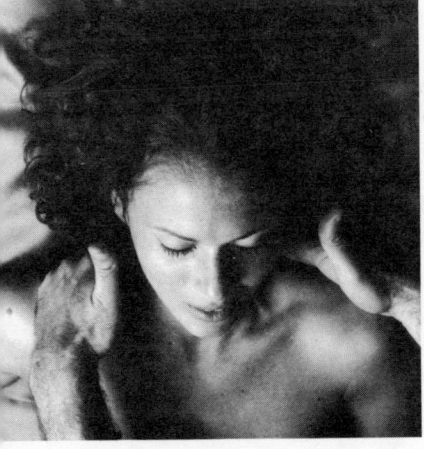

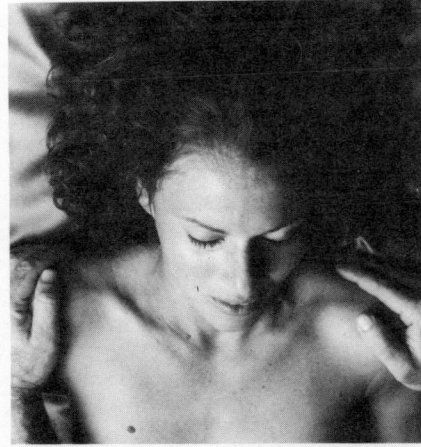

itself. Once you're off the bone and onto these muscles, you can use much more pressure. Again, the exact amount will vary depending upon how well muscled the shoulder is.

6. Turn at the shoulder, and return across your partner's chest, fingers together and hands perfectly flat. When you reach the sides of the neck, press forward into Position No. 3 on the back of the neck. Once you're back on the neck, it's easy to reverse the direction of the first two movements in the sequence. This will complete the circle and leave your hands pressed, once again, against your partner's eyes.

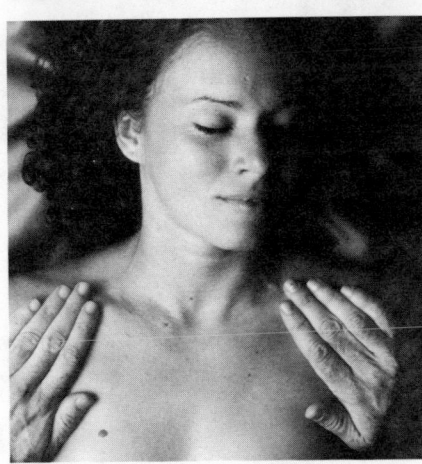

Each one of the body's extremities needs to be stretched at some point during a full body massage. The head, wrists, and feet all have natural handles that make these stretching movements easier. On the head you will find handles at the chin and near the base of the skull right at the point where the skull curves in to meet the neck. Pull back at both of these points simultaneously, and the neck will stretch evenly without jerking the head forward or backward. Cup your partner's chin with one hand (as shown), and at the same time pull straight back on the base of the skull. Pull until there is moderate tension on the neck, and hold that tension for a silent count of ten. You can,

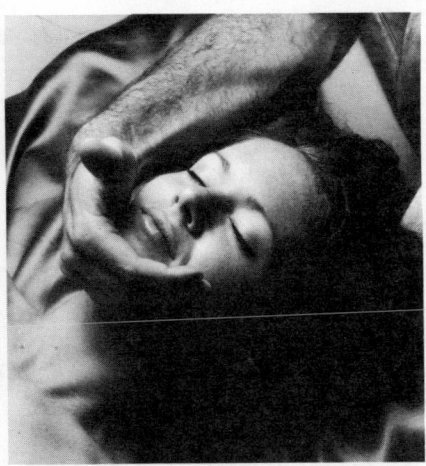

if you like, turn the head slowly from side to side while you pull.

101

Before you lift the neck, you may want to move your partner's hair. Wipe the oil off your hands one at a time so you don't have to break contact. Hair should be stroked, not pulled, back to where you want it. Always be sure to leave a bit of slack at the roots so that later movements won't pull on your partner's scalp. Hold your hands so the fingertips meet and interlace slightly, basket style. Lift until you feel resistance. Your partner's head will fall back in a voluptuous arc. The hand position used in this movement involves an exception to the full-contact rule. Be careful not to press your thumbs down on the front of the neck. There's a very complex blood vessel system

your hands in tiny circles, pushing up against the neck muscles. Women experience a great deal of tension on this part of the body, and if your partner has complained of stiffness, you might want to reassure her that you will be returning to the neck later on in the massage. Some of the neck muscles are more easily reached from the back.

This movement allows you to feel the strange and wonderful devices inside your partner's neck. Most people enjoy being explored in this way as long as you keep the pressures very mild. Grasp the trachea (or Adam's apple) between your thumb and opposing four fingers. Anchor this movement with your free hand behind your partner's neck. The most pleasing movement here is just a gentle vibration. Don't try to move the tissues below the surface.

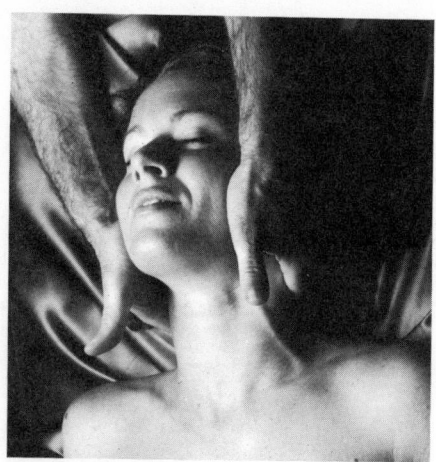

right under the surface, and if you press down on it, your partner could pass out.

Hold the neck up for a silent count of ten, and lower it slowly. Once it's lowered, you can move right into stroking movements with four fingers of each hand. Here again your thumbs should be elevated throughout the movement. You can stroke back and forth on the neck, one hand up while the other is down, or rotate

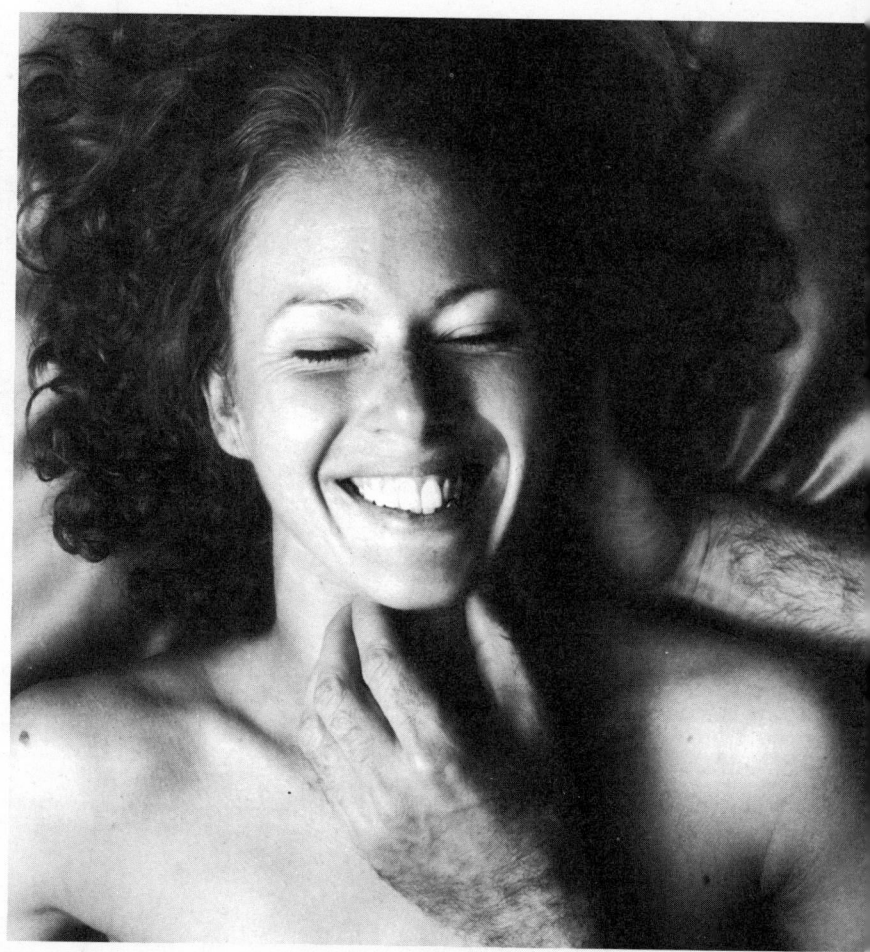

The Front of the Legs

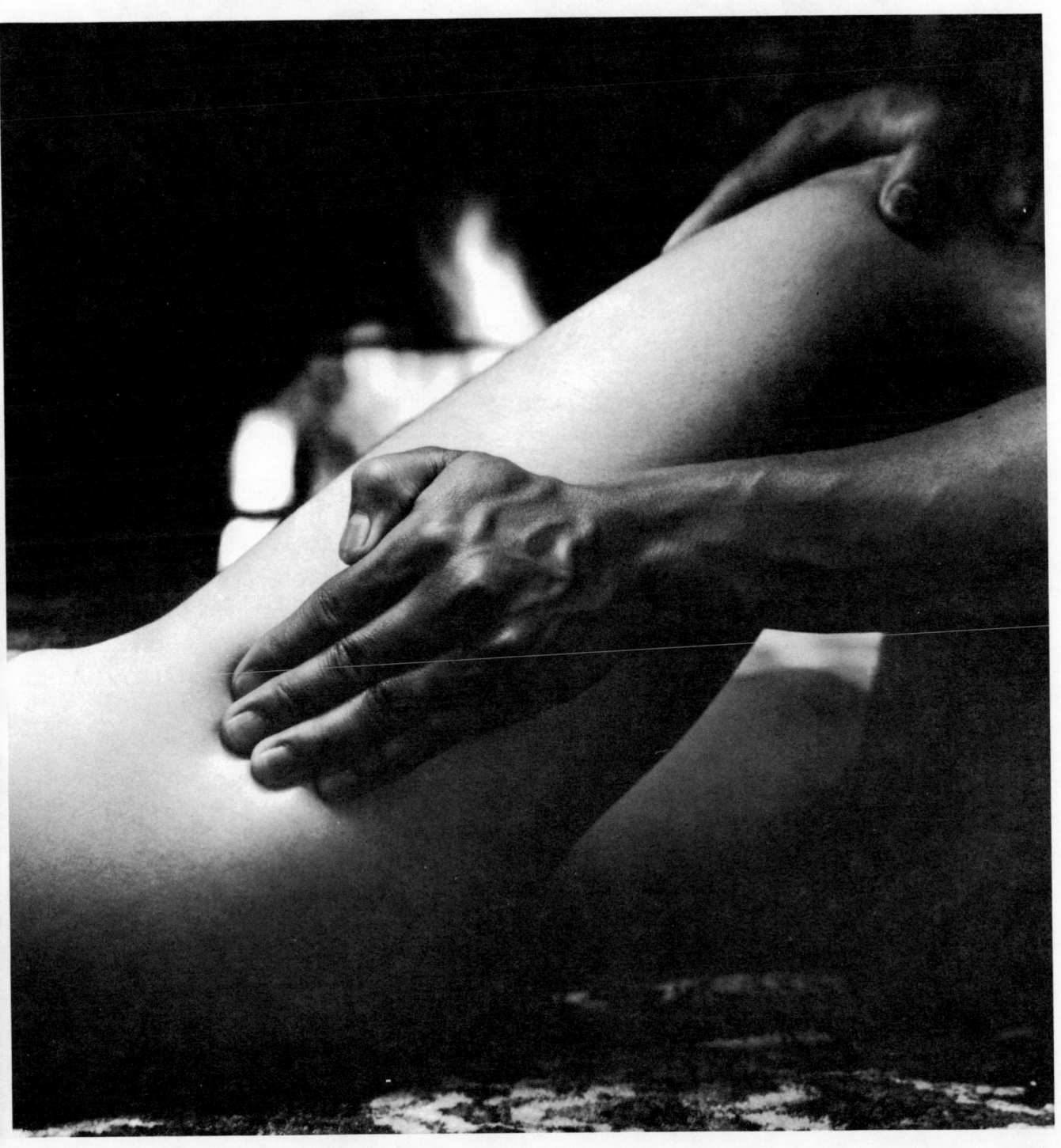

The Front of the Legs

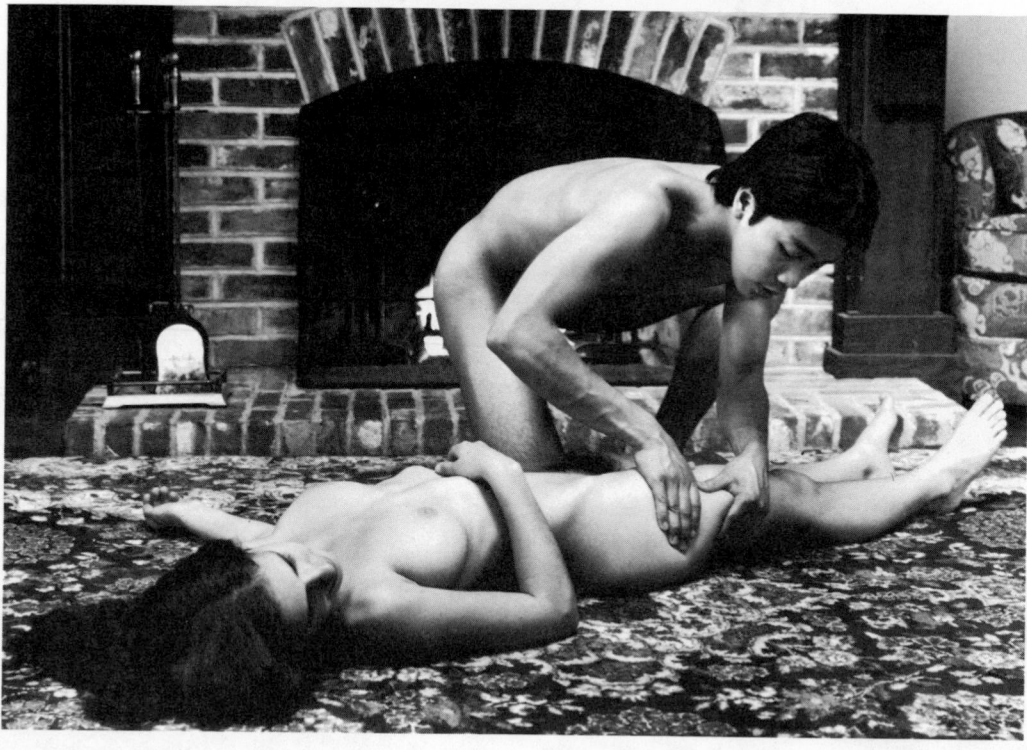

The body's largest joint is also the most unpredictable one. Instead of acting like a simple hinge in the middle of a limb, the knee is constantly tempted to slide sideways, tearing internal ligaments, cartilage, and tendons. Each one of these injuries is sufficient to immobilize almost anyone. Many dancers and skiers end their careers with sudden knee injuries. Runners find themselves hardly able to walk, and people who avoid serious exercise to protect their knees can injure themselves while lifting a shopping bag. Knee injuries always seem to strike without warning. The only thing certain about them are the huge medical bills which always follow.

Must modern life become an inexorable journey from infancy to arthritis filled with giant knee pads and monster bandages? Since this is not a desirable (or fashionable) approach, the best alternative is to find ways to stabilize the naked knee. Masseurs who wish to consider this problem will do most of their work on the front of the leg. The four muscles that extend the knee joint and make it possible for you to rise from a chair are on the front of the thigh. All these parts connect to the knee via a single tendon. The kneecap actually grows out of the center of that tendon and many delicate internal parts of the knee are directly linked to this large four-sectioned muscle (called the quadriceps). If any part of the muscle is under- *or* overexercised, the knee is likely to suffer. Frequent massage will leave the quadriceps flexible and relaxed, the best possible state for healthy knee operation.

But Socrates, sitting up in bed, drew up his leg, and rubbed it with his hand, and as he rubbed it said: "What an unaccountable thing, my friends, that seems to be which men call pleasure. . . .
—PLATO, Phaedo

Most arteries run deep within the body's tissues close to the bone. On the protected inner thigh there is a notable exception. The large femoral artery runs down the length of the inner thigh so close to the surface that it can sometimes be seen clearly. Intense pressure over this artery should be avoided. If you wish to knead the inner thigh, be sure to keep your contact almost superfi- cial. The outside of the thigh, however, presents one of the best opportunities for really deep kneading anywhere in the body. Always reach across your partner's body, and knead the opposite thigh (as shown). Remember to use your thumbs to pick up the flesh as your hands circle. Work up and down the outside of the thigh from knee to hip. After you've completed the side of the leg, move onto the top of the thigh, and knead it exactly the same way from knee to hip. This sequence will cover all of the quadriceps that operate the knee.

If the knee joint is more exposed than the other large joints, it is also the easiest to massage. Near the surface on both sides of the kneecap, the knee joint is equally accessible all the way around to the back of the leg. At the core of this joint, between the bones, is a large semilunar cartilage that constantly changes shape as the knee is moved. Massage of the knee will reach the sides of this cartilage, the eleven ligaments that connect internal bones, and the local tendons. It will also stimulate the production of fluids that lubricate the whole joint and remove internal wastes. Because the knee is so complicated, an injury that makes walking difficult should really be checked by a doctor. The most important role of massage in knee injuries is to restore the knee to full function after structural damage has been repaired. Stiffness in the knee often lingers for months or even years after an accident. Two weeks of daily massage can make the most remarkable difference for a mending knee. People who have had trouble going up and down stairs find that they can ride a bicycle effortlessly for miles.

Inside the knee

Femur
Ligament
Fibula
Tendon to quadriceps
Patella
Lubricating fluid
Cartilage
Patellar ligament
Tibia

Back-of-the-Knee Vibration—A Friction Variation

Thumb Friction to the Knee

This vibration movement will reach the important blood vessels that cross the back of the knee and stimulate circulation throughout the area. It's always a good way to begin your knee massage because it warms the joint from the bottom up. Flatten your hands, and press your fingertips toward each other under the knee until they almost touch. Holding this position, the hands can move up and down very quickly without having to reposition. Pump the hands up and down on the back of the knee; when one hand is up, the other should be down.

The body is full of little crevices and corners that love to be rubbed. Just below the side of the kneecap you will find one of the most interesting ones. Flexing your partner's leg slightly gives you easy access to the whole area for a wide range of knee movements. Thumb friction can be effectively anchored just below the knee on your partner's thick calf muscle. Reach around the kneecap with your friction hand (without pressing down), and press your thumb into the soft, fleshy depression next to the kneecap. Work in a tiny corkscrew pattern as you circle the knee. Above the knee you will

feel the depression disappear as you cross the thick tendons of the upper leg.

Depending on the size of the relationship between your hand and your partner's knee, you may want to try full-hand friction movements here also. If your hands are small and your partner's knee is fairly large, you can press around it with four fingers of one hand. Sometimes it's helpful to anchor this movement on the calf with your free hand.

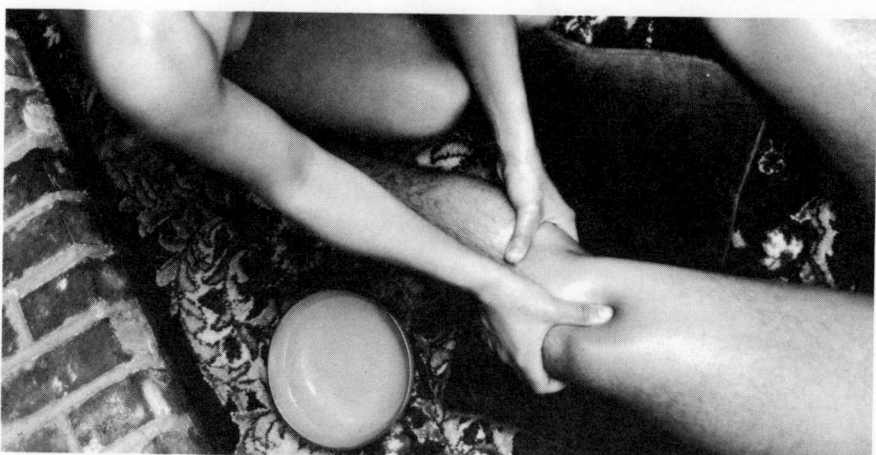

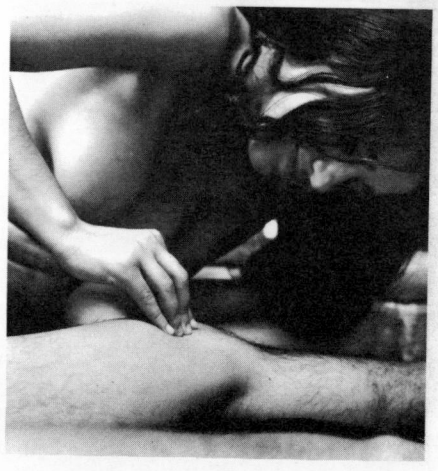

The kneecap (or patella) is one of the most unusual bones in the body. Instead of contacting another bone directly, it is actually suspended between two tendons above the soft inner tissues of the knee joint. The kneecap protects these inner tissues from injury, but in doing so, it becomes particularly susceptible to injury itself. The bone literally grows out of a large tendon that descends from the quadriceps muscle of the thigh. Below the kneecap the patellar ligament attaches directly to the tibia, the thickest bone in the body. On both sides this tiny bone is anchored to some of the body's most massive structures, which are capable of wrenching it into the most painfully compromising positions.

Like the kneecap, all the internal structures of the knee are subject to powerful forces. While the knee supports and balances the entire weight of the body above, there are constant vertical and horizontal pressures which must be absorbed. Five external and six internal ligaments absorb these forces and connect the large bones that meet at the knee. The movement of pressing under the kneecap reaches the internal tissues of the knee.

Begin by pressing both thumbs together at the bottom of the knee with your four fingertips pressed together on the back of the knee. Your thumbs will travel around the knee in opposite directions. At the top of the knee and again at the bottom, they will cross each other (as shown). Use easy pressures until you've had some feedback from your partner.

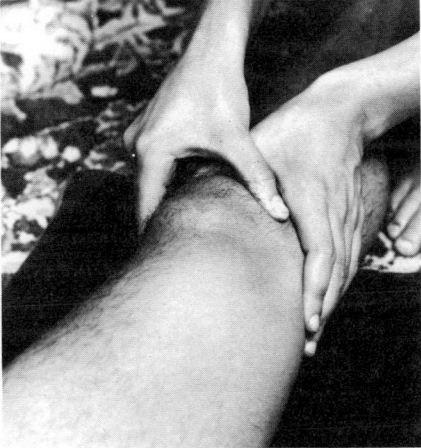

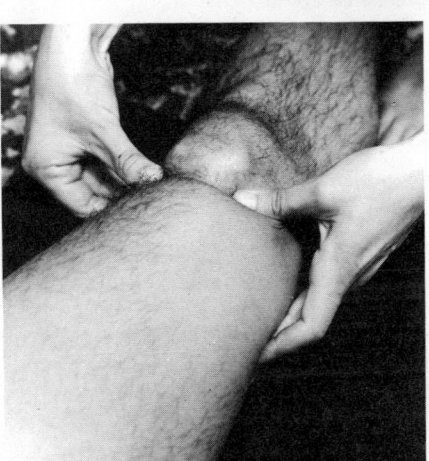

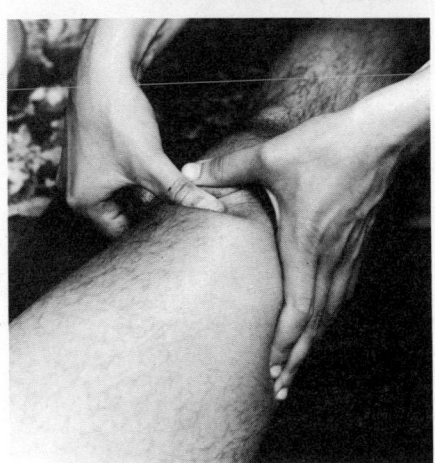

When you massage the knee, it's a good idea to support it with a small pillow. This bit of extra support will prevent you from stretching the muscles at the back of the knee when you press down. Gently lift your partner's leg above the knee, and slide a pillow under the knee. Stroking works on the sides of the knee and should always be anchored with your free hand just under the knee. Stroke back and forth and in small circles, being careful not

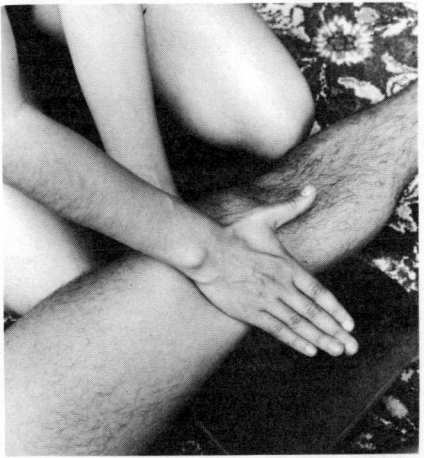

to press on the kneecap itself. Work onto the leg about six inches above and below the knee. When you finish the inside of the knee, reverse your stroking and anchor hands, tilt the leg slightly away from yourself, and stroke the outside of the knee.

Thumb Stroking the Sides of the Knee

Kneading the Knee

Testing the Sciatic Nerve

This movement covers the entire surface of the leg on both sides of the knee, from the kneecap down. Keeping your four fingers together, allow your thumbs to press into the depression on the sides of the knee. Stroke up and down along the knee, and as you stroke, allow your thumbs to creep down slowly along the sides of the leg. You'll have total finger contact at all times with this movement from the side of the kneecap to the massage surface. Moving your thumb down will allow you to emphasize pressure with this finger at different points on the side of the leg. You can also experiment with different speeds during thumb stroking, from very slow to moderately fast.

This is the familiar full-hand kneading movement used on the torso and arms. The only difference here is that your hands will work just a bit farther apart than usual. Kneading above and below the kneecap at the same time, you can use the whole surface of your hand. The top hand kneads the important quadriceps while the bottom hand works right up to the lower edge of the kneecap. Generally it's easier to pick up more flesh above the knee than below.

Although this is a front-of-the-leg movement that twists the top of the toes, almost all its effects will be felt on the back of the thigh. By supporting the leg straight out and twisting back the top of your partner's foot, you stretch the hamstring muscles on the back of the thigh. These large muscles are used to flex the knee during walking, running, and lifting.

Buried deep within them is the crucial sciatic nerve that runs down the back of the leg from the spine. Pressure on this nerve can be quite painful and will often lead people to assume they have seriously damaged the lower back. If the nerve is pinched, however, massage can be used to relieve the problem and leave your partner smiling. This movement will detect tension anywhere along the nerve by stretching it without putting pressure on the lower back. Go slowly because if the nerve *is* pinched, your partner will feel it as you flex the foot. That reaction indicates that you need to focus on the sciatic nerve area when you massage the lower back of the leg and the lower back.

Lift your partner's leg at the heel of the foot, and wrap your arm around the leg (as shown). Your fingertips should press up on the inside of the thigh, thus allowing the forearm to act as a diagonal brace above and below your partner's knee. Once you have firmly supported the leg, go ahead and grasp the foot over the top of the toes (as shown). Bend the top of the foot back all the way to the point of resistance. As you press into this resistance, you will create the necessary tension on the hamstrings and the sciatic nerve.

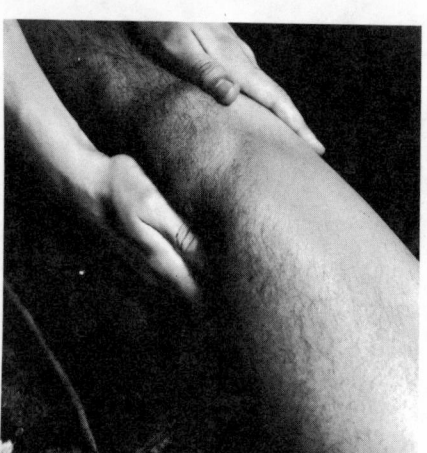

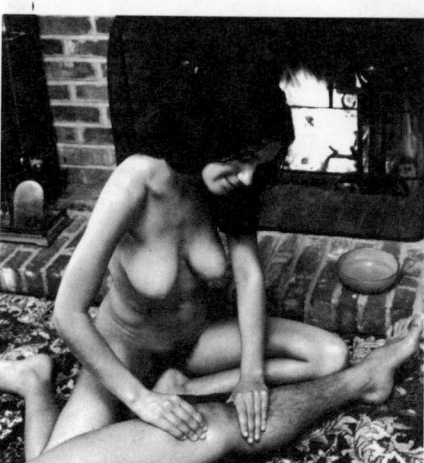

Down Stroking the Leg

This exceptional full limb movement blankets the entire leg with warm sensation. All the stroking is down the leg away from the heart. It's important to allow your hands to mold to the constantly changing shape of your partner's leg as you descend. Begin pulling down at the top of the leg with one hand. When that hand reaches your partner's knee, do the same thing with your other hand. Then start just a bit lower on the top of the leg with your

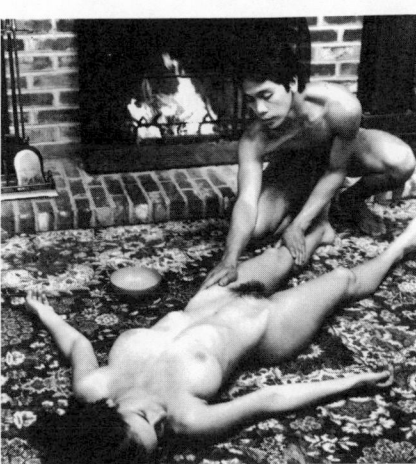

first hand. Work down the leg this way, covering every part of the leg at least once with each hand. Toward the foot your strokes will become very short: you can end the down stroking on the ankle or move out onto the foot itself.

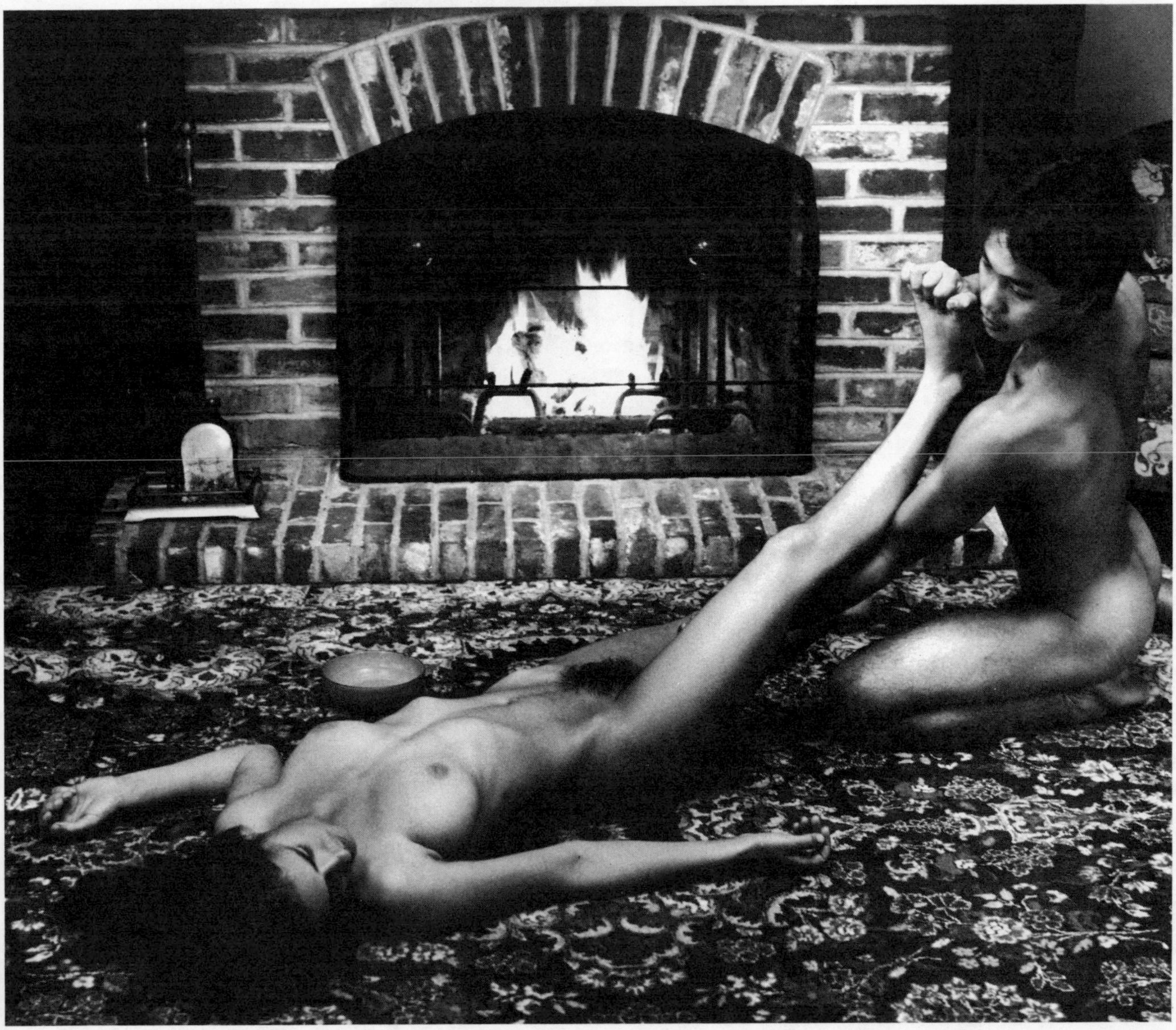

The bones of the lower leg are so close to the surface that you will need to reach around them to work on the muscles. This is easy to do if you flex the leg first and support it with your knees. Kneel on either side of your partner's foot, and bring your knees together until they press firmly against the foot and ankle. This clamping action will anchor your movements on the thick calf muscles. Reach around the calf with four fingers of each hand. Keep your fingers together, and press them up while you knead with your thumbs. Circle with both thumbs against the calf muscle. Even though you're working on opposite sides of the leg, this movement will work exactly

the same way as it did when your thumbs were touching on the top of the leg: One thumb is up while the other is down. Work up the leg to the bottom of the knee, then down until you run out of muscle to knead.

Knead the top part of the calf with the flat part of your thumbs. On top the thumb kneading movement is exactly the same as the one you used on the arms (see page 62). The difference here is the large bone right at the surface of the leg. Light pressures over it feel best. The leg doesn't need to be flexed for this movement. When you set it down, you may want to support your partner's foot on your thigh.

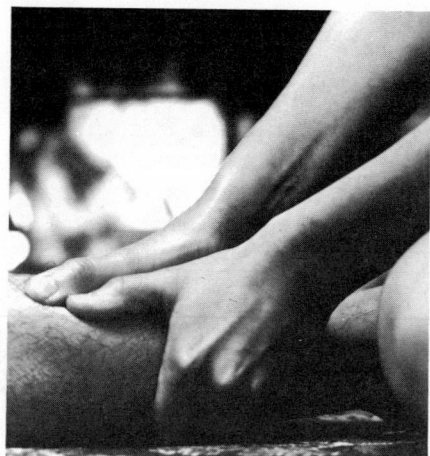

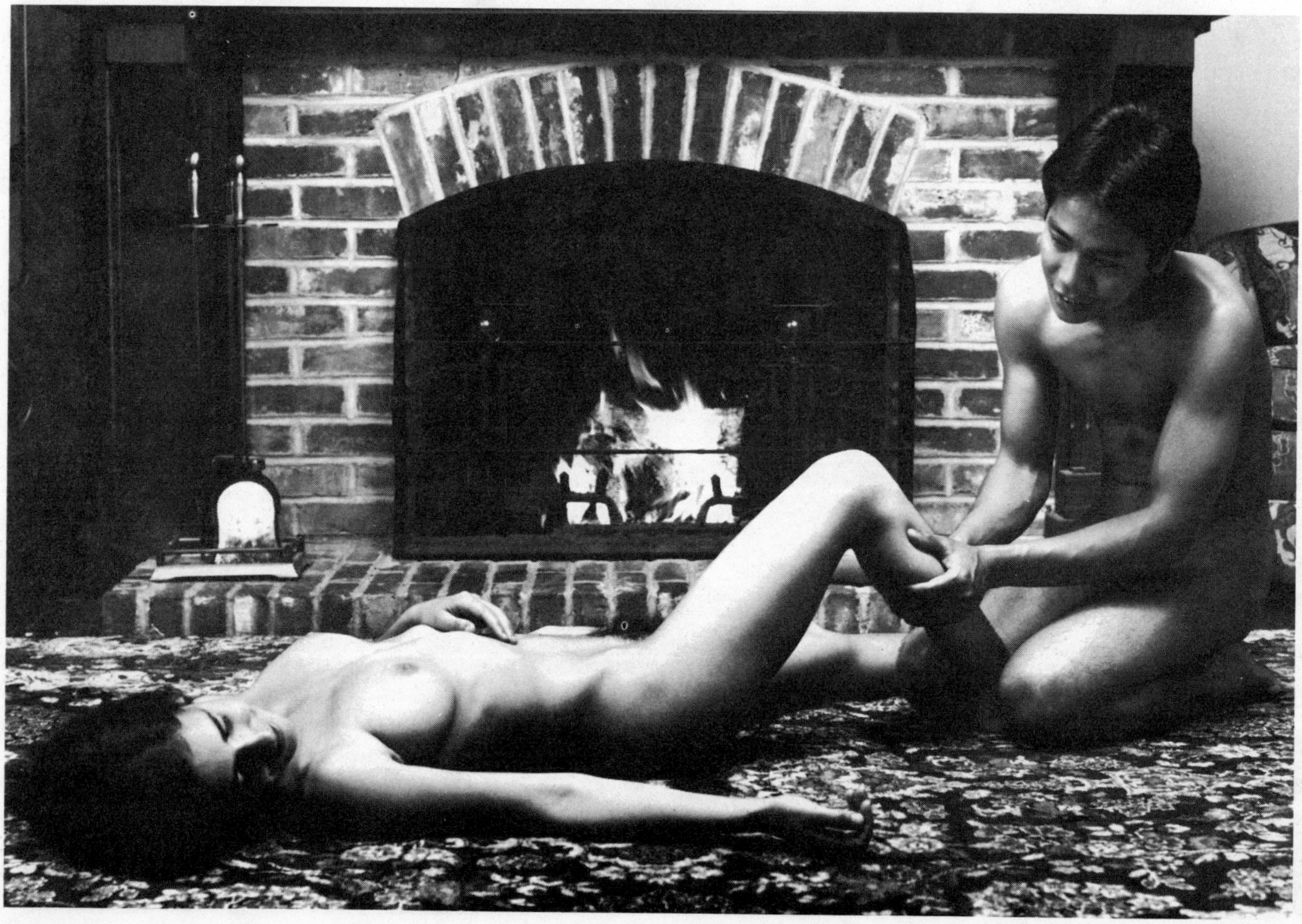

Press your hands together around your partner's ankle. Your thumbs should overlap the top of the leg. As you move up toward the knee, squeeze the leg hard enough so that a roll of flesh appears in front of your index fingers. This movement will visibly empty the veins of the lower leg for a few moments. It not only aids the action of the heart but presses lymph up the leg and clears the entire system.

Fingertip Hacking the Calf: The popular notion that percussion movements are supposed to be a ferocious barrage of blows reveals one of the most basic misconceptions about massage. Tensed muscles and nerves will remain that way no matter how long they are pummeled by some witless oaf. Like friction strokes, percussion movements aim to stimulate the tissues just below the surface, and you don't need enormous pressures to do that. A gentle rain, not a thunderstorm.

Use your body to cushion part of the blow during every percussion movement. Instead of bringing your whole arm to bear when you come down, break the movement at the wrist as though you were swinging a golf club or baseball bat. Let your little finger hang down so it further cushions the blow. Each time a hand comes down you will hear a tiny snapping sound as the fingers

come together. This can be an exciting moment. Some people get carried away with hacking and begin pretending they are playing the congas. Fortunately there are excellent music stores everywhere these days where they can practice on real congas while the rest of us practice real massage.

Fingertip hacking will certainly work well at slow speeds. If you're careful not to skip any part of the leg, your partner will scarcely notice the difference. Move up and down the calf three times.

Hacking can be used on firm muscle tissue throughout the body. Always be sure to stay off bony areas. Turn the leg slightly so the calf muscle can be reached more effectively. The palms of your hands should brush each other as your hands move up and down your partner's legs.

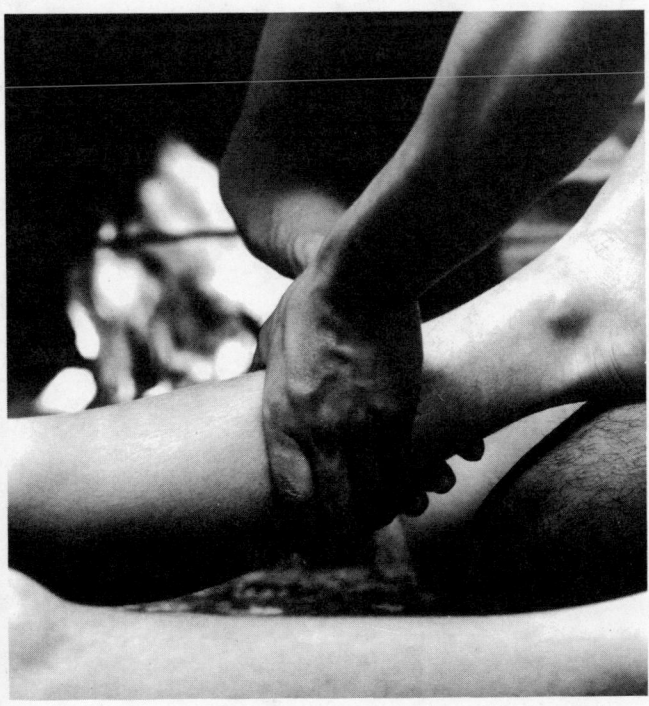
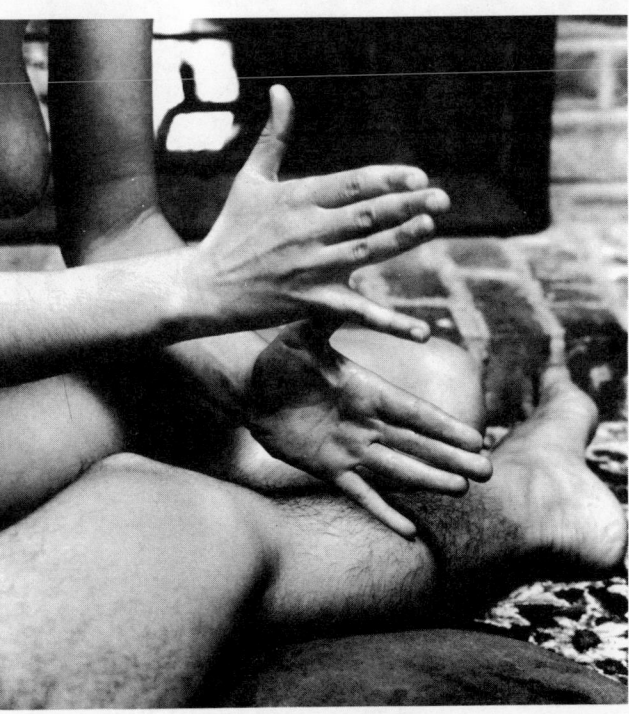

Circling the Thigh with Your Forearm—A Stroking Movement

Clapping the Thigh: Clapping is a simple percussion movement that can also be used almost anywhere on the body. Keep your fingers together, and work from the wrists. Your thumbs should brush each other as your hands move up and down the leg. Allow both hands to mold themselves to the shape of your partner's thigh. Here again, you should make contact from the heel of your hand to the fingertips. Work back and forth three times from the knee to the hip. Like all percussion movements, clapping brings blood to the surface and stimulates circulation throughout the area.

It's easy to relax with this movement and continue it for a long while. This is a stable position which will allow you to rest your back for a few minutes when you're working on a floor. If you rotate your forearm while you're resting, your partner will remain quite happy. The important thing here is to anchor the leg firmly enough so that you can concentrate all your attention on the thigh and forearm connection.

Lift your partner's leg above and below the knee, and move it out so there's enough room for one of your knees when you kneel. Flex the leg at the knee, and kneel on both sides of it, pressing your legs together against your partner's calf (as shown).

Grasp the leg at the knee with your free hand to anchor the movement further. Remember to oil your forearm along with the thigh. Use moderate pressure, and turn the entire forearm in small circles, pressing down on your partner's thigh. Begin at the top of the leg, and work down to the knee. Move your arm back and forth so that the whole surface makes contact from elbow to wrist as you work up and down the thigh.

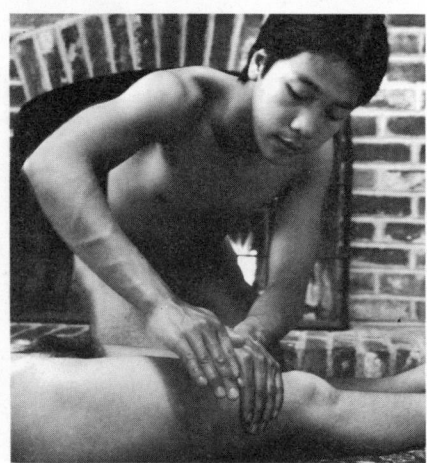

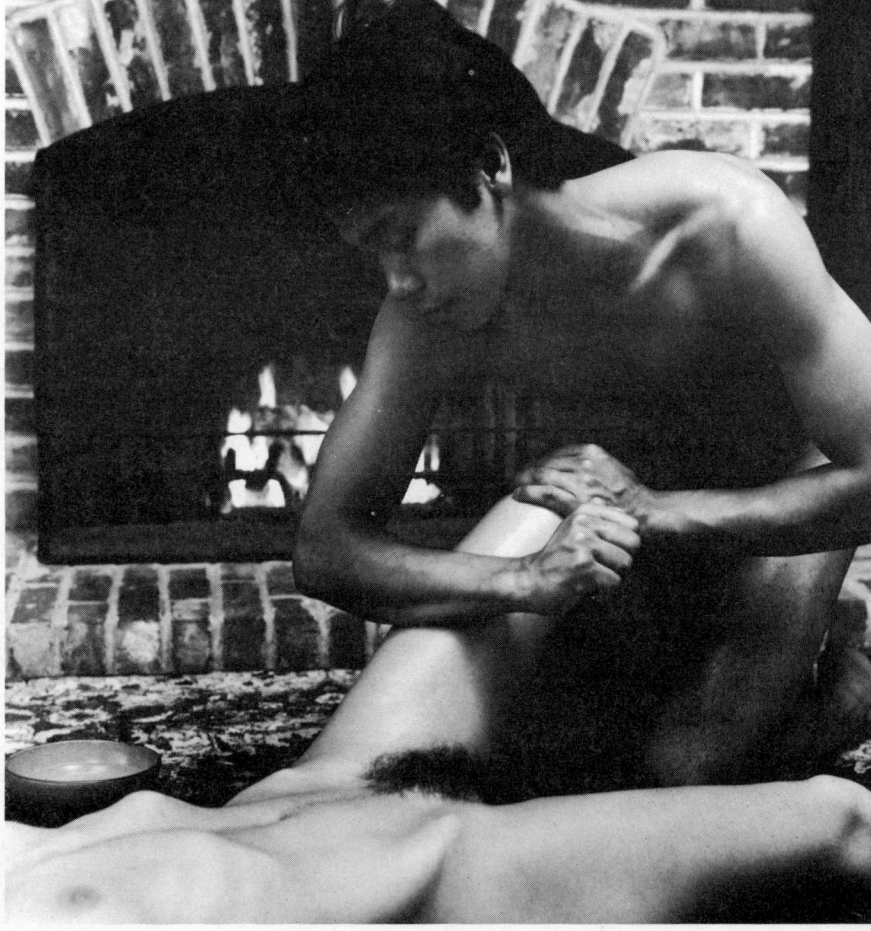

The formidable joint at the hip is deep and well protected by powerful ligaments. Although you cannot actually touch this joint the way you could the ones at the wrist, knee, and elbow, you can reach it through strong friction movements around the top of the leg. At the top of the leg the femur, the longest bone in the body, turns in toward the pelvis, where it ends in a large ball joint. You can easily feel the top of the femur just below and slightly behind the sharp, protruding edge of the pelvic girdle. Hip friction works all the way around the thick knobby top of the bone.

Anchor your partner's leg with your free hand at the knee (as

shown). You may also want to kneel on both sides of your partner's leg and to anchor this stroke further by using your legs to press up against the calf. As always, friction movements should be either circular or straight back and forth. Keep your pressure constant, and work all the way around the top of the bone. In the area between the top of the femur and the pelvis you can press in and almost reach the hip joint.

Work on each hip for about half a minute.

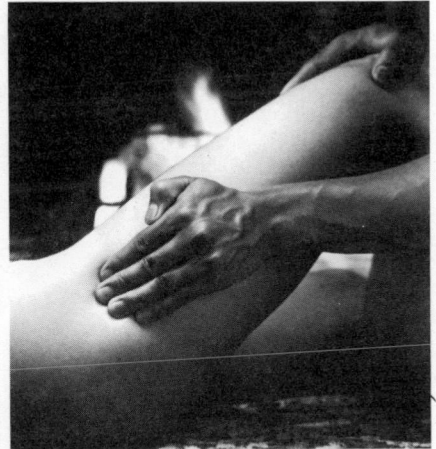

Femur

Fibula

Tibia

Operation of the ball joint at the hip

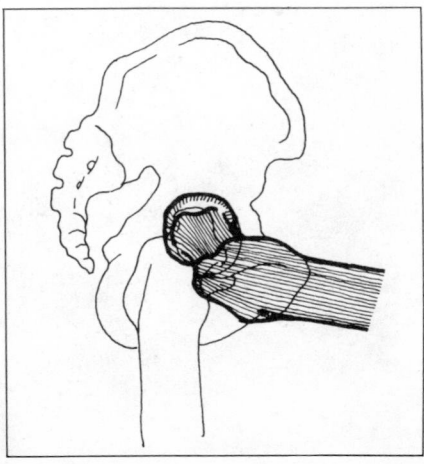

On the top part of the body, venous return of blood to the heart is assisted by gravity. The legs, of course, cannot depend on this force, and the veins are equipped with a series of valves to prevent blood from backflowing on the way up to the heart. All these valves will open only toward the heart. When they fail, the blood vessels of the leg swell up and the condition known as varicose veins develops.

There are two venous systems in the leg, one deep inside and the other right at the surface (and often visible). Since both systems are connected through smaller veins, any massage movement that reaches the surface veins will penetrate to the deep system. The two venous systems allow the blood traveling back toward the heart to take many different routes. This full limb movement will reach the entire system. It will assist the heart by

pumping large amounts of "old" blood out of the leg while, at the same time, clearing the lymph nodes from ankle to hip. This massive circulation effect will tone all of the leg's blood vessels and help keep the valves within the veins operating smoothly.

Begin stimulating circulation in the legs by clearing the lymph center on the lower torso (see page 43) that is closest to the leg you are massaging. Use the same combination of friction, vibration, and fingertip kneading movements with which you massaged the torso. When you finish, move down the leg, without breaking contact, all the way to your partner's foot.

Cup both your hands around your partner's leg at the ankle. The hands should be opposed (as shown) and in full contact with the leg from fingertips to the bottom of the palm. The full-contact aspect of this position is particularly important because it allows you to reach veins on the sides of the leg. Press all the way up to the top of the leg, keeping your hands in exactly the same

position. Use moderately firm pressures. On the thigh you may see flesh rolling in front of your lead finger. The only times you will have to ease up on your pressure a bit are over the kneecap and at the protruding pelvic bone near the top of the leg. At the top of the leg, you will find that there's a definite advantage to be gained by leading with your left hand on the right leg and with your right hand on the left leg. This will allow your top hand to turn just under the pelvic bone while the bottom hand turns at the top of the leg (as shown).

Returning to the ankle, make superficial contact on both sides of the leg. Turn your hands once again at the ankle without breaking contact. With practice, the whole sequence, complete with turns at both ends of the leg, will flow without hesitation or interruption. Repeat the sequence ten times.

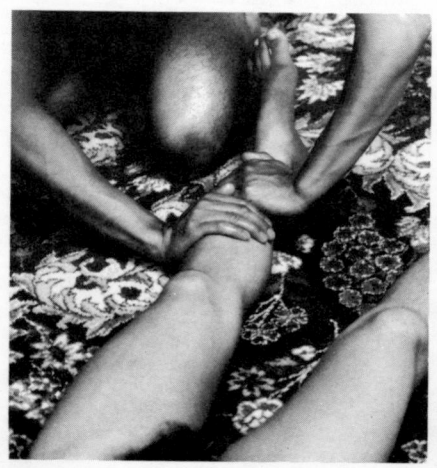 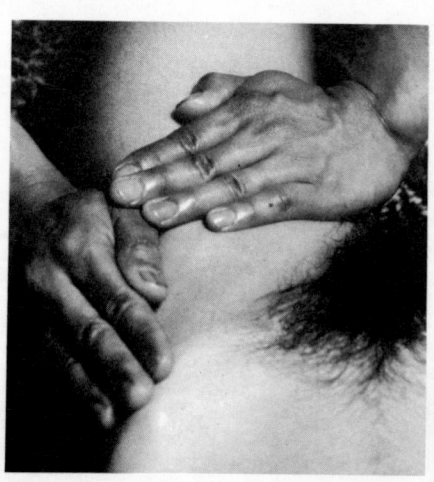 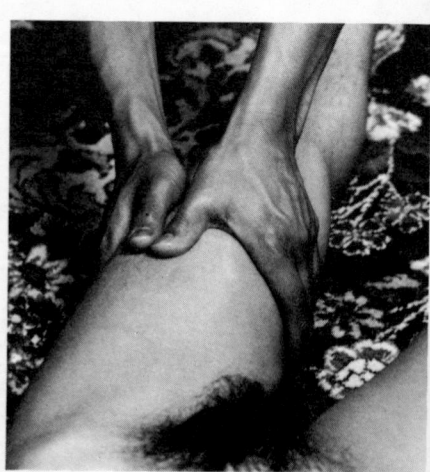

The Feet

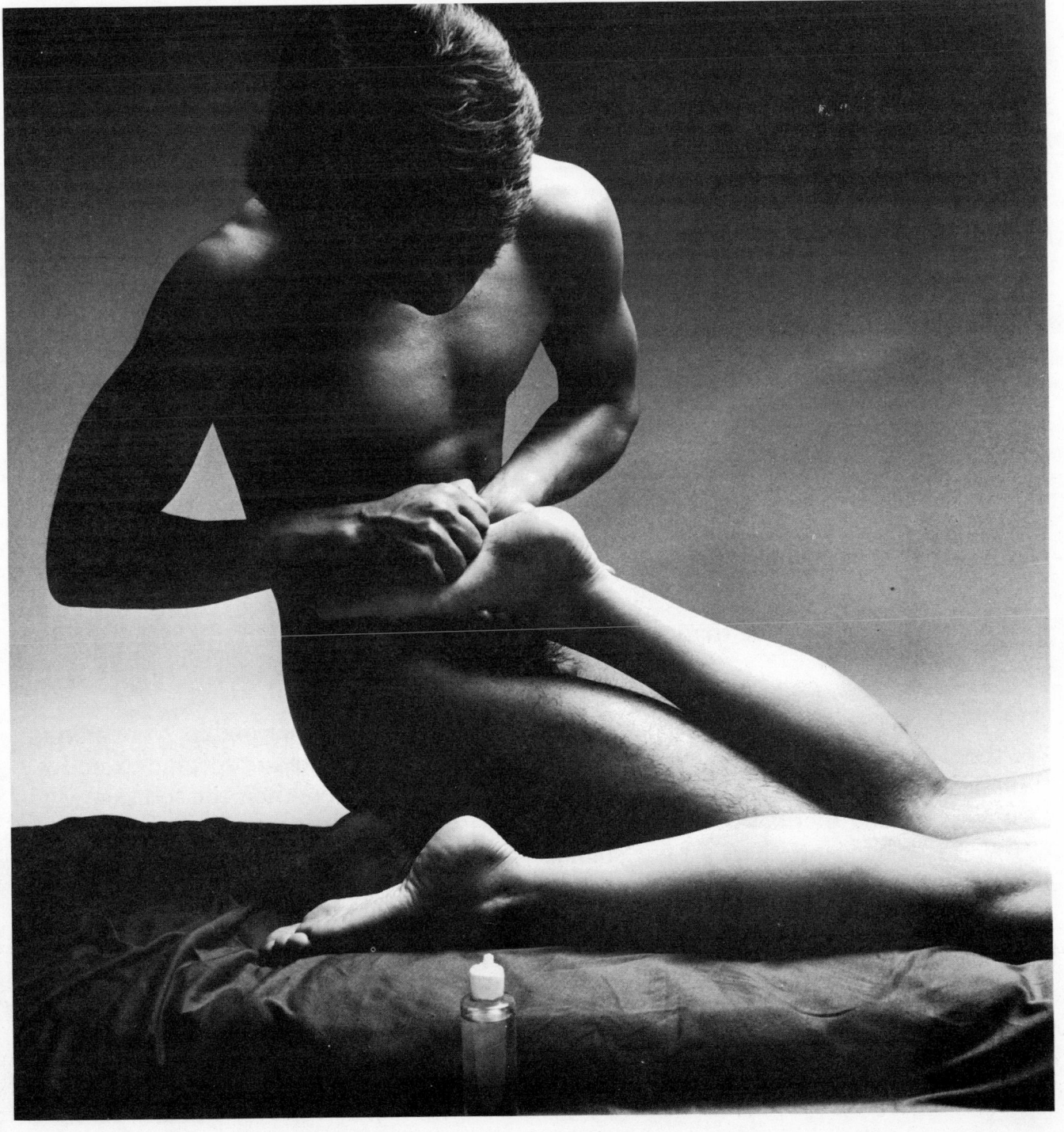

The Feet

A decent foot massage is one of the few simple pleasures left in life. Although it's always best to relax the whole body when you massage any part of it, you can certainly do some good on the feet while your partner relaxes in an easy chair. (Work on the floor, and be sure to allow the leg to bend at the knee.) People who are afraid of massage or regard it as a waste of precious time will almost always let you fool around with their feet while they relax and watch TV. Shoes tend to isolate the body from the world and prevent people from actually enjoying their feet. But since most nerves from the lower spine end there, the feet can be a source of great pleasure. Once in a while they deserve more than the inside of a shoe.

The inside of your hand, for example, is far more sensual than the inside of a shoe. Your partner will recognize this immediately because massage has a way of relaxing and then awakening the feet. When this happens, there's a fair chance you can turn off the TV and get into a full body massage.

When *Homo sapiens'* ancestors descended from the trees, the bone structure of the foot developed two arches for walking on level ground. Anatomical studies speak of "the architecture of the foot" simply because the interior rela-tionship between twenty-six bones and two massive arches is so precise. There are, of course, medical specialists who focus exclusively on this part of the body. Nevertheless, people with constant foot pain often head right for the neighborhood shoe store, checkbook in hand. Would these same folks buy a new hat to cure a headache? The latest flashy shoe fad always seems to promise a new concept which will miraculously trans-form the foot. Unfortunately the only people who benefit from shoes with no backs and toe straps, narrow toes and high heels, or wide toes with no heels are those in the shoe industry. Rather than seek advice from trendy shoe salesmen, people with aching feet might do better to return to the trees for a few hours every day. It's easier on the feet and the pocketbook.

If your partner prefers to remain on the ground, there are specific exercises which will strengthen the foot along with every other part of the body. Your partner can work on the foot with exercise while you use the Fluid Release sequences in this chapter to ease the transition from a weak, unsteady foot to a strong, healthy one. Everyone you work on, whether he exercises or not, will appreciate the way massage leaves the feet feeling supple and almost weightless.

Toe stretching is a good way to exercise passively the complicated lever joints at the toes and on the bottom of the foot that make walking, running, and jumping possible. While you passively exercise the joints, you can also stretch the crucial ligaments that connect them and help the foot work smoothly. To do this, you need to press almost straight down from the toes without bending the whole foot back and flattening the arch.

Lift your partner's foot onto your thigh, and support it with one hand below the ankle (as shown). Your partner's heel can rest lightly on your thigh, if you like, and the toes should almost touch your chest. Keep your fingers together, and press down over your partner's toes, bending them all the way back to the point of resistance. As you press down on the toes, the foot will arch gracefully under your fingers.

If your partner has complained of cramped muscles on the sole of the foot, you may want to vary this movement so that it flattens out the arch. Hold the foot exactly the same way, but press up on the ball of the foot just below the toes. Instead of pressing down toward the ankle, press up toward your partner's head. Stretch the arch out, and hold for a silent count of twenty. Repeat this movement three times.

Like the metatarsal arch of the foot, ankles support the entire weight of the body. Because they must also turn while providing this support, ankles get more attention than any other joint on a runner's body during a massage except the knee.

When you press around the ankle with the tips of your thumbs, you can empty the joint of accumulated fluids. These fluids, sometimes generated during exercise, cause the occasional swelling that can slow down or even completely halt an exercise program when the rest of the body feels fine. Hold your partner's heel basket-style with four fingers of each hand, and press into the thin depression just below the ankle with your thumbs. Circle each ankle three times in each direction. Sometimes you can feel fluid draining from the joint as you work.

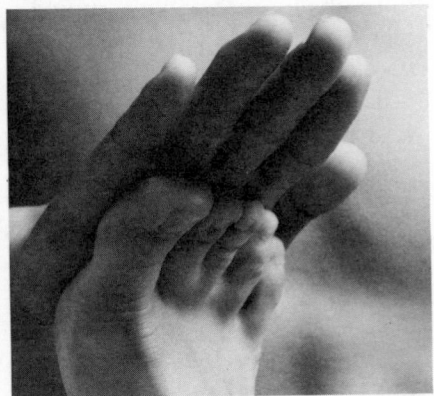

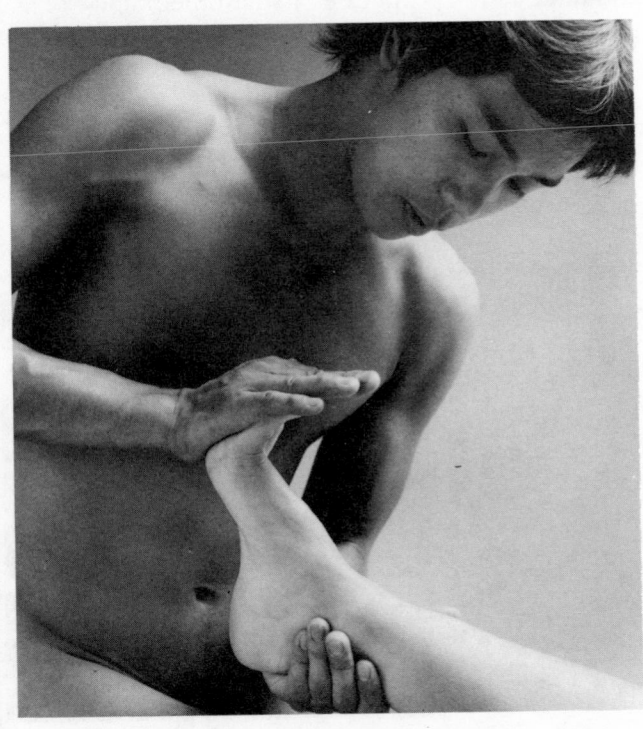

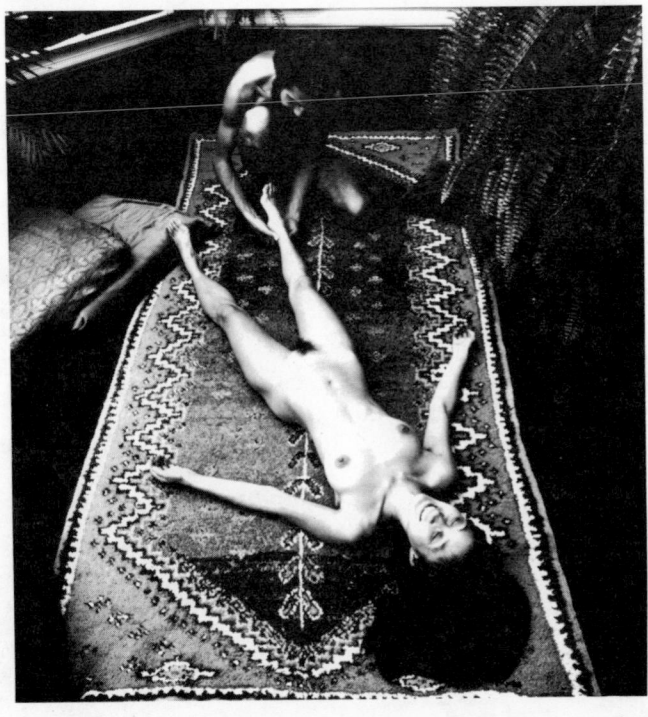

Every massage is a close study of the entire body from scalp to toes. On the toes you may discover corns and blisters that your partner is trying to ignore. Large corns can easily be filed down, but it's best not to do this during a first massage. Unless your partner is ready for it, an abrasive little file will definitely interrupt the peaceful mood you've been working on for such a long time. Toe care has a lot to do with shoe choice; nobody has to live with corns and blisters. No matter how stylish the shoe, if it binds your toes, your partner will soon be hobbling around most inelegantly.

Unless they are really persistent and therefore require medical treatment, most corns will soften enough to be rubbed off after a few hot-water treatments. The following preparation, taken from a forty-year-old medical text, sounds more interesting than hot-water and modern drugstore remedies.

Acid salicylic, 1.
Extract of Cannabis Indica, .50
Ether, 3.
Flexible Collodion Q.S., AD., 10.
apply with applicator or camel's hair brush •

Cannabis indica, an extremely potent strain of marijuana, is, of course, still illegal in most states. If the police find some in your car, you can judiciously explain that it is used for soaking corns.

• Frank D. Dickson, M.D., and Rex L. Dively, M.D., *Functional Disorders of the Foot* (Philadelphia: Lippincott, 1939), page 246.

Anchor the middle of the foot with one hand, and pull up the sides of each toe (as shown). Because the toes are often very small and hard to grasp, you can pull rapidly, almost snapping your fingers off the tip of each toe, before you go on to the next one. The idea is to put pressure on the sides of the toe without actually pulling hard on the toe itself. (For more on toe care, see "A Pedicure," page 185).

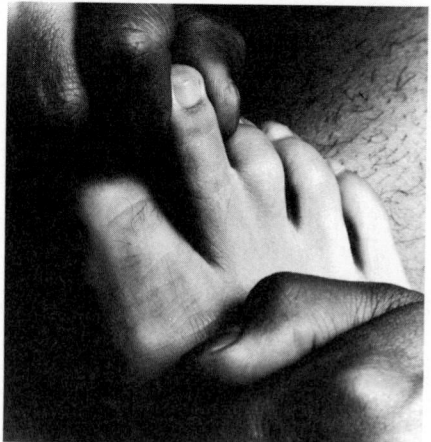

Toe flexing can be felt just below the knee on the outside of the leg where the great muscles that operate the foot begin. Even if you're planning to massage only the feet, you will want to knead up the leg to the knee a few times to relax these muscles. At the feet, the muscles branch out and run across the top of the foot. A generous circular kneading with the full surface of the thumbs will cover all the branches. Press down from the tip of your thumb to the base. Both thumbs should follow each other the same way they did on the arms and hands.

To increase the pressure, fit your partner's foot against your knee and thigh (as shown), and use your knuckles. Position yourself so the foot fits easily without straining. That way you should be able to provide support from the heel all the way up to the toes. Anchor the foot against your thigh with one hand, and press down with the flat part of the knuckle of your other hand. Be sure that all your contact is with the flat part of the knuckle and that you avoid digging in with the pointed part on curved surfaces. Press down, and work in tiny circles from above the ankles to just above the toes. If this

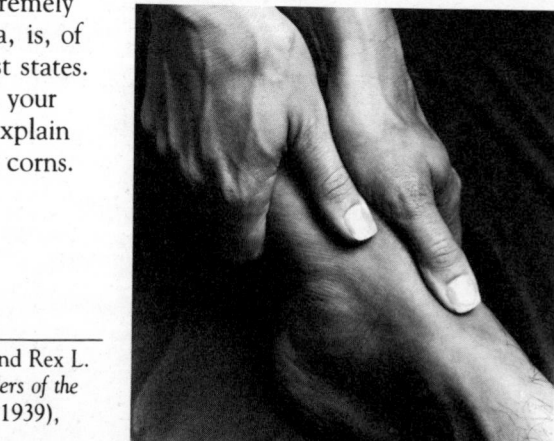

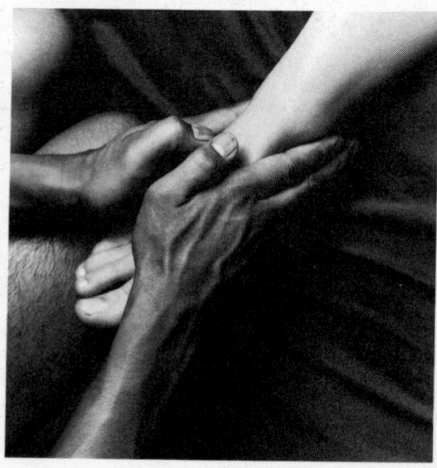

movement is delightful for most people, it is absolutely irresistible to runners. The most taciturn marathoner will usually smile despite himself.

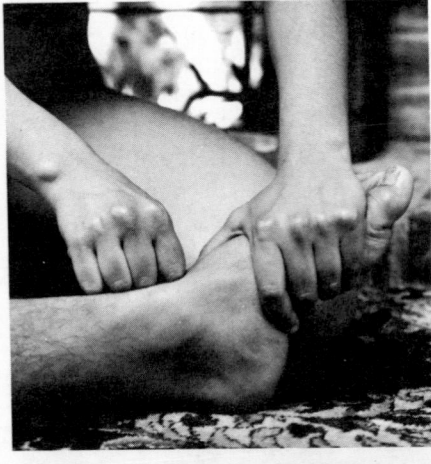

Every full body massage should include a minute or so of friction to both sides of the complex joint at the ankle. In the case of sprains, this movement can be decisive in reducing swelling and restoring mobility to the foot (see "Sprains," page 171). You will feel a very irregular surface when you circle the ankle; press down into the soft valleys, and go a bit easier over the bony ridges. Anchor the foot by holding it around the arch (as shown).

You'll need to hold the foot firmly here. Be mindful of the foot's surface blood vessels, and concentrate your anchoring pressure on the bottom of the foot with your thumb and four fingers.

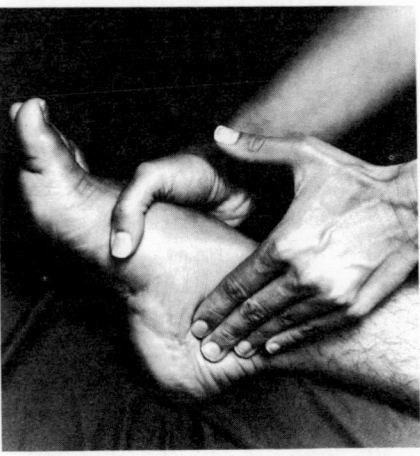

As you work around the ankle, your friction movement should alternate between tiny circles and the familiar rapid back-and-forth motion. Press down with all four fingers. Feel into the joint.

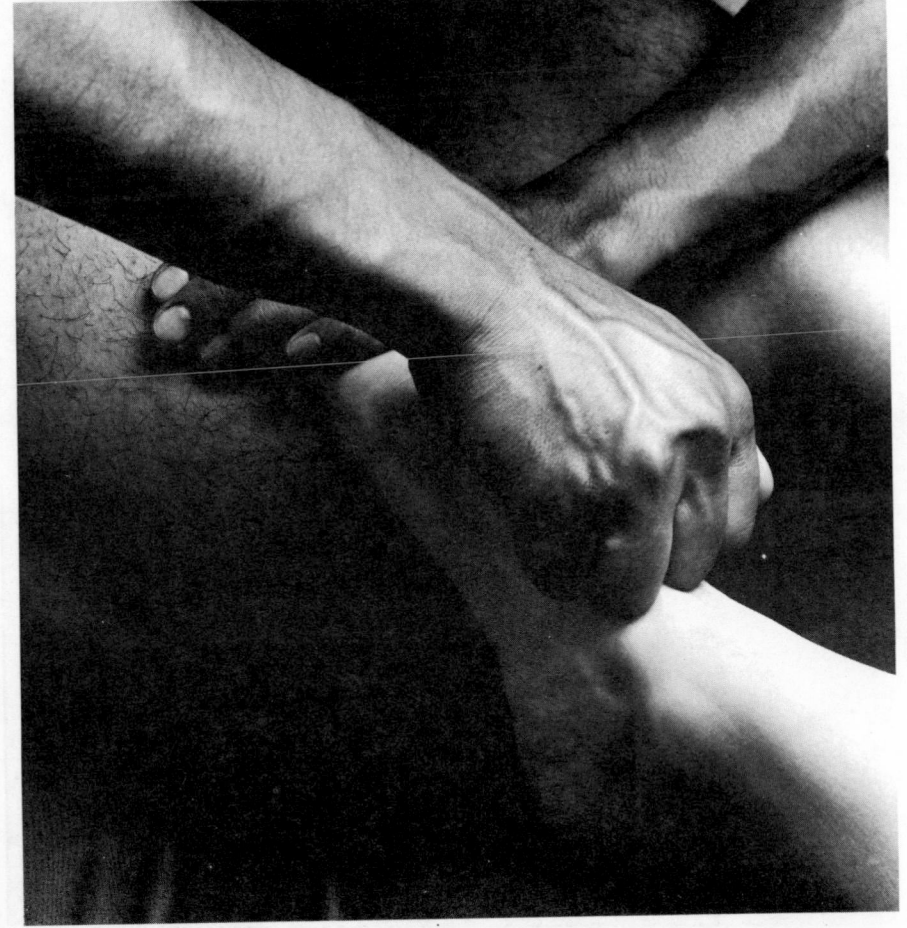

Once you've completed ankle friction, it's a good idea to press the blood and lymph back toward the heart. Whatever toxins you have stirred up during friction will be dispersed quickly, and your partner's foot will begin the gradual awakening process that characterizes every decent foot massage. This is the most effective circulation movement on the whole body simply because you are a long way from the heart and the veins of the foot are very close to the surface.

Cup your hands so they fit the contours of your partner's foot. Oil thoroughly, and press one hand down the foot from the base of the toes to the calf above the ankle. You can go even higher if you like. When you reach the top position, begin at the toes with your other hand pressing up the same way. As the second hand begins to ascend, the first hand returns to the starting position. Because this is a hand-over-hand movement, your partner often

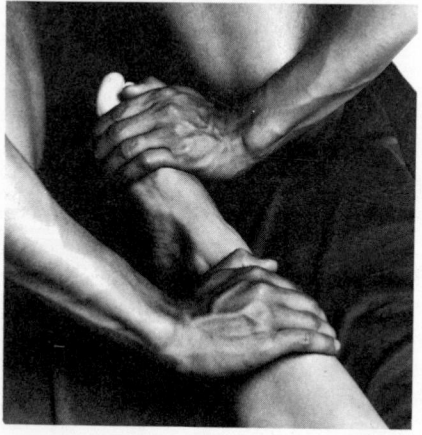

feels as though many hands were stroking each foot. It's a wonderfully pampered feeling, exactly the sort of thing people want in life but seldom find.

Feet support the body, supply leverage, and cushion shocks. The arch is directly involved in all three of these vital services. Even when you are seated, it supports the weight of the leg from the knee down. Because of the way it shapes the surrounding tissues, the arch allows the foot to balance the rest of the body. If the naturally curved structure of the arch is overloaded, the connecting ligaments between bones will be stressed.

People have found an amazing number of ways to overburden their arches, thus straining the ligaments and muscles of the foot. Your partner may have over-enthusiastically embraced a new exercise program and discovered that arches accustomed to spending the evening facing a television screen may not adapt smoothly to several miles of hard earth track. You may be massaging people who are overweight and whose arches are always overburdened. Or your partner may spend too much time every day standing motionless. This will stretch out the muscles and ligaments of the bottom of the foot without allowing them to relax.

Unfortunately arches and feet cannot be traded in every 30,000 miles like radial-ply tires. Your partner will have to live with the way he treats his feet, and you can make it a lot easier. The next four movements deal with the muscles, ligaments, and bones of the great longitudinal arch.

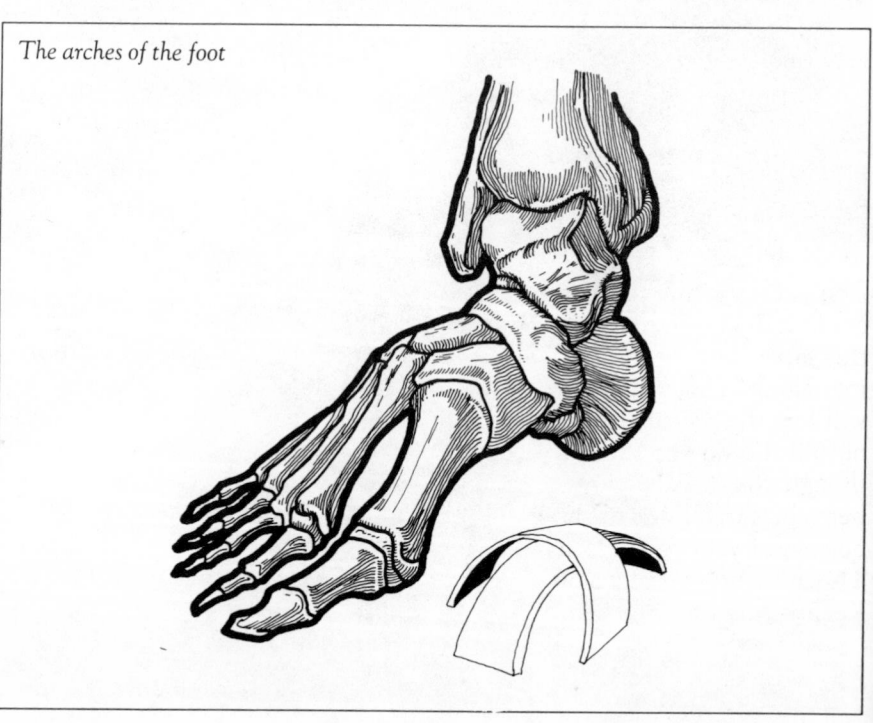

The arches of the foot

Arch Compression—A Stroking Movement

Passive Exercise for the Foot

Hand-over-Hand Circulation for the Achilles Tendon—A Stroking Movement

The bottom of the foot is the toughest part of the body and has the thickest skin. No massage movement uses more pressure than this compression stroke to the arch. When you're learning this movement, pay particular attention to the amount of pressure that feels good. Depending on the size difference between you and your partner, it may be possible to use just about all the force you can muster without causing pain.

Begin pressing with the heel of your hand just under the ball of your partner's foot where the arch starts. Press very hard into the arch, following its contour. Anchor the movement just above the ankle with your other hand.

Every runner comes to recognize the importance of choosing the right shoe. Just a few miles in the wrong shoe will punish the foot and leave a runner feeling exhausted. If your partner is struggling with the wrong shoes, you can use massage to ease the strain. This passive exercise movement will relax overtensed muscles and help keep the foot supple.

Support the leg with one hand, and hold your partner's foot just above the arch (as shown). As the foot is turned, this position will allow you to move two important interior joint structures: the ankle and the joint at the middle of the foot. Turn the foot in a complete circle. The

Lift your partner's foot (as shown), and pull toward yourself with the flat part of each hand. Press up into the tendon as you pull. As you pull down with your hands, be sure the foot is well supported. Some people like this stroke to move very fast. As long as you don't overoil the foot, there's really no danger in experimenting with high speeds here. But no matter how fast you go, remember to pull, not slap, at the tendon.

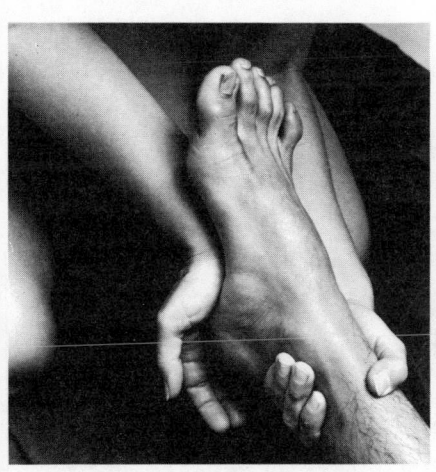

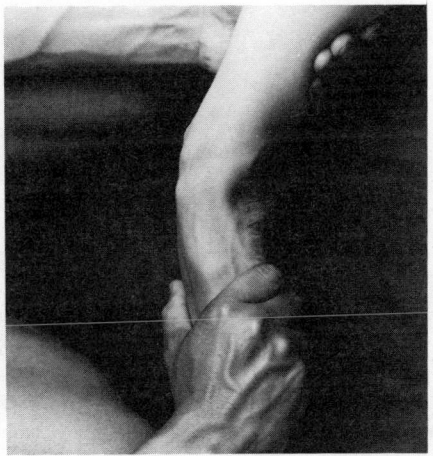

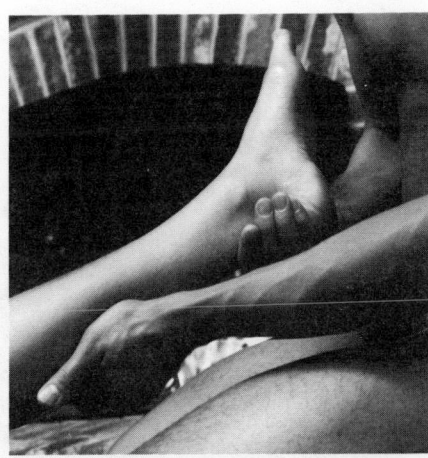

The anchor hand will help you confine the powerful effects of this movement to the foot you're massaging. That way your partner will feel the pressure at the arch, not all the way up the leg. Even though you're using extra pressure here, be careful not to shove the bottom of your partner's foot. This is a stroking movement. Keep it smooth and even.

circle should be as wide as is comfortable for your partner. In the up-and-down position of the circle you will be working primarily on the ankle, while in the side-to-side part you can flex the center joint (as shown). Circle three times in each direction.

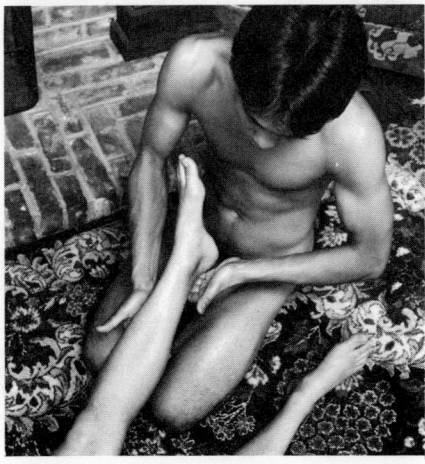

None of the body's natural handles is more convenient than the heel and the top of the foot. By pulling there, you can articulate all the joints below your partner's waist. Lift the foot at the heel, and grasp it around the top. Pull back simultaneously on both places, using pressures that are equal. Be sure to hold the top of the foot far enough down toward the ankle so you don't bend it when you pull. Once you've had some feedback on the pressures involved in this movement, you can easily judge the amount to use for different body types. In the meantime, moderate pressures are safe. Hold your maximum pressure for a silent count of ten, and release gradually.

Arch compression is the first movement on the bottom of the foot and the last on the front of the body. It always gives your partner a powerful incentive to turn over and continue the massage. At this moment turning over is the easiest thing in the world for your partner to do. As always in massage, conversation gestures, and clocks are entirely unnecessary. One or two words will do. Touch both your partner's legs, and keep contact as the legs turn.

Some people will lie down with their hands under the chin, thus flexing the shoulder blades and making back massage very difficult. Lift one arm above and below the elbow, and *suggest* (you never give orders in massage) that it might feel more comfortable with the arms lowered to the sides. Move the arms as you make this suggestion.

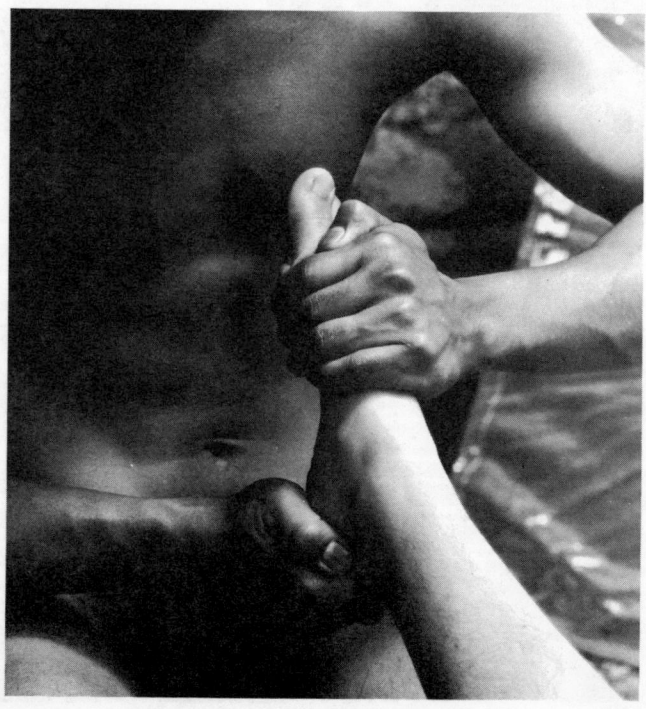
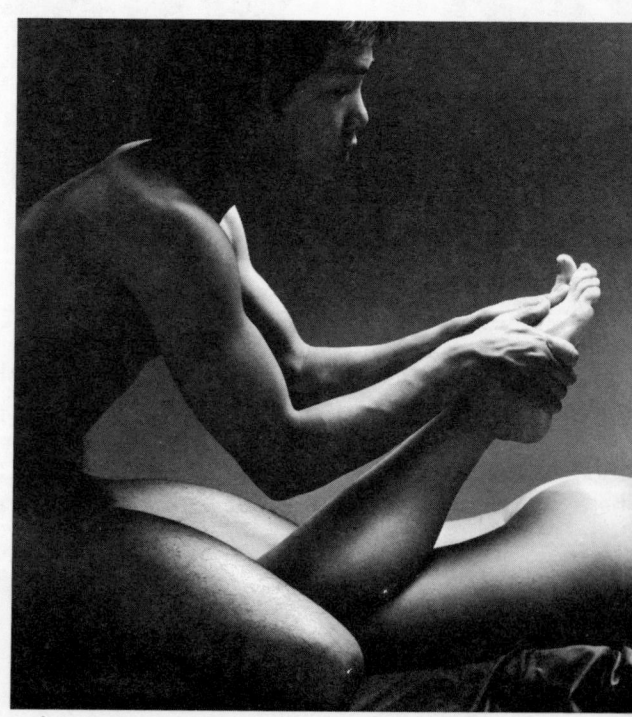

This is the familiar fingertip kneading sequence that you have used over the body (see "The Arms," page 59). Here is your chance to bear down and see what you can do with it. Remember to use the whole surface of your thumb from the tip to the ball. Both thumbs remain in full contact with each other as they circle up and down on the arch and the bottom of the foot.

Here again, you can use more pressure than any other friction movement as long as you anchor the foot correctly. Hold the foot across the top, opposite the arch, and concentrate the pressure of your anchor hand on the sides of the foot to avoid restricting circulation. Press into the bottom of the foot with the four fingers of your friction hand. Keep your fingers together while you shake the internal tissues. You will feel the tendons and ligaments of the foot ripple against your fingers.

Knuckle kneading, like all the arch movements, uses lots of pressure. For that reason it's always a good idea to anchor the foot and leg firmly before you begin. You can support the leg lightly against your own thigh and hold the foot with your free hand. This way you can press down directly either onto your hand or onto your thigh. Circle with the flat part of your knuckles around the arch and up onto the heel of the foot. You may want to combine this circling with a straightforward up-and-back movement across the entire bottom of the foot. Whatever you decide, concentrate most of your effort and pressure on the arch.

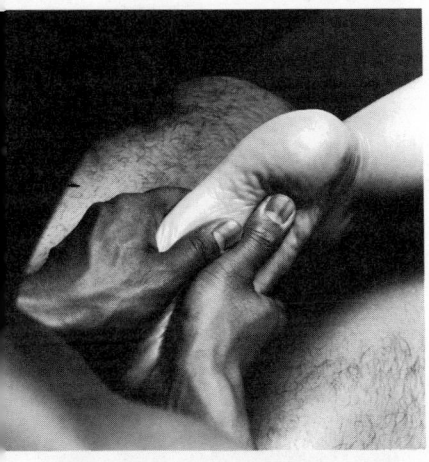

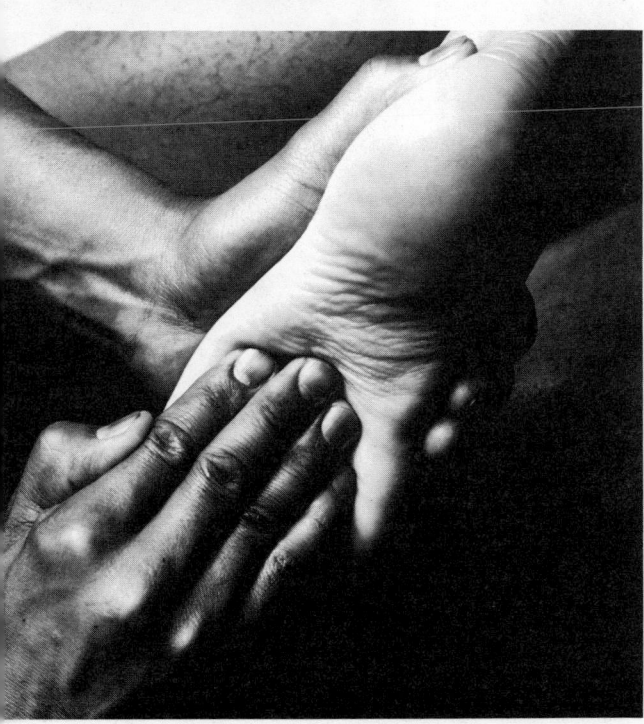

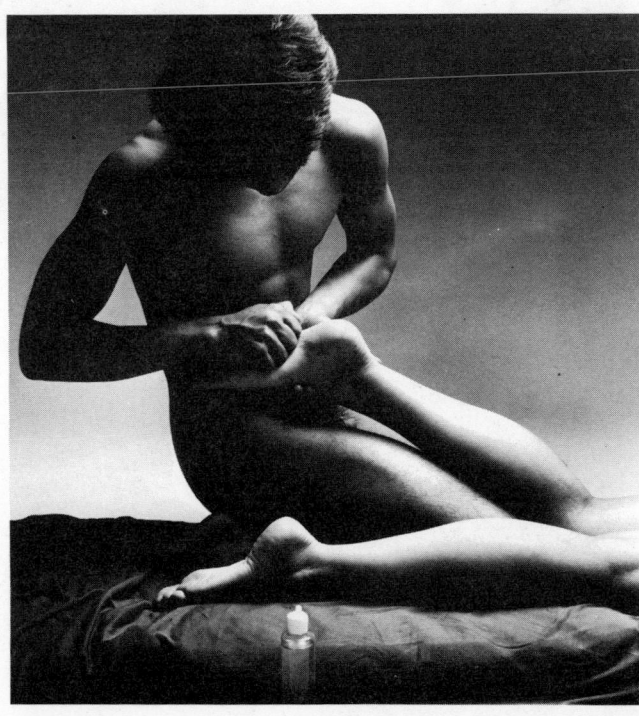

Since the foot must support the entire weight of the body, its interior construction is very strong. The twenty-six bones of the foot are bound together by a complicated network of powerful ligaments. One of the most pleasant aspects of foot massage is the way these ligaments are gently stretched when you rotate the bones of the foot.

Grasp each side of the bottom of the foot with the balls of your thumbs (as shown), and press up

The muscles of the leg connect to the heel of the foot via the Achilles tendon. This tendon, the largest in the body, can easily be felt as it runs down the back of the lower leg and wraps around the heel. No other tendon is more important to runners and other athletes because without it there is no way to lift the heels of the feet when they walk. Since the Achilles tendon is used so vigorously in all sports, athletes are forever having problems with

it. If you tear it, you're going to be out of action for quite a while. Lesser problems, like strains and bruises, can be effectively minimized by regular massage to this area. The idea is to keep the tendon relaxed and supple rather than allow tension to accumulate here. The following three movements deal with the Achilles tendon from its insertion point at the heel up onto the lower leg, where it merges with large muscles.

Kneading: Grasp the foot with four fingers just below the ankle (as shown), and knead the tendon with both thumbs from the heel up to the center of the calf. Work slowly in small circles, and be sure not to skip any part.

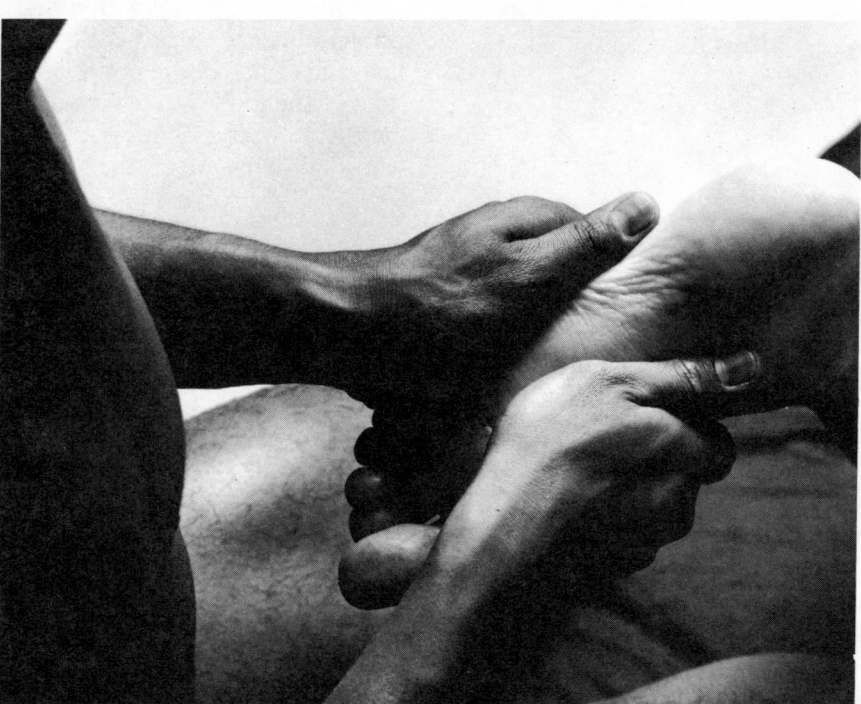

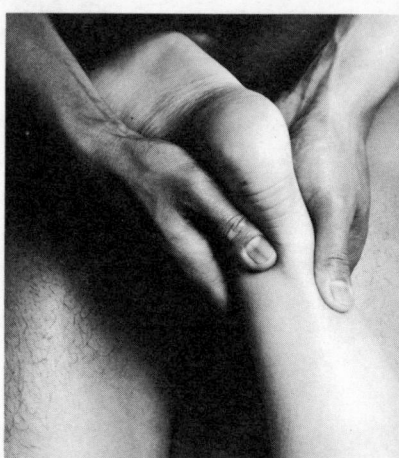

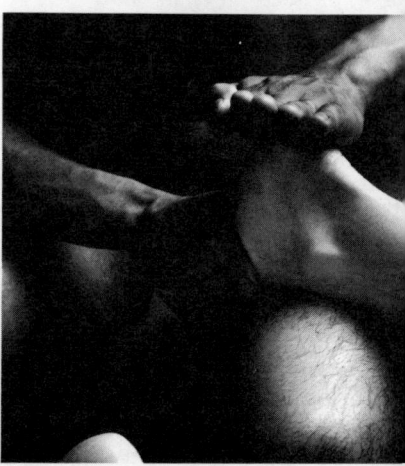

against the top of the foot with four fingers held tightly together. Your grasping position should be firm because the hands do not move across the foot during this movement. Rotate your hands in small opposing circles. As the ligaments stretch inside the foot, you will feel the long, fingerlike metatarsal bones changing position.

Circling: Circle the heel slowly with the flat part of your palm. Hold your fingers together and straight out throughout this movement. Anchor the foot by supporting it on your thigh and pressing down on the arch with your free hand. This extra support will allow you to use plenty of pressure when you circle on the heel. The bone at the heel is the largest one in the foot; the Achilles tendon sweeps right around it and inserts (connects to) the far side. Cover the whole bone with the soft inner part of your palm.

Friction: The friction movement anchors the same way as circling except that you can advance your anchor hand so that it presses

From the middle of the foot to the toes, the foot will bend back and forth and from side to side. Support the heel and ankle with one hand, and grasp the whole top of the foot over the toes. As long as you hold your anchor hand steady, you can move the top of the foot independently of the bottom. You can also bend the toes back and forth (as shown).

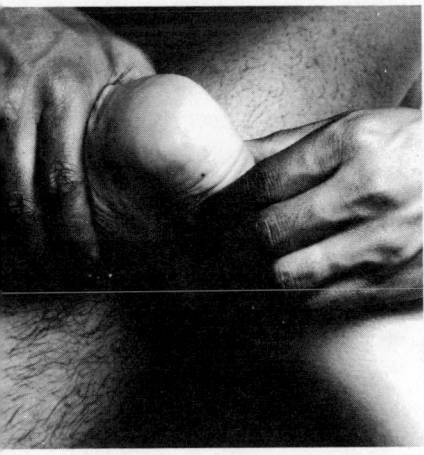

against the heel. Because the tendon is thick and not part of an intricate network, you can actually grasp it between the thumb and four fingers of your hand. Friction movements here should alternate between tiny circles and a straight up-and-down action. Work from the heel to the center of the calf; be sure to open your fingers to follow the shape of the tendon as it thickens and merges with the muscles of the leg.

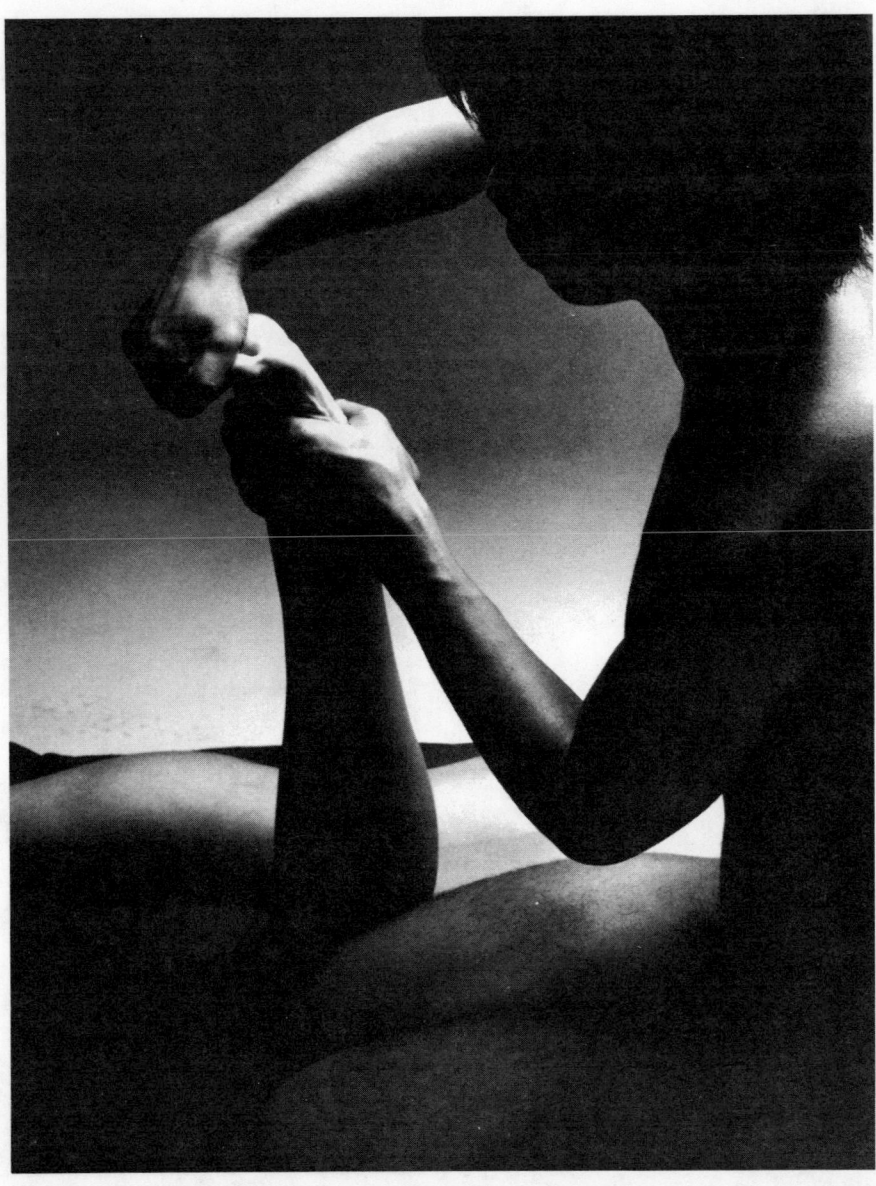

Passive Exercise for the Back of the Foot

Brushing the Feet and Toes

The passive exercise movement you used on the front of the feet works equally well here on the back. It's certainly worth repeating, especially if your partner has been having foot trouble during an athletic workout. Support part of the leg with your thigh, and anchor the movement, once again, just above the ankle. Turn from the ball of the foot (as shown).

In the course of a full body massage, the back of the feet get brushed more often than any other part of the body. Since nobody ever complains about this extra brushing, it is certainly one of the best ways to make transitions from one part of the body to another. Begin at the middle of the calf, and be sure to contour your brushing to the shape of the foot and heel. Break contact slowly at the toes, and immediately begin massaging the back of the legs.

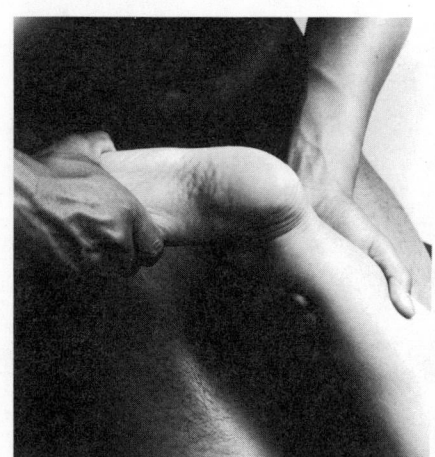

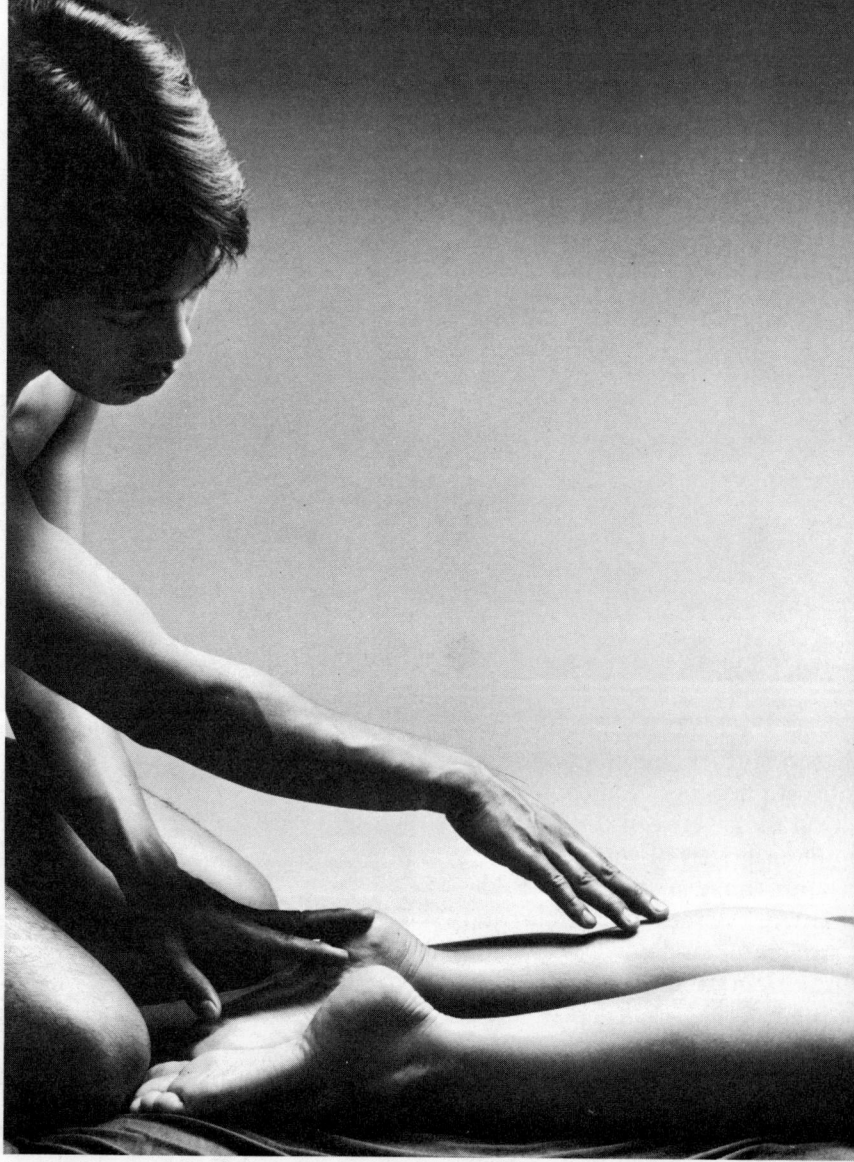

The
Back of the Legs

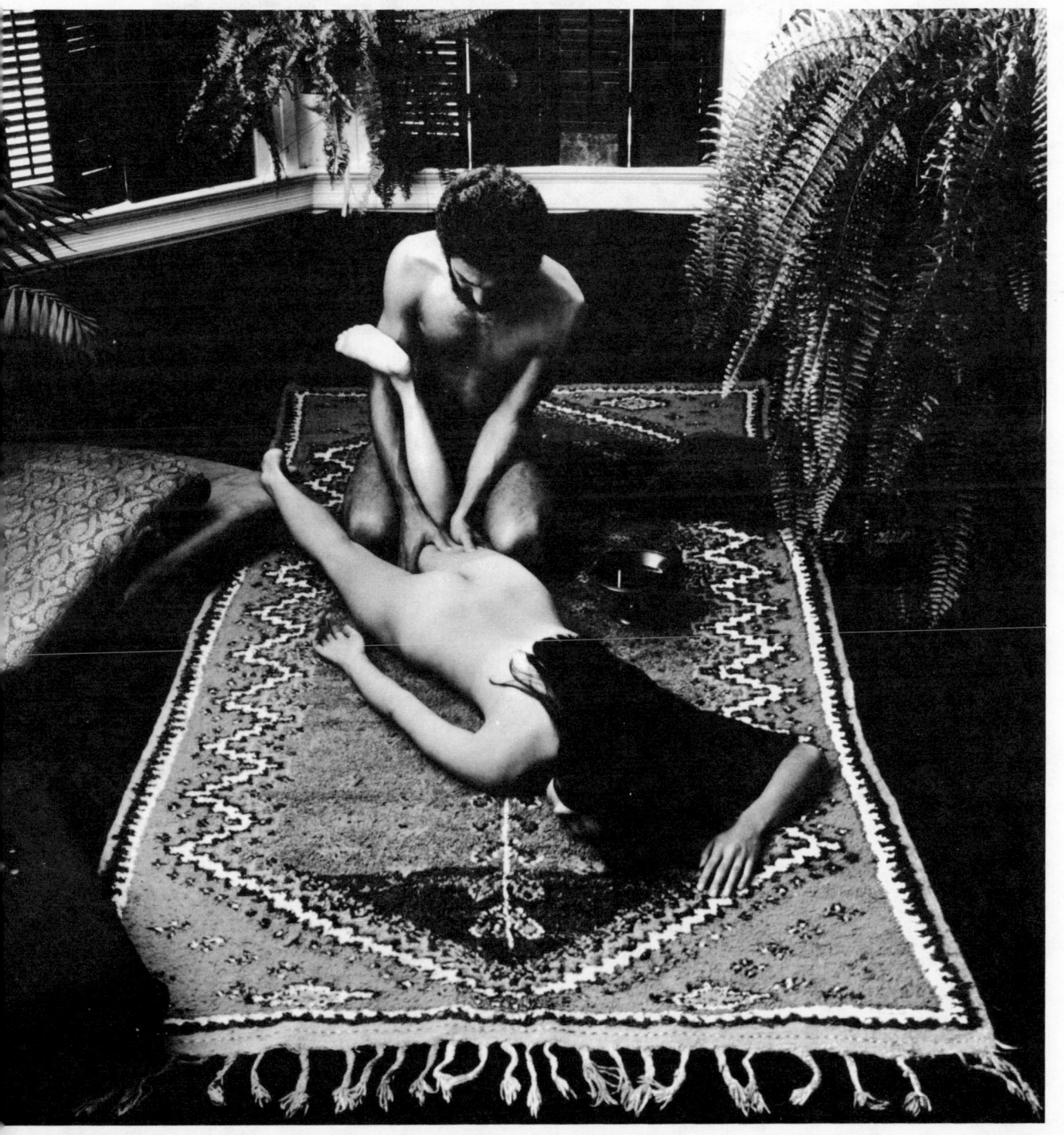

The Back of the Legs

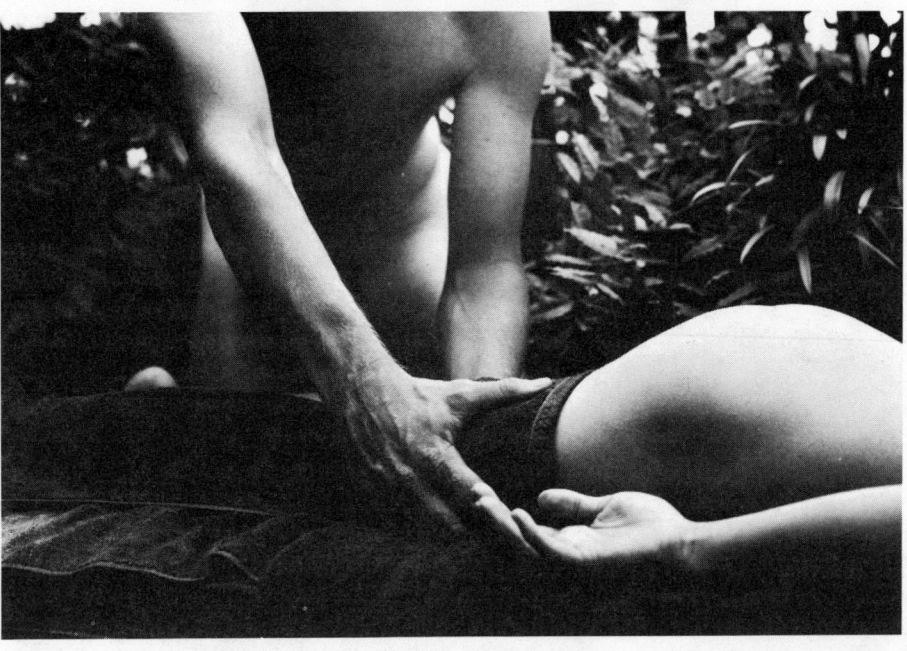

The sciatic nerve, one of the body's most important referred pain indicators, can be massaged on the back of the thigh. Pain here almost always indicates some sort of problem in the lower back and will serve as an important guide for you to plan your approach to the back itself.

Like headaches, lower back pain motivates millions of people to reach automatically for aspirin and other mildly addictive nonprescription drugs that knock out the whole nervous system. Massage proposes another route. Whenever possible in referred pain situations, begin by relaxing nerves around the site of the pain, and work back slowly to the source of the problem. Of course, there's no way to reach the center of the diaphragm after massaging its referred pain center at the top of the chest. But on the back of the leg you have an excellent opportunity to reach the sciatic nerve, its tributaries up and

down the leg, and finally the lower back itself. There are three simple ways to isolate and detect sciatic nerve problems, and two of them work from the *front* of the leg. Pulling the leg and flexing the foot (see page 108) will almost always indicate sensitivity in the sciatic nerve area. The gluteus muscles that run across the buttocks and down onto the back of the legs have their insertion point on the front of the leg (see diagram, page 35). If, when you press around this insertion point, your partner feels shooting pains down the leg to the foot, you can be sure the sciatic nerve is irritated. The third point to check is toward the center of the thigh on the back of the leg. Right there the sciatic trunk is very close to the surface. Moderate pressure will usually tell you whether the nerve is going to require extra attention during your massage work on the back of the leg.

The nervous system

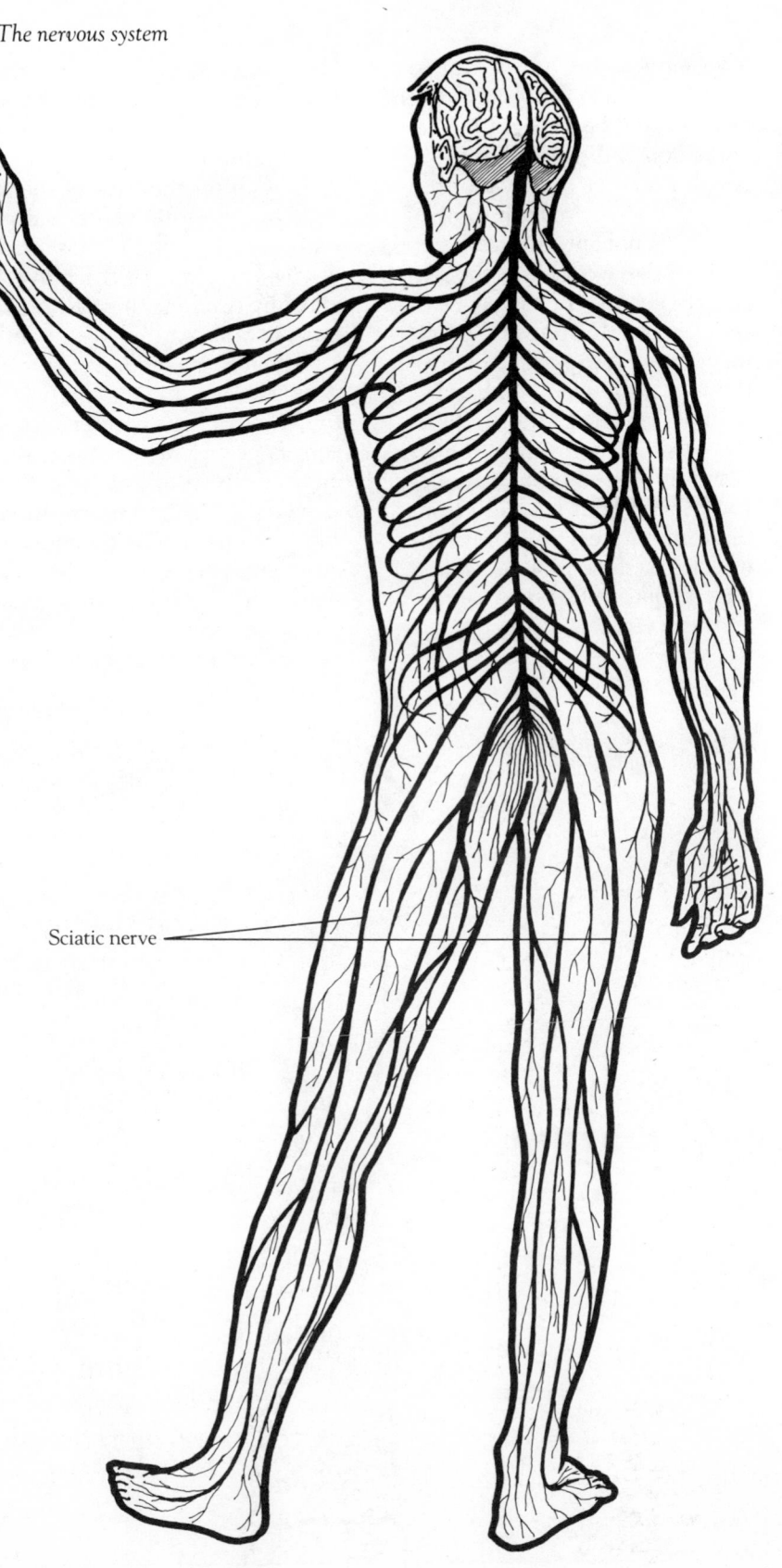

Sciatic nerve

If you have any indication that the sciatic nerve is irritated, you can begin relieving your partner by relaxing the entire back of the leg. Begin at the end of the nerve's tributaries near the foot, and work on every other part of the leg before you touch the tender spot over the nerve again. Very often you will find that by the time you reach this point again the pain has diminished quite a bit or vanished altogether. Still, it's best to heed this warning and pay special attention to the lower back, probably the source of these nerve problems on the back of the legs.

There are really three upper limits to this movement, and it's sometimes fun to try them all during a single massage. Each one begins like the pressing movement that follows, and should be repeated ten time. The first upper limit, the easiest one to reach, is at the top of the leg just below the buttocks. Your hands turn here and return to the ankle exactly the same way they did on the front of the legs. If you feel you can comfortably reach a bit farther, let your hands continue over the buttocks and make your turn at your partner's waist. Unless you're much bigger than your partner, the third position will involve moving up the side of your partner's body as you stroke. Begin at the back of the ankle. When you are near the top of the leg, move up to follow your hands without breaking contact with your partner. Follow your hands up the side of your partner's body so that you can actually extend this movement up onto the back. When you reach your partner's waist, instead of turning at the top of the leg, simply change your hand position so that you can continue up the back to the shoulders and finally return to the leg as in Two Super Relaxation Movements for the Back (page 140). That way, by moving up the body as you stroke, you can actually cover the whole body from heel to shoulders in one long, uninterrupted motion. Stroke down the back until you reach the waist. At that point your hands continue down the legs to the heel in the leg circulation position.

Your movements on the calf to press blood and lymph toward the heart should begin right at the ankle and end just below the lymph nodes at the back of the knee. Venous circulation, of course, is not interrupted here; once you've worked on the lymph centers behind the knee, it's easy to return to this pressing movement and extend it all the way to the top of the leg. The hand position is identical to the one you used on the front of the leg. Working on the back of the leg, you can tilt your hands so that the thumbs press down into the muscles of the calf while your fingers squeeze the sides of your partner's leg.

Here, once again, is the familiar thumb kneading movement you used, for the first time, on the upper arm. There's more flesh to work with on the back of the leg, and your pressures can be substantially greater without causing discomfort. Anchor the movement by reaching around to the front of your partner's leg with four fingers as you move up and down the leg. Depending on the thickness of your partner's leg, your fingertips may not actually meet. Even so, moderate contact as you glide up and down the leg will serve to anchor the movement and keep your thumbs steady. It's important to consider the position of the thumbs on the back of your partner's leg. The

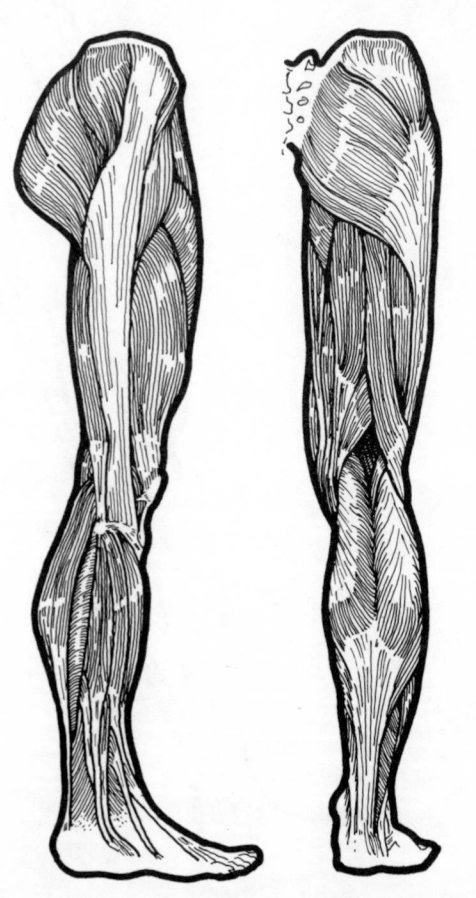

Large muscles that operate the foot begin at the knee.

chor fingers should always be
ld loosely enough so the
umbs can contact each other
ong their entire length.
Begin at the ankle, and work
ll the way up to the top of your
artner's leg. Even on thin legs
s unlikely that you will be able
reach all the way around your
artner's thigh. Reach far enough
anchor the thumbs comforta-
y, and knead up and down the
igh until you have thoroughly
overed the circles; when one is
p, the other should be down.
se the whole surface of the
umb, and avoid digging in with
e tips. Since this movement
ill not contact any bones on the
ack of the leg, pressures can be
rm and even over the entire limb.

Thumb kneading is an important part of any Fluid Release
sequence and is particularly valuable in reaching parts of the leg
that cannot be effectively
kneaded with your full hand.

The intricate web of muscles,
tendons, and ligaments on the
back of the knee will completely
relax when you flex the knee and
support the lower leg with your
arm. Relaxing that area also

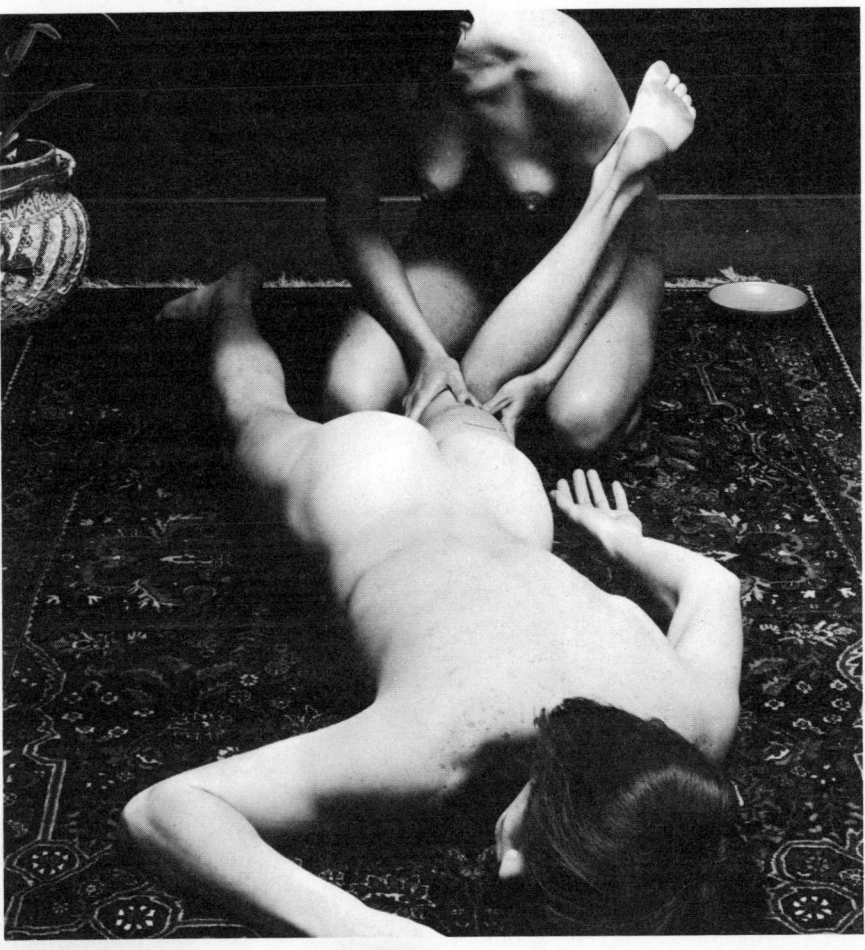

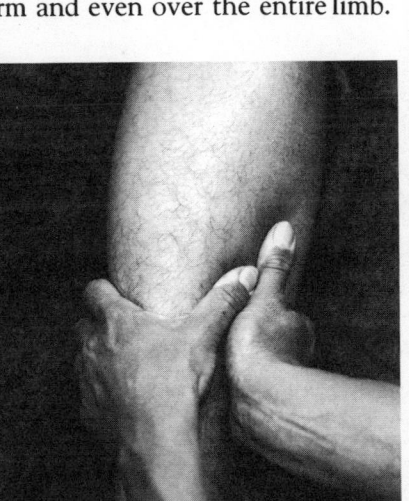

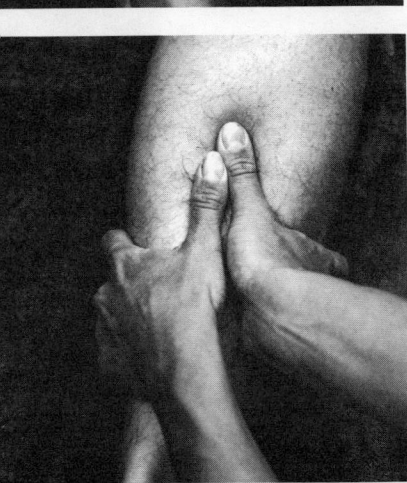

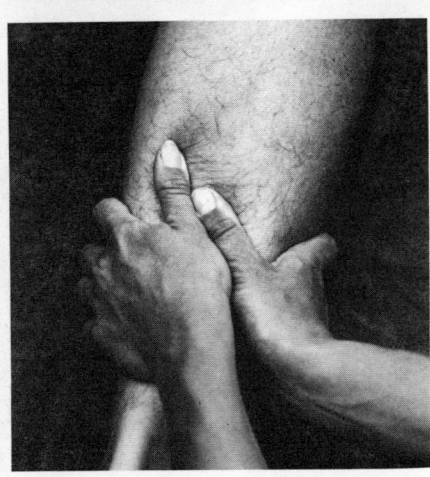

allows you to reach the lymph nodes around the knee which drain the lower leg and foot. Use your partner's foot to anchor the lower leg against your arm (as shown). Steady your hand by loosely grasping your partner's leg just below the knee with four fingers while you knead with your thumbs. Although your thumbs meet the back of the knee at an angle, it's best to avoid pressing down on the tips. Use the broad flat portions of your thumbs, and rotate as in other thumb kneading movements. Depending on the thickness of your partner's legs, it may not be possible to bring your thumbs all the way together. Knead up from the center of the knee to the muscles of the lower thigh.

Occasionally when you're doing a full body massage, you reach a point where you want to rest for a while. Rather than break contact and abandon your partner altogether, you can use this simple compression movement to focus your energy almost anywhere on the body while you lean forward gently onto your hands (see page 190). Working on small areas of

the body, be sure to maximize your contact. The top of the leg is the widest area on any limb. Two large parallel muscles dominate this part of the body. You can massage them both at once by stroking down the thigh. If you use your thumb (as shown) it's easy to press between these muscles about halfway down the thigh. Thumb pressure here will reach the sciatic nerve and begin to relax it. Soothe this nerve and you release tension not only in the lower back but also down the leg all the way to the foot. Stroking down the thigh from the hip, cup the side of your partner's leg with one hand while you press between the muscles of the thigh with the other. Short, smooth strokes moving slowly down the

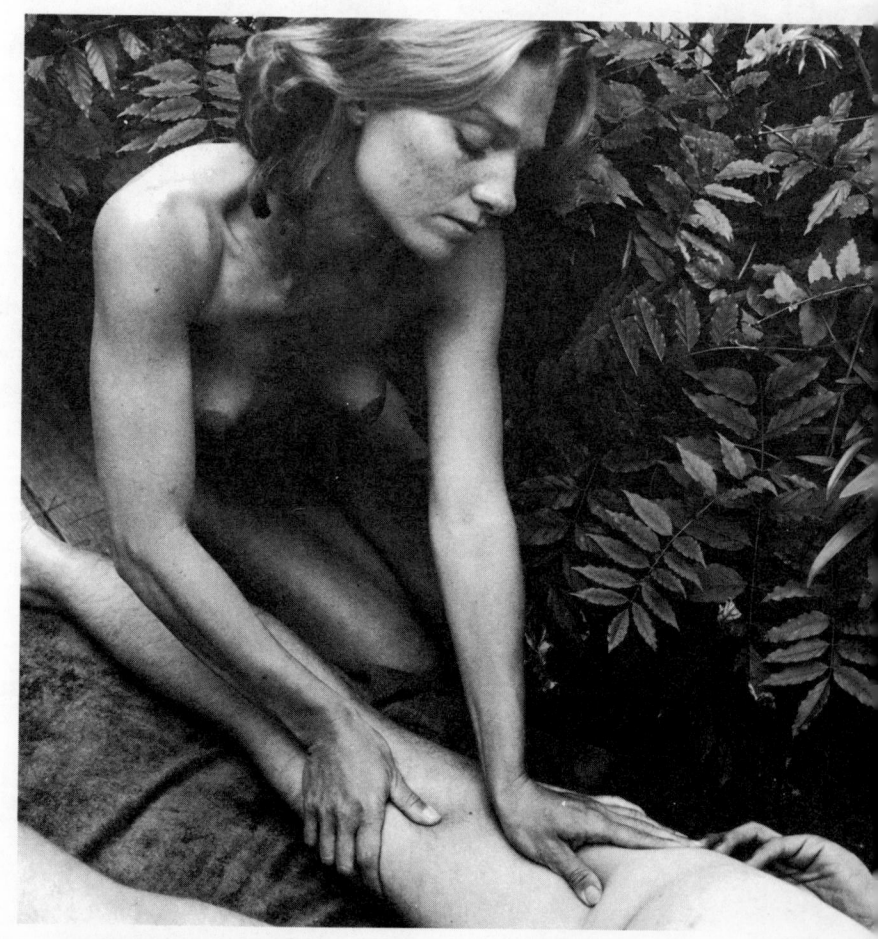

high work best here. Your hands break contact one at a time to return to your partner's hip and stroke down to the knee.

Percussion can have either a stimulating or a sedative effect on a nerve. Mild superficial percussion movements will excite and awaken the nerves. If your partner complains of feeling sluggish and has been depending on large amounts of caffeine to get through the day, this is the sort of percussion that's called for as part of a general massage. But if the problem is pain, soreness, or irritation, you may want to use more pressure to relax the nerves. There's a kind of generally nervous temperament that keeps the nerves in a state of constant irritation. We all recognize "the overwrought, highly strung, nervous type, which is so commonly seen in the cities of the United States. Here life not only demands the most in human efficiency, but constantly keeps the nervous tensions high, whether it be in professional, commercial or social life. Even in athletics this tension is marked." •

Those words, written by an English masseuse, just after World War I, seem appropriately modern. Since she wrote, frantic attempts to solve this problem have produced the tranquilizer, an ominous little pill that forces people to relax (for a while) by inducing chemical changes in the brain. How much easier and safer to sedate the nerves with percussion movements that will not leave your partner depressed and anxiety-ridden a few hours later.

Nerve percussion is really a variation of slapping. By bending the ends of the fingers (as shown), you can direct the force of this movement so that specific nerves can be reached. It's not necessary to dig in with your fingertips. Your contact point should be around the fleshy balls of your fingertips. Like the other percussion movements, nerve percussion will flow more smoothly if you relax your hands and let them bend at the wrists. Work up and down the center of the leg three times.

• *Practical Massage and Corrective Exercises*, Nissen, op. cit.

133

Working from the top of the leg where muscle groups overlap around to the side (as shown), you can stimulate ligaments and tendons around the massive ball joint at the hip. The joint itself is off the center line of the leg bones toward the center of your partner's body. Working with friction movements, you can feel a depression at the side of the hip. There's plenty of room here for you to press inward and bring friction right up to the tissues around the joint. On this side of the leg, friction movements to the hip joint should move in a slow arc from the top center of the leg to the depression on the side of the hip and back again.

You can use the entire leg as a lever to exercise your partner's hip joint passively. This will work quite well as long as you remember to hold your partner's leg *above* the knee when you lift by grasping the lower part of the thigh. Be sure that no part of your hand presses against the delicate joint at the knee. Use your other hand to press down firmly (as shown) over the small part of the back. This will prevent your partner from rolling when you lift the leg and will maximize the movement you're creating at the hip joint. This movement is really limited by the flexibility of muscles on the front of the thigh. Working just to the point of tension, you can use it to stretch these muscles while you exercise the ball joint at the hip.

The inside: Since you don't have to avoid the femoral artery here, kneading pressures can be much greater than on the front of the leg. Don't be afraid to dig in with the full surface of both hands. Work up and down the leg three times—more if reducing is part of your partner's massage program. The thick hamstring muscles, used in walking, running, and dancing, almost always need toning during weight loss. Press down into them with your fingertips as you knead and be sure to use your thumbs. Knead all the way from the top of the leg to the foot, working in slow rhythmic circles. Pay special attention to the well defined muscles on the back of the knee. Stop there occasionally as you move up and down the leg and knead them with your fingertips. Runners and dancers will thank you for the extra care.

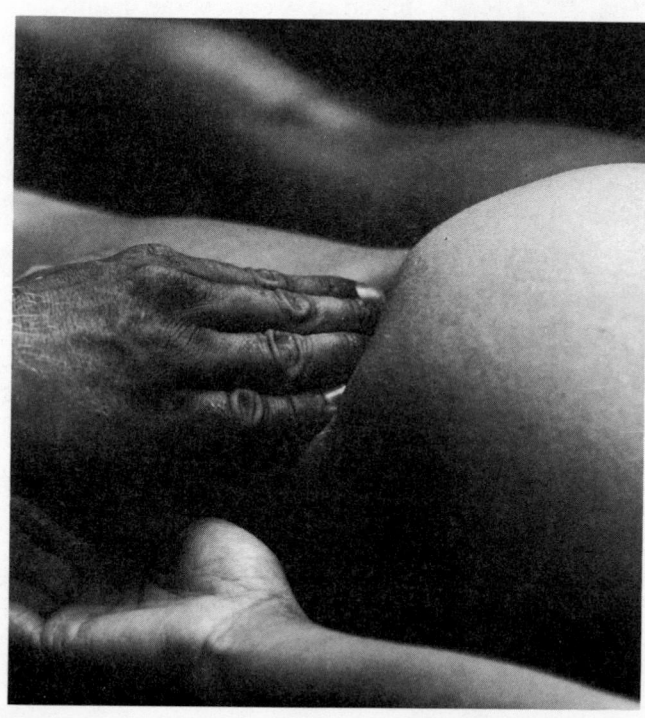

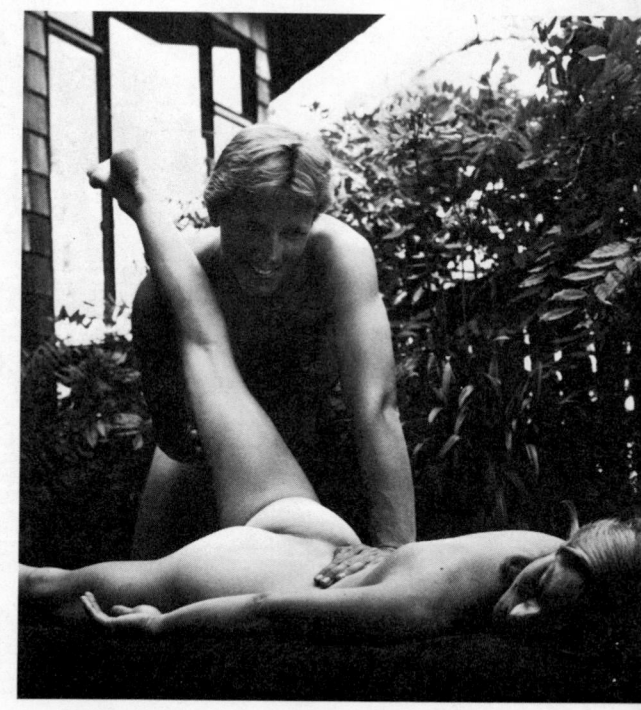

The outside: It's most comfortable to knead the outside of the leg the same way you kneaded the sides of the torso, from the opposite side of your partner's body (as shown). This movement

and it's a good idea to increase your pressure when you knead them. Again, pay special attention to the back of the knee.

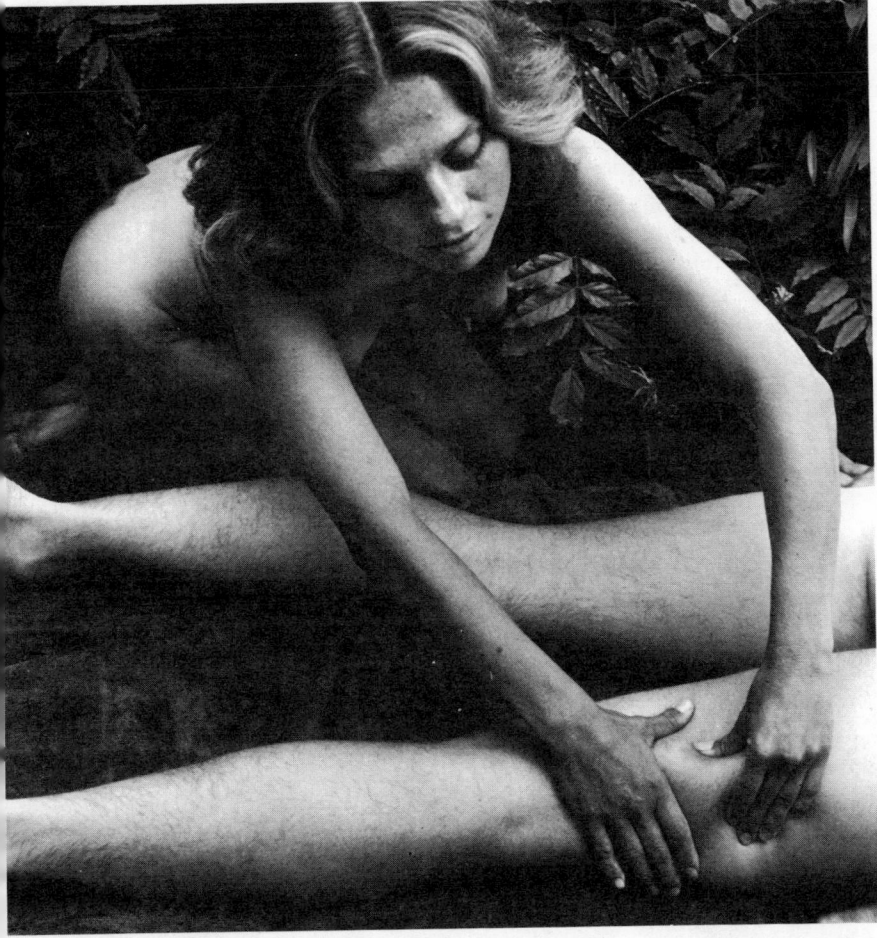

will also provide an excellent transition when you're ready to move from one leg to another. You can do this by kneading up and down the inside of one leg, across the buttocks, and down the outside of the other leg. Stay in contact with the outside of the opposite thigh as you step across your partner's body to begin work on the leg. Tissues on the outside of the thigh are relatively firm

If your partner is in good shape and has been exercising regularly, you may find that the muscles on the back of the thigh seem hard even when they are relaxed. This is not necessarily a sign of tension but rather an indication that the body is not storing a great deal of surplus fat. Muscles that feel tight *under* a layer of fat are usually a sign that your partner is tense. As you work with massage, the difference between tense muscles and toned muscles becomes more readily apparent. You will usually find toned muscles on a fat-free, well-exercised body. They may feel tight, but only by comparison to muscles which are positively flabby.

If you can't find flesh to pick up with your thumb when you're kneading with the whole hand, it's time to try knuckle kneading. This movement allows you to exert much more pressure on the deep tissues of your partner's leg than fingertip or full-hand kneading. Press down evenly with the flat part of your knuckles (as shown). Rotate the hands in alternating circles the same way you would in any other kneading movement. Because the pressures are deep, you may want to add a bit more oil during this move-

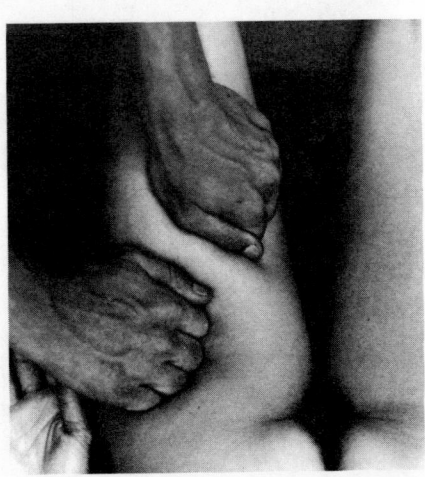

ment, particularly if your partner has hairy legs. Circle over the whole top of the thigh and onto the knee. Your right hand will always be down when your left hand is up.

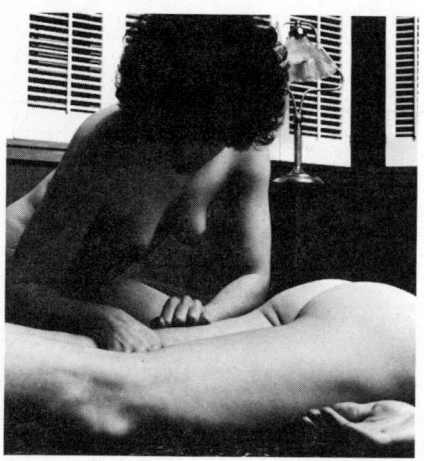

Because they offer such a fine opportunity for kneading, the buttocks are always a great favorite with masseurs. If you're using massage along with exercise to help your partner lose weight, it's important to remember that many exercise programs unwittingly exclude these large muscles. The muscles of the buttocks will contract only against strong resistance like climbing stairs. Running and walking on level ground will not effectively tone them. Overweight runners who stubbornly refuse to recognize this fact begin to assume alarming pearlike shapes after a few weeks of running.

Knead the buttocks the same way you kneaded the sides of the legs: in long vertical motions. Depending on your partner's size, these kneading strokes may also include parts of the upper leg and lower back. Move slowly all the way across your partner's body over the buttocks. Work in parallel lines up and down the body, but when you reach the bony center, be careful not to press down on the spine. Buttock kneading allows you to pick up more flesh than any other kneading movement. Your partner will feel the difference when you cross over the entire center of the body, kneading deeply.

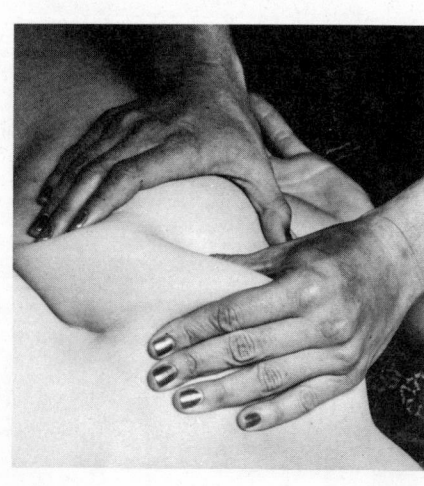

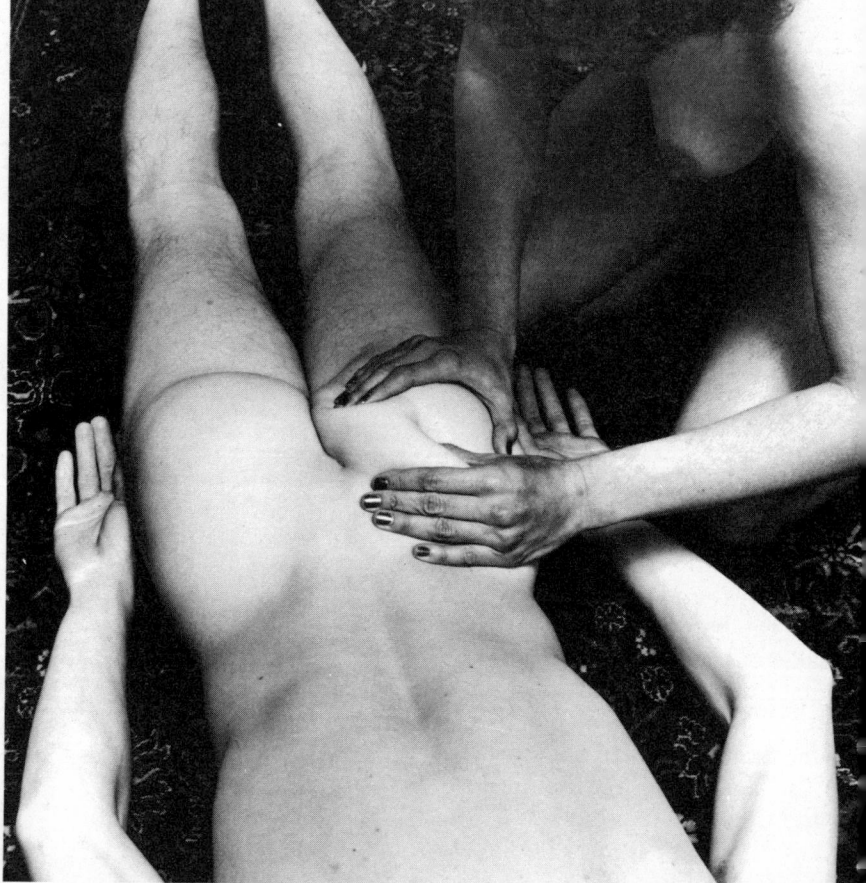

The Back

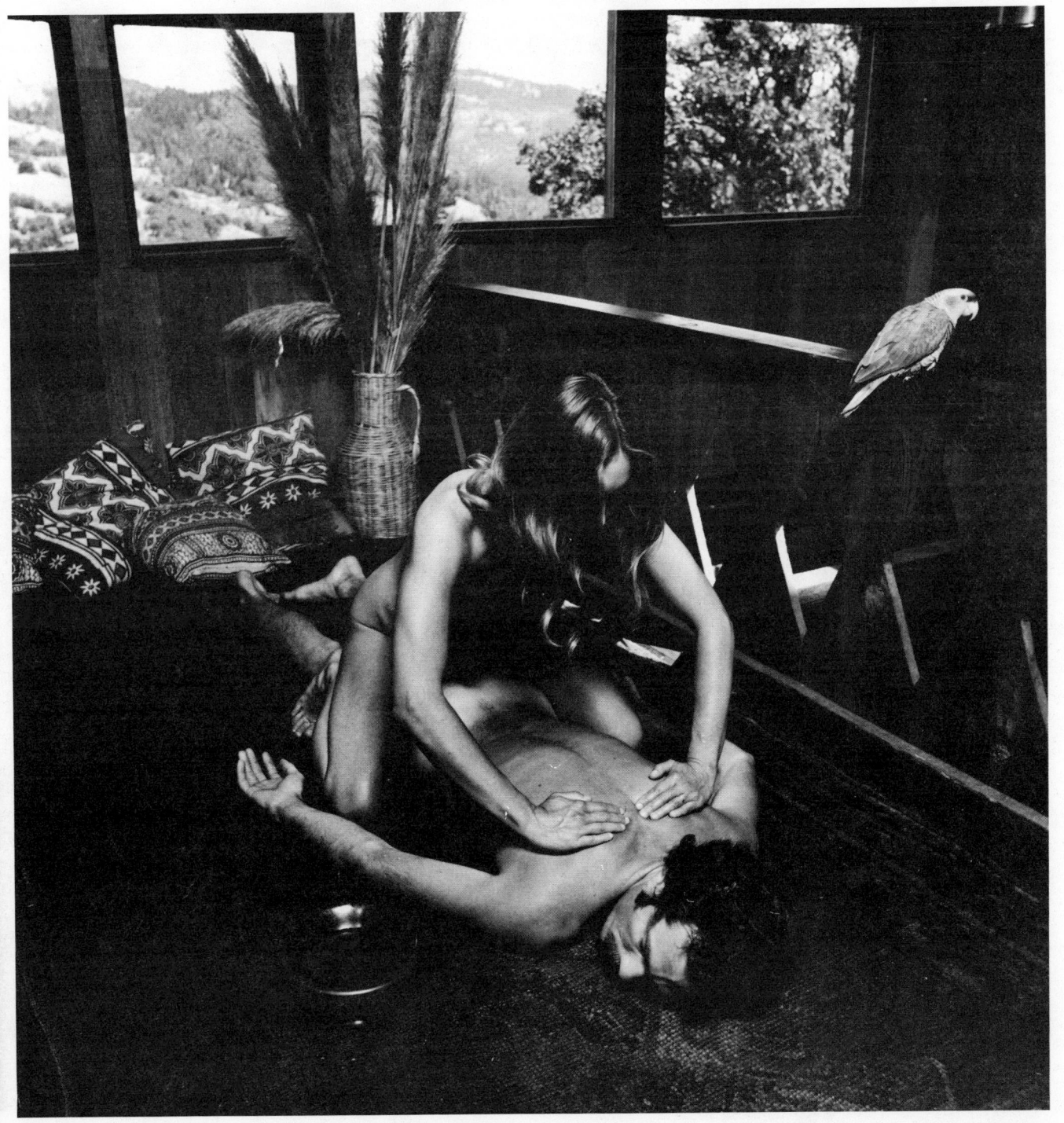

The Back

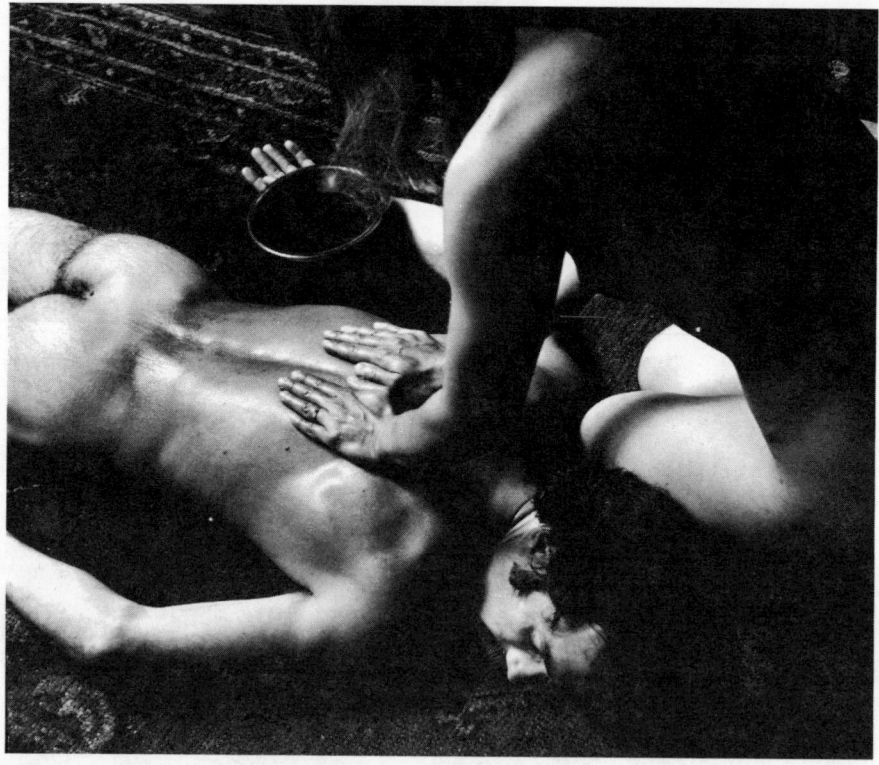

As a general (but by no means universal) rule, masseurs find that men and women experience tension in different parts of the body. Women are bothered by stiffness across the top of the back and at the base of the neck. Men complain of tension that develops into sharp pain around the lower back. People who suffer from aches and pains at either end of the back usually spend a lot of time worrying about it. Worrying tends to worsen the situation and create a vicious cycle since nervous anxiety may be causing the problem in the first place. This does not mean that the excruciating pain which strikes the lower back when something heavy is lifted improperly is imaginary. Rather, many sprains and muscle tears can be avoided if the back is massaged regularly. Internal tension, even in well-developed muscles, reduces the range of response that is available to a relaxed muscle. By relaxing a muscle during massage, you restore its range of response and help protect your partner from similar accidents in the future.

Back problems, like circulatory diseases, are far more common now than they were 100 years ago. The sedentary middle-aged executive who suddenly breaks into a dead run while carrying three suitcases at the airport may also try lifting a refrigerator from a full standing position. People who live like this will soon find themselves far beyond the powers of any masseur. Almost any exercise program teaches one the limitations of the body. Intense back pain, particularly lower back pain, is definitely a signal that the body has been pushed beyond these limitations.

The Spine and the Nervous System

There are several signals which should be heeded before your partner actually tears the ligaments of the lower back or damages a disk. Some people complain of constant stiffness even after exercise. Others will take for granted persistent lower-back pain as a "normal" sign of aging. They may worry secretly about the pain while reminding themselves that back problems are unimportant. There is, however, no part of the body which is more crucial to an overall sense of well-being than the lower back. Since the spine itself is ultimately affected by muscle and nerve problems, it's always best to take lower-back complaints seriously. Deal with them promptly before they become nasty.

Almost nothing happens anywhere in the body without somehow involving the nervous system. Since the nervous system determines exactly how people will feel, relaxing it is the single most important concern in any full body massage. An hour of massage can have a spectacular effect on nervous people who have been dependent on the neighborhood drugstore for rest and relaxation. Dr. Douglas Graham, normally a conservative writer, described the effects of massage on his patient's nerves this way in his *Massage: Manual Treatment; Remedial Movements:*

Upon the nervous system, as a whole, massage most generally exerts a peculiarly delightful and at the same time profoundly sedative and tonic effect. While it is being done, and often for hours afterwards, the subjects are in a blissful state of repose; they feel as if they were enjoying a long rest . . . and quite frequently it makes optimists of them for the time being. An aptitude for rest or work usually follows, though generally those who submit to this treatment feel gloriously indifferent, and needless apprehensions are dispelled.

On the back, the body's main nerves are close to the surface and easily reached. By relaxing them, you can lower stress levels throughout the body and materially improve the health of every internal organ.

The nervous system is organized into a pattern that looks like an upside-down tree. Thirty-one pairs of spinal nerves branch out neatly across the back from the shoulders all the way down to the waist. These nerves supply all the internal organs and can be regarded as direct pathways to the interior of the body. At both ends of the back, other, longer branches spread out onto the limbs. Vertical nerves close to the spinal column control blood circulation, glands, and the crucial vasoconstriction response (see page 176). All these nerves form a massive communications network that connects directly to the 12 billion cells of the brain.

The spine is held erect and in place by two long groups of muscles that run parallel to it on both sides. If your partner is under a lot of pressure or just simply tense all the time, one of these muscle groups may become very tight. Not only is this tightness easily felt by a masseur,

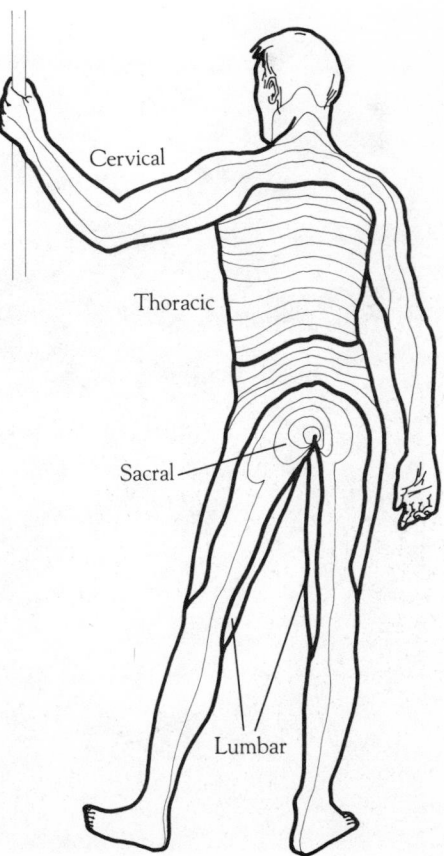

How spinal nerves service the body

but it is often actually visible. What you see are the muscles on one side of the spine pulling the spine and pinching nerves that supply the lower back and legs. The pain your partner feels may extend from the lower back right down the sciatic nerve onto one of the legs.

Although this sort of thing can be very painful, it's not necessarily that serious. If the doctor has decided that there's nothing wrong internally, you may find that back massage will bring your partner exactly the kind of immediate relief he craves.

If you want a simple way to introduce a friend to the joys of massage, try the following two movements twenty-five times each from both ends of the back. Between the two points you will reach every major muscle, nerve, and bone in the area. This 100-stroke sequence will leave your partner more relaxed than most two-week vacations.

The easiest, most balanced way of doing this stroke is by straddling your partner (as shown) and leaning forward with your whole body. Unless your partner is much smaller than you, it's OK to press down very hard as you move up the back. These are strong muscles; you won't overwhelm them. One thing you do want to avoid on the back, though, is direct pressure to the spine. With the exception of a few well-cushioned, very controlled movements, back massage works around the spine, not on it. Before you begin, make sure

you've oiled the whole back, including the shoulders and sides.

Press straight down on the base of your partner's back with the whole surface of both hands. You should just barely feel the edge of the spine between your fingers. Your hands follow the contour of your partner's body as it drops away from the spine. You will feel a smooth, even flesh contact from the base of your palms to the fingertips. The whole stroke moves up the back, maintaining this contact. Work all the way to the top of the back and out over the shoulders as you turn your hands. Pull down the sides of your partner's body, maintaining that full-hand contact. Pressures on the sides need not be as great as the ones you used going up the back. Pull all the way to the waist, and turn your hands so

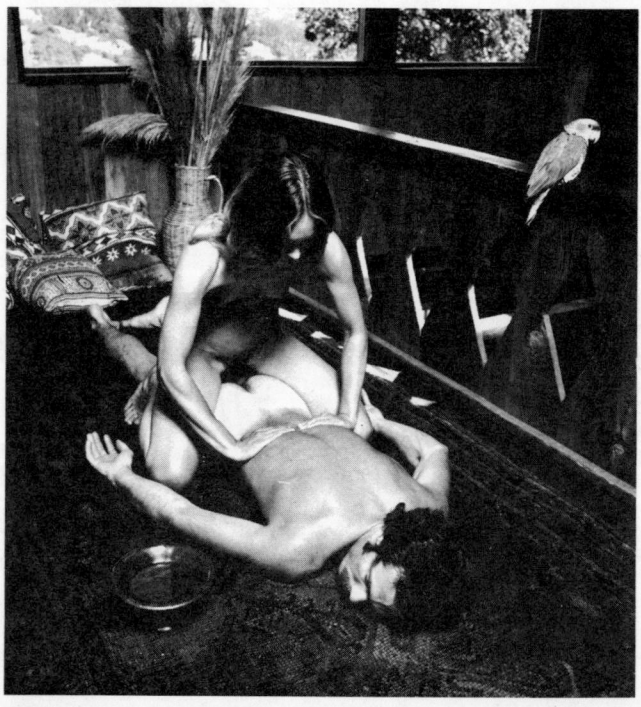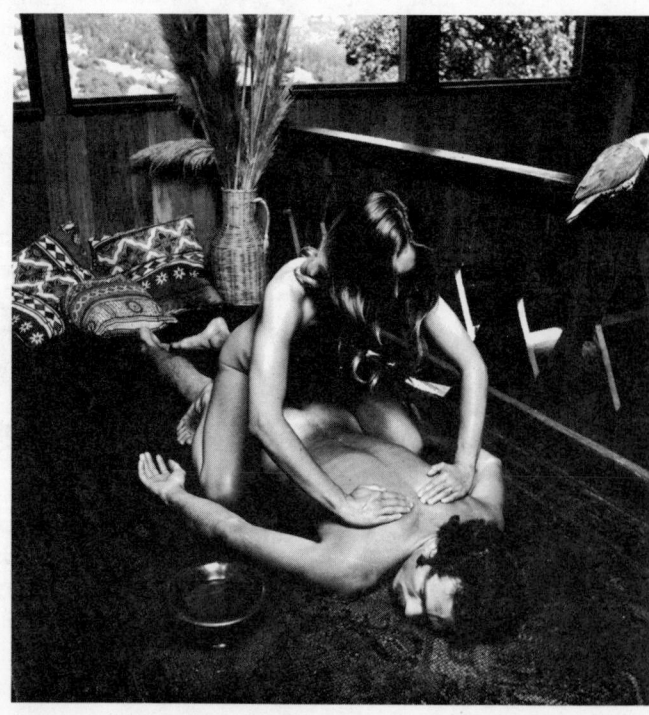

they can glide into the original position. Turns at the shoulders and waist should flow without any hesitation in the overall movement.

This flowing sensation is even more important in the next movement, in which greater pressures are brought to bear on the muscles along the spine. Working from the head with both these movements, you may want to kneel next to the head with your knees touching your partner's shoulder. This time your thumbs should brush the spine as your hands travel down the back. Keep your fingers tightly closed, and press down hard on the base of your hands. While you perform this movement from either end of the back, the pressure on the base of the palm should remain steady. Lean forward onto your hands.

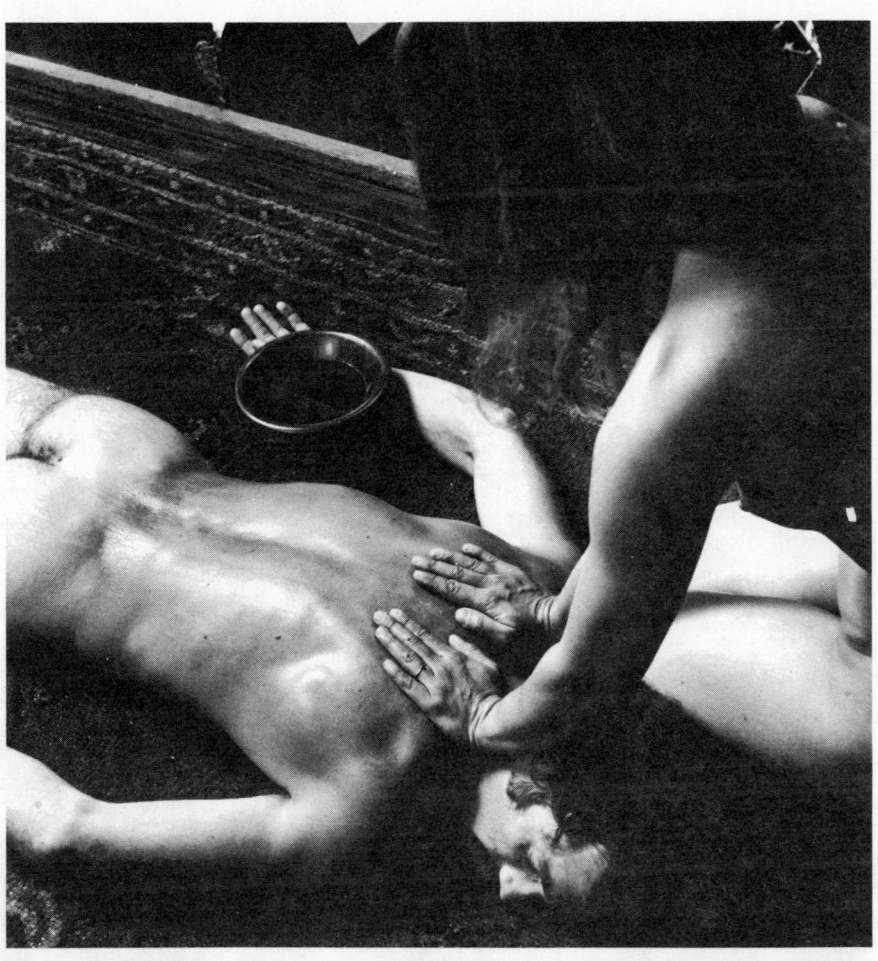

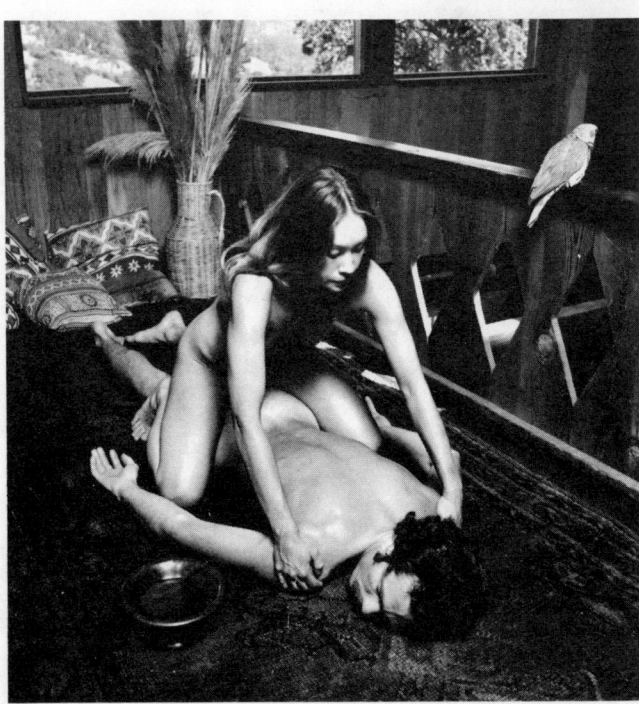

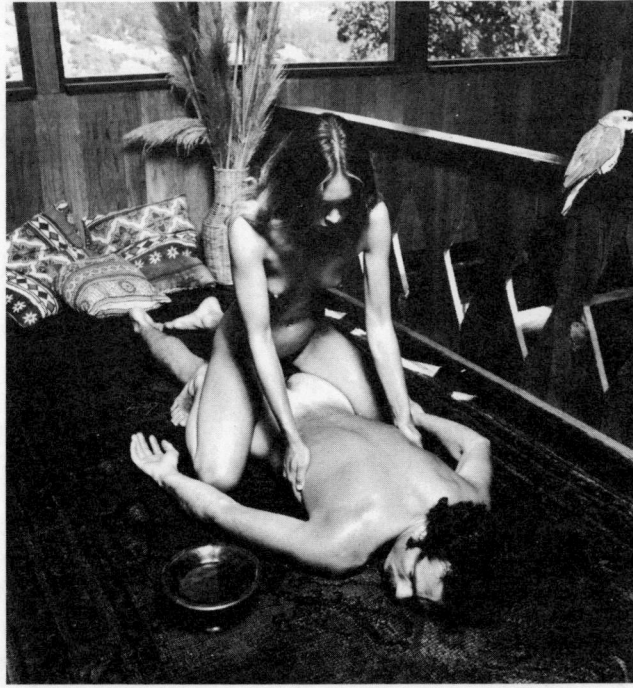

If you're working down from the shoulders (as shown), reach as far as you comfortably can before you turn and pull up the sides of the body. As you move from the side to your partner's shoulders, your arms will be turned fully ninety degrees from the starting position. Simply rotate them in place without breaking the rhythm. This is a powerful movement, and people love it. You can actually feel the back relaxing under your hands.

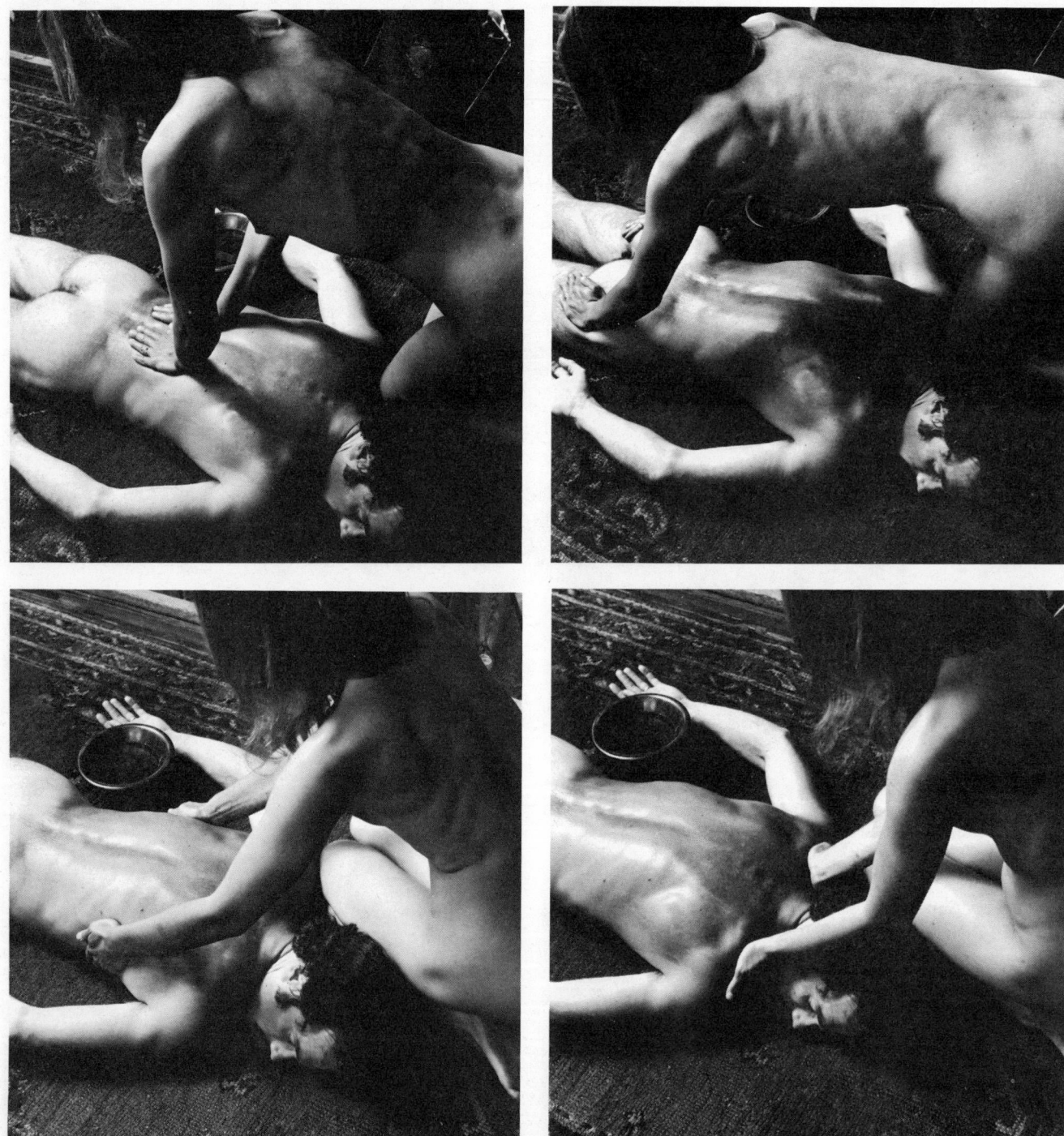

Crossing the Back—A Stroking Movement

If you finish massaging the long muscles along the spine down at the bottom of the back, there are a few more movements you might want to consider while you are still in the straddling position. One of them is the opulent back-crossing stroke that concentrates pressures on the upper back and shoulders.

Cup your partner's shoulders on both sides of the neck, and pull back slowly to the center of the back. At that point turn both hands sideways so the fingers point toward opposite sides of the back. Press down evenly, keeping full-hand contact all the way until your fingertips touch the massage surface. That's where you reverse everything you've just done until your hands reach the shoulders again.

Despite the unusual turn at the center of the back, this movement should flow just as evenly as the full back strokes. Each time you cross your hands move them up the back just a bit until, finally, you're actually crossing right at the top of the back. If your partner is female, be sure to focus on the broad muscles that stretch horizontally across the top of the back. Women feel a lot of tension here, and this part of the movement is especially important to them. It's likely to encourage more of the luxurious sighing you heard earlier during the back massage. That's good reason to continue what you're doing, and follow up with kneading movements to the top of the back muscle groups and to the back of the neck.

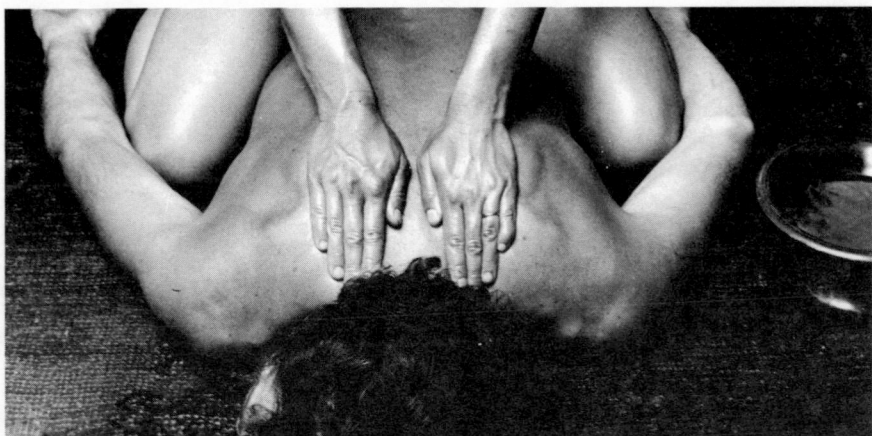

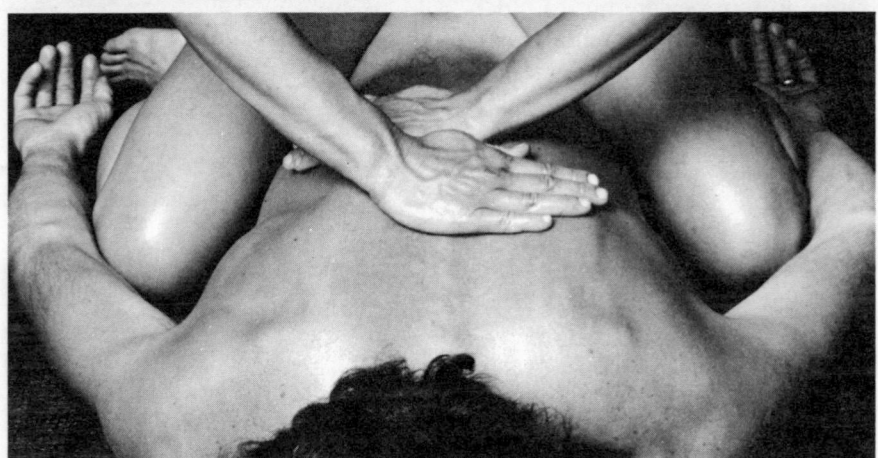

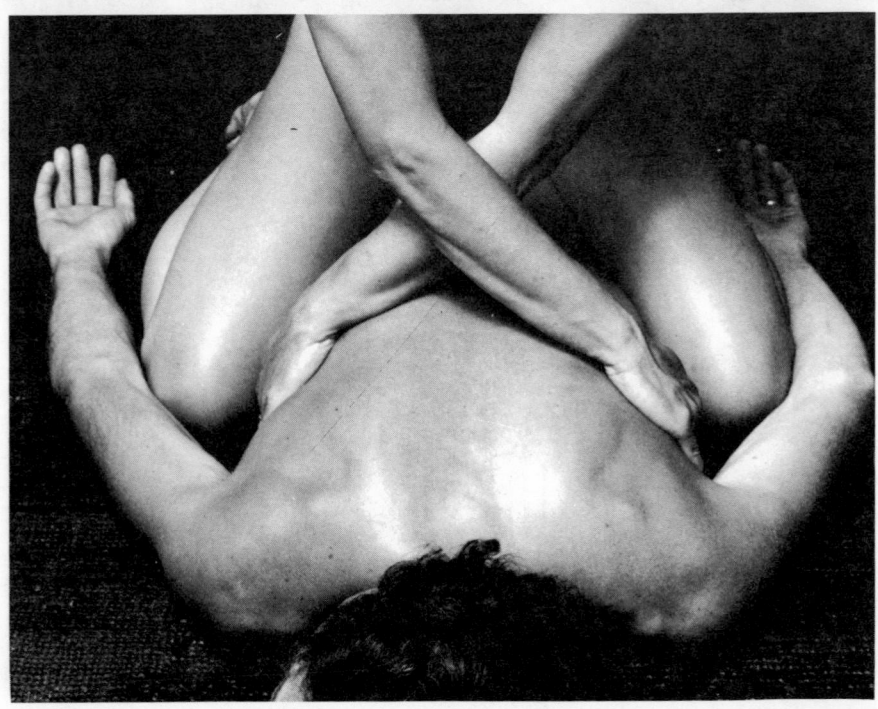

143

When people feel fatigue across the top of the back, they often reach up and rub the angle between the head and the shoulders. This, of course, is the very spot where the upper-back muscles rise to support the head. It's also a natural place for friction because it's narrow, entirely muscular, and easy to reach.

Anchor the movement at the center of your partner's back with your free hand. Grasp the shoulder firmly before you begin friction, but be sure not to pinch the flesh. Shake the muscles back and forth and in small circles.

The shoulder, like the other joints in the body, is not usually affected by most massage movements. If the joint feels really tight, you may want to fold your partner's arm back (as shown).

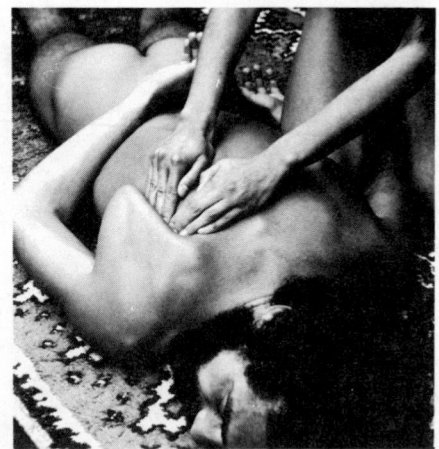
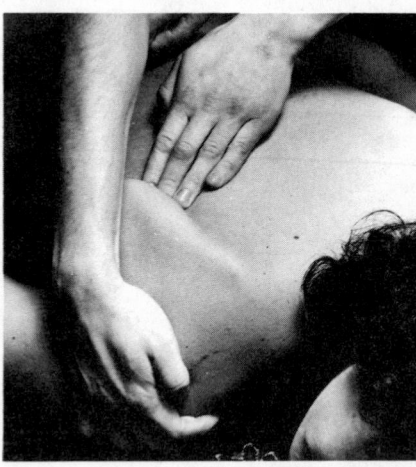

Friction rates and the amount of pressure you use have a great deal to do with the effect of this movement on your partner. Light friction over a nerve center will stimulate your partner, but if you increase your rate and pressure, friction has a sedative effect.

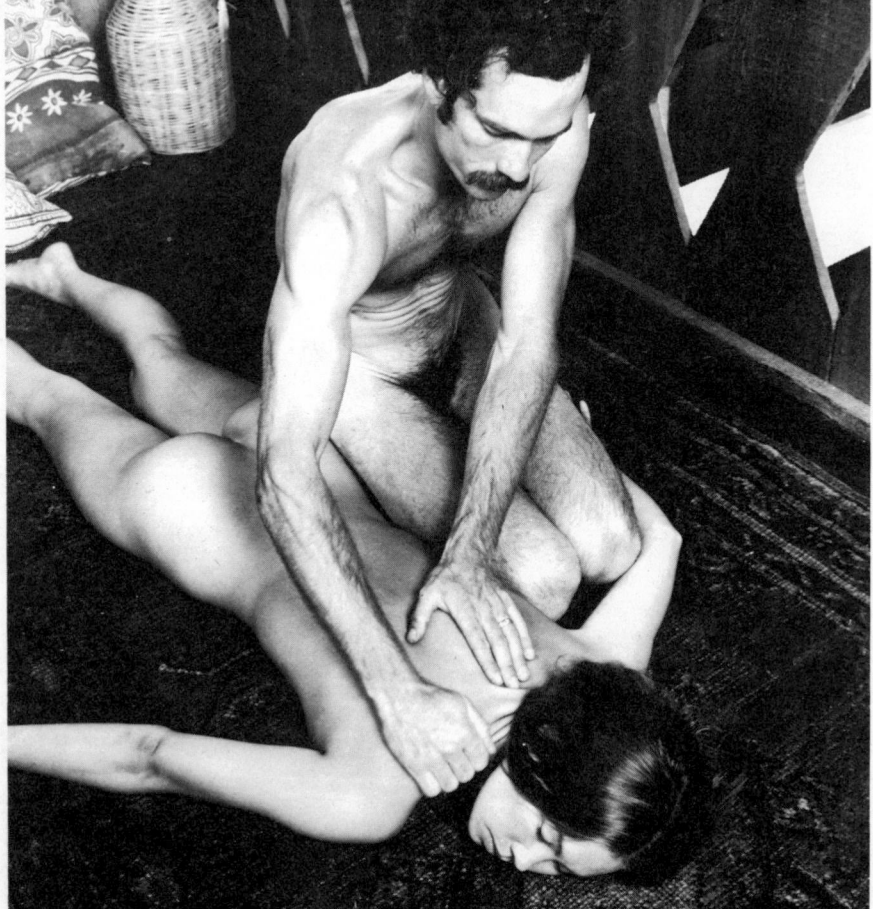

Back walking is one of those movements in which little people finally have a great advantage over big people. There's no other way to exert this much steady pressure on your partner's body, and there's no part of the body that cries out for it more than the back. As a general rule, anyone who's going to walk on your back should weigh at least 50 pounds less than you. He will also need a decent sense of balance and clean feet.

If you're going to try back walking, be absolutely sure the bottoms of your feet are spotless. You'll be following this movement with a general back massage, and every speck of grit will show up on your partner's back. Hold out your arms for balance, and step onto the long muscles that run parallel to the spine just below the shoulder blades. If your partner is capable of speech, he may be able to direct you to different parts of the back. Otherwise, move slowly up and down the spine on the long muscles, being careful to stay off the spine itself. When you get a bit more confident, try kneading those same muscles by circling lightly with the ball of one foot while you balance with the other. A great deal of movement is not necessary. You have no idea how good it feels just to have you standing there.

People who are dieting always appreciate the extraordinary way this movement can be used to tone the skin. The skin is actually lifted away from the mass of internal tissue and rolled between the fingers. Occasionally you will massage a back that is just too thin or tight to allow for extra folds of skin. If you suspect this is the case, go ahead and test the tissues by gently picking them up between two fingers. Like any massage movement, rolling should never be forced. There are two ways of doing this movement, and it's always fun to alternate between them as you move up and down the spine.

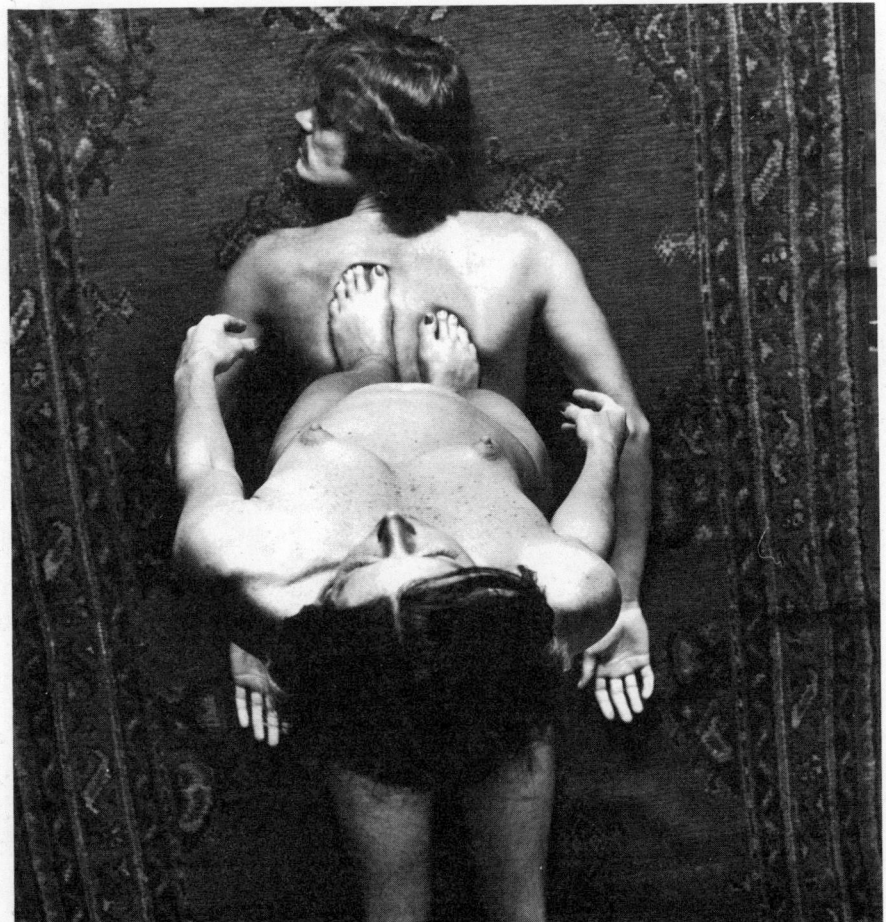

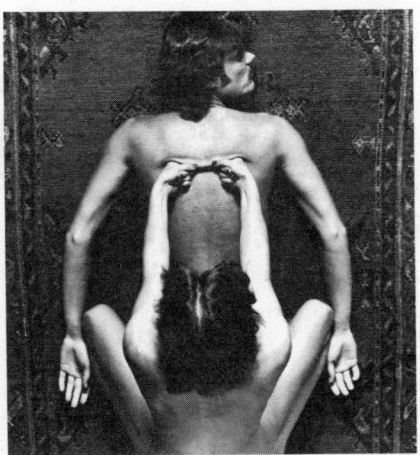

Thumb Rolling: Lay your hands flat on your partner's back with the thumbs on either side of the spine. Press up toward the shoulders with your thumbs until a fold of loose flesh appears. Grasp the fold with four fingers of each hand, and roll the flesh gently between your fingers. You can begin this movement at the bottom of the spine and work up slowly all the way to the top of the back.

Forefinger Rolling: Lay the knuckle side of both fists down on your partner's back, and extend both forefingers until they almost meet at the spine. The fingertips should actually brush the sides of the spine. Press down and forward until a horizontal fold of flesh appears. That's the fold you're going to grasp and roll with your thumbs. Once you have lifted the fold, you can roll it quite easily between your thumbs and forefingers. Move up and down your partner's back, lifting and rolling the flesh every few inches. Some backs will be tight near the waist but much easier to work with near the shoulders.

Some people demand lots of pressure on the back, and why not give it to them? The knuckle press will allow even very small people to concentrate great amounts of pressure on the most enormous back. There is, in fact, no movement, short of the specialized back walking, that focuses so much pressure on one spot. Grasp your contact hand around the wrist with your other hand, and press down hard. Your contact is on the flat surface of the knuckles. Once you establish the desired pressure, you can circle with the contact hand, maintaining pressure at the wrist. Go up and down the long muscles along the spine and across the shoulder muscles three times.

The back is the largest single part of the body that will permit continuous kneading. There is no reason to limit your kneading to the physical edge of the back. Lower-back kneading is a large

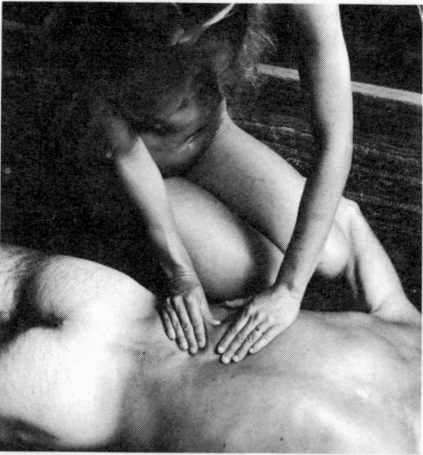

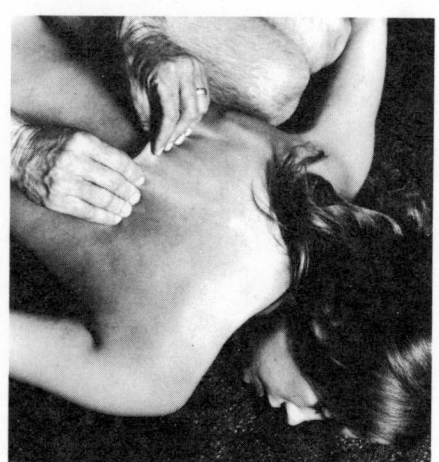

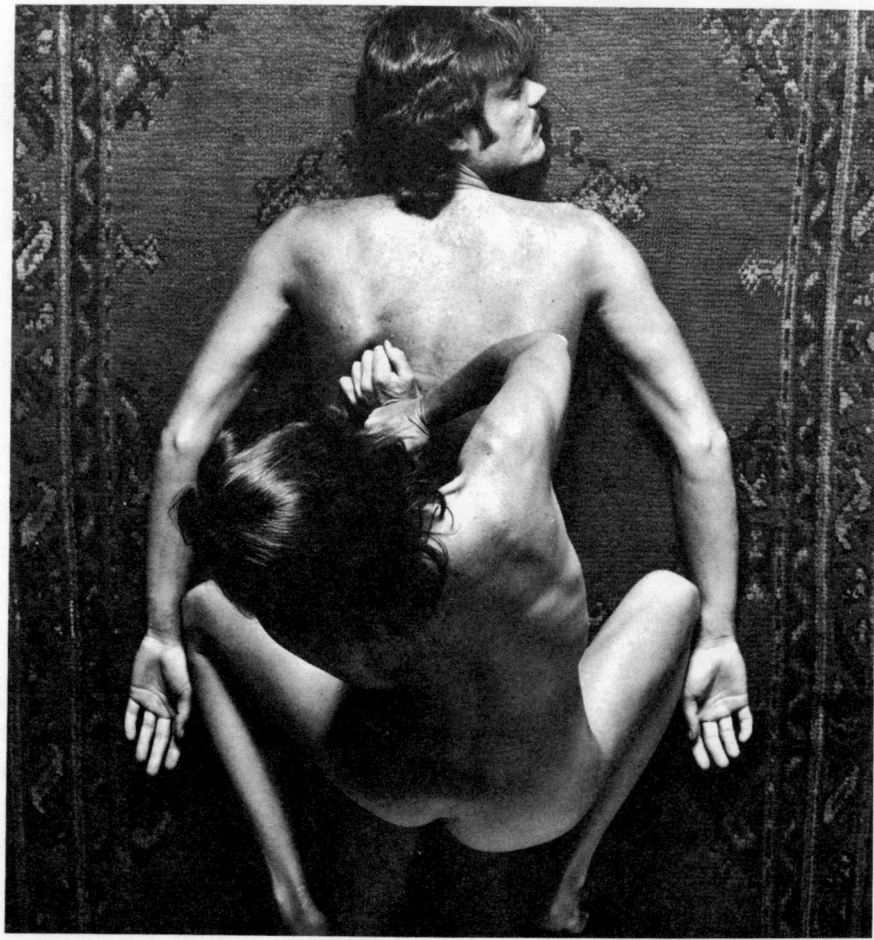

generous movement that can certainly extend across the buttocks and onto the thighs. Sit comfortably alongside your partner, and make body contact at the arm and chest with your knees. That way, if you should accidentally lift your hands while reaching across the body or down the legs, contact will not be broken. Knead up and down the back in overlapping vertical lines. Most of the muscles will accept deep pressures. These pressures will increase nutrition to the muscles and help strengthen them.

Muscles at the top of the back merge with the neck and support the head. Anyone who appreciates head massage will thoroughly enjoy these top-of-the-back kneading strokes. If you're doing

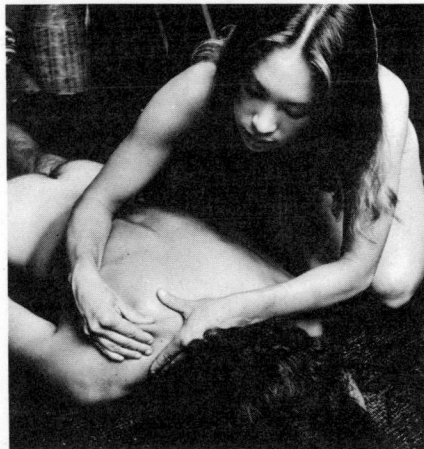

a full body massage, quite a bit of time may have passed since you worked on the head. Even so, since you relaxed the head these top-of-the-back muscles have been crying out for contact. Knead them into the same sweet oblivion the rest of your partner's body has already reached.

Work from the face side of your partner's head so you can reach around to the back of the neck. Begin kneading at the far shoulder, and move slowly across the top of the back. When you reach the back of the neck, knead up onto it to the hairline. When you run out of neck to massage, move down to the back, and cross over to the shoulder next to your knee. Remember to knead the neck each time you cross over your partner's back. Fingertip movements that were broad on the back will become very tiny when you reach up behind the ears. But like all movements in your full body massage, whether large or small, the rhythm remains the same.

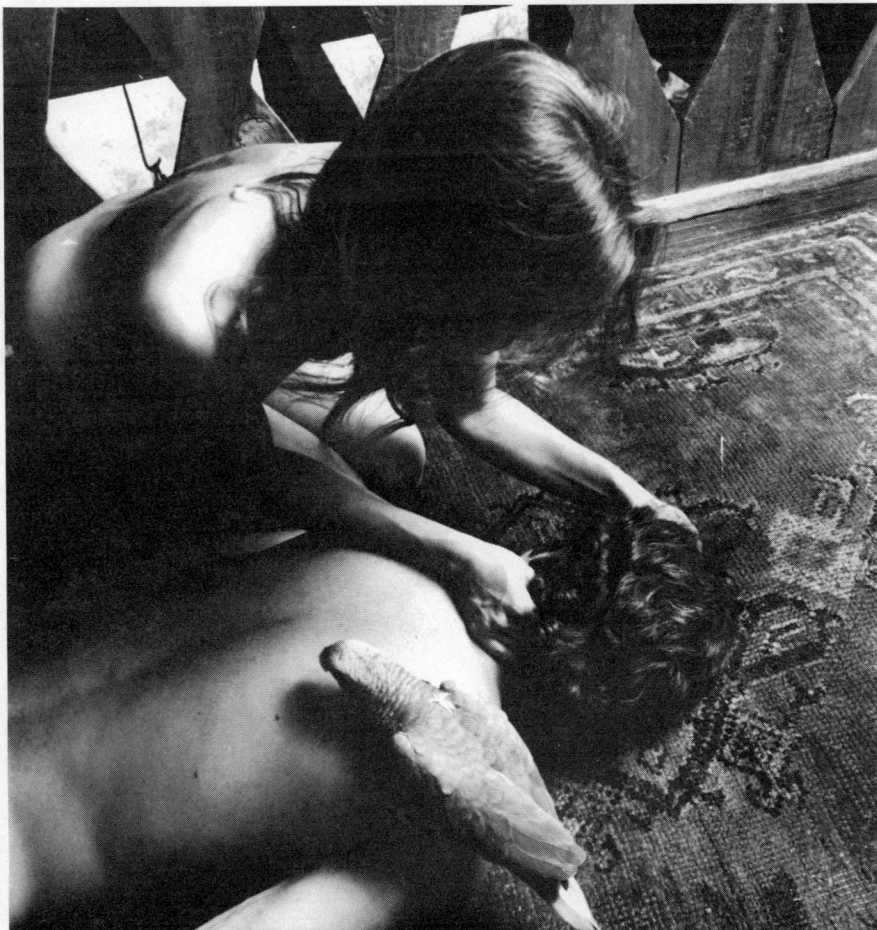

Back friction movements work on one side of the spine at a time. To localize and focus this potent stroke, the hands work at right angles to each other. The anchor hand will press down parallel to the spine, while the friction hand circles at right angles to the spine. Pressing down with your anchor hand, hold the flesh firmly in place. Your friction hand can then turn in small circles on the opposite side of the spine without moving the flesh around your anchor hand. Move up the back slowly one hand width at a time. When you reach the top of the back, cross over to the other side, reverse your hands, and repeat the movement.

Friction takes time and lots of effort. But your effort here is well spent because the back will accept some of the most intense friction movements of any part of the body. This movement by itself will greatly boost nutrient and oxygen supplies to all the internal tissues. This internal change is not one of those theoretical moments which are observable only in a laboratory. Your partner will feel the difference immediately. Rather than ask for proof, you need only observe the helpless grin that almost always follows back friction.

Your partner may ask that you focus the friction movement on a specific spot. People make these requests, and in massage, if not in life, everyone gets exactly what he wants. Press down right over the special spot with your anchor hand, and apply friction with your free thumb.

Like friction, the vibration movement should be anchored on the opposite side of your partner's spine. Move up and down the back this way with both hands, and reverse your position when you cross over. No reason to stop at the bottom of the back if you can comfortably reach beyond. Vibrating buttocks is always fun.

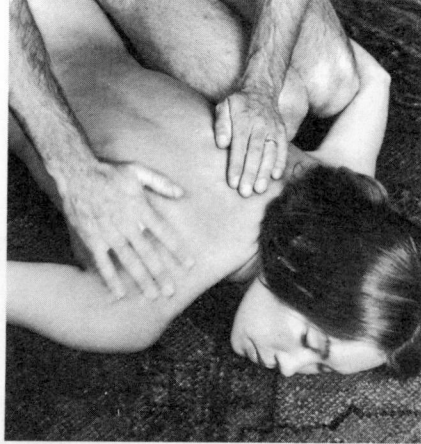

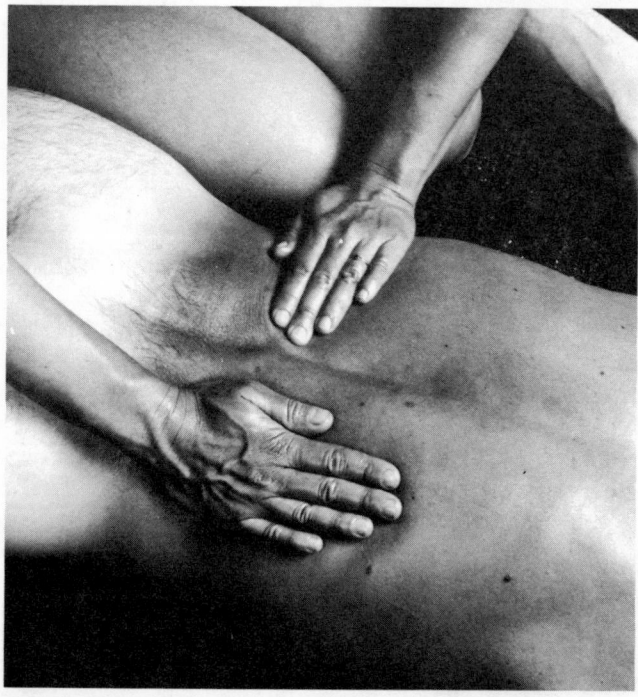

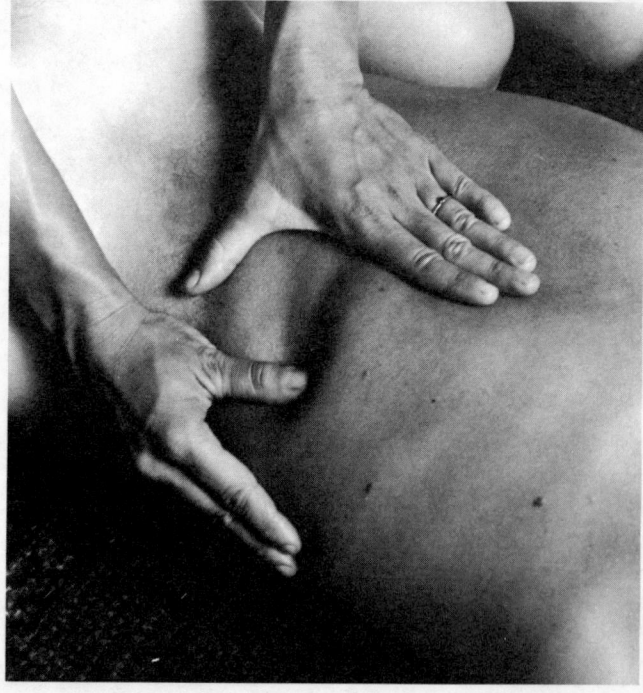

Two Super Contact Movements That Use the Whole Forearm— Stroking Movements

These massive forearm movements are perfectly suited for the broad flat planes of the back. Depending on your partner's size, you can often cover the whole back from wrist to elbow without even moving your arm. Oiling both your forearms up to the elbow is lush and extravagant, but merely a suggestion of what your partner feels when you press both arms across the back. Keep your arms straight out and parallel until the very end of the arc is reached. You can usually press down quite hard while you move up and down the back.

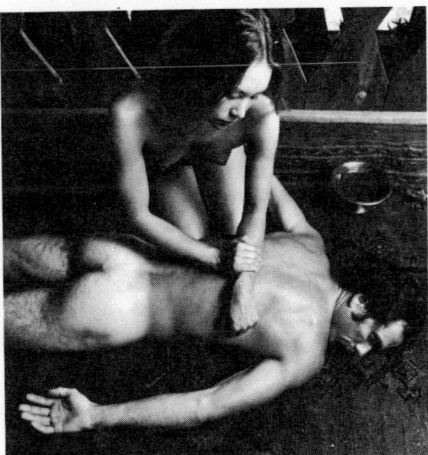

Forearm compression will allow you to direct your pressures much more precisely. On the back, this movement works exactly the same way it did on the torso. Concentrate, once again, on the long muscles that parallel the spine. Remember to lower the flat part of your knuckles occasionally to maximize contact.

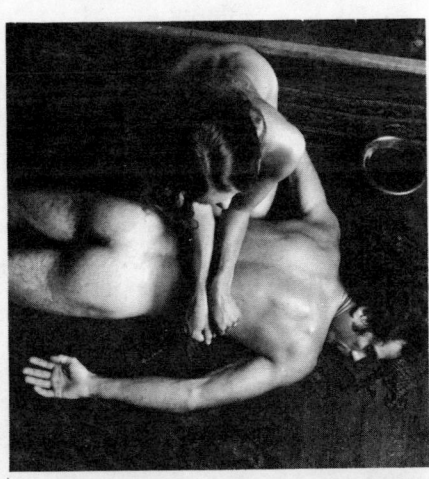

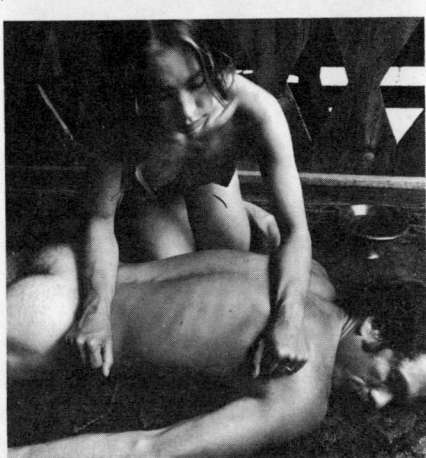

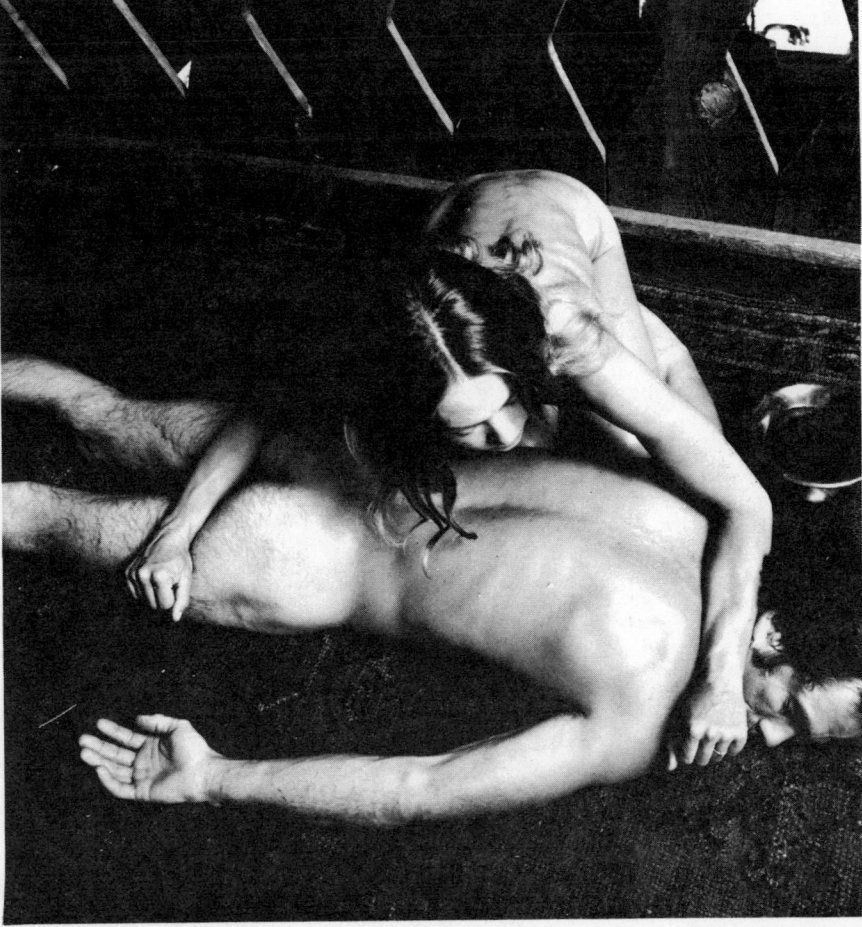

Here, again, is one of those rare massage movements in which physical strength is a factor. Unlike back cracking (see page 160), this passive exercise *can* be duplicated by your partner alone. Still, if size and strength permit, this is a fantastic addition to any back massage. Dancers absolutely crave it.

Gently slide your hands under your partner's shoulders, and grasp (as shown). Raise your outside leg, and plant the foot firmly. Lift your partner slowly, and as the torso rises, rest your elbow on the outstretched leg. This way your leg can act as a natural tripod to support your partner's body. Hold for a silent count of twenty, and lower your partner slowly and evenly.

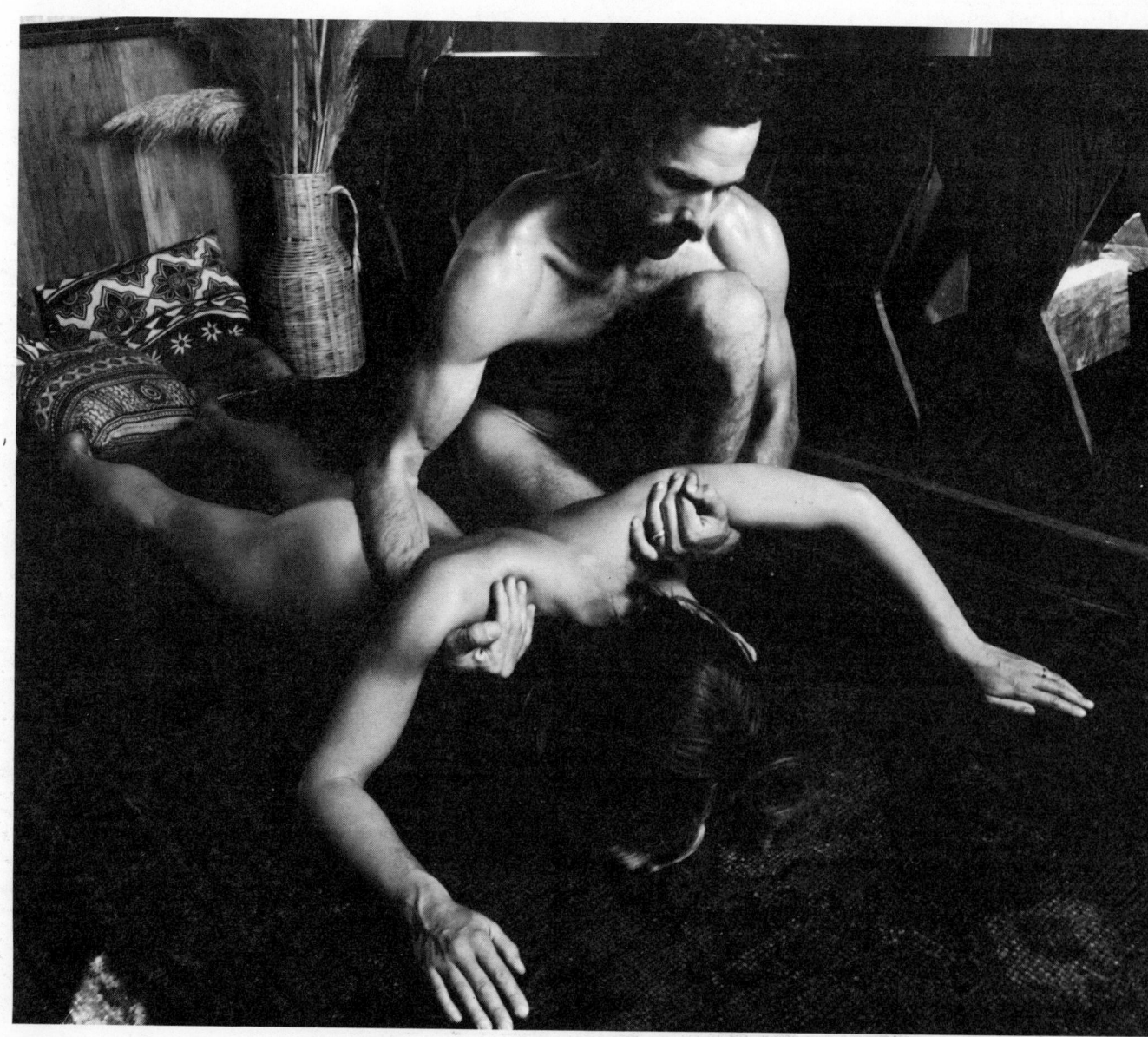

Pressure on the spine means direct stimulation of the central nervous system. There are two ways this stimulation can affect your partner: You can either excite the nerves with brisk movements or sedate them with slow rhythmic strokes. If your partner has been depressed, quick movements up and down the spine will promote a feeling of exhilaration and well-being. If, on the other hand, you're dealing with insomnia, spasticity, nervousness, or hypertension, slow rhythmic strokes will produce a feeling of drowsiness and relaxation.

The closed-finger movement allows you to press down directly on top of the spine while the flesh of your hand cushions the contact. Although the fingertips are at the forward edge of this movement, you should actually lead with the base of your palm. That's where the pressure is concentrated. The fingertips simply go along for the ride. Press down

on your contact hand by crossing it (as shown) with your free hand. Reverse this movement at the shoulders, and move back to the waist without breaking contact or rhythm.

The open-finger contact movement moves up and down the back the same way. The difference is in the way pressures are distributed at your hands. The contact hand will touch your partner's back only at the fingertips and the base of the palm. The center of the hand and fingers remains arched throughout the movement. Try to equalize your contact pressure between the heel of your hand and the two contact fingers. The spine will fit neatly between the two contact fingers as you press up and down the back.

Nerves that supply the heart branch off the spine between the shoulder blades. This is the area on which to concentrate if you want to soothe the heart. Two or three minutes of vigorous massage will usually reduce the pulse rate by about 10 percent. Vigorous, of course, does not mean violent. Work between the shoulder blades right up to the spine with friction, kneading, and vibration movements. The spine itself can be massaged with a combination of the two previous movements. A light percussion movement, like the hacking stroke you used on the leg (page 111), will nicely complement the sequence. Use it on the thick muscles around the spine, but stay off the spine itself. These movements will soothe the cardiac nerves and the heart muscle itself.

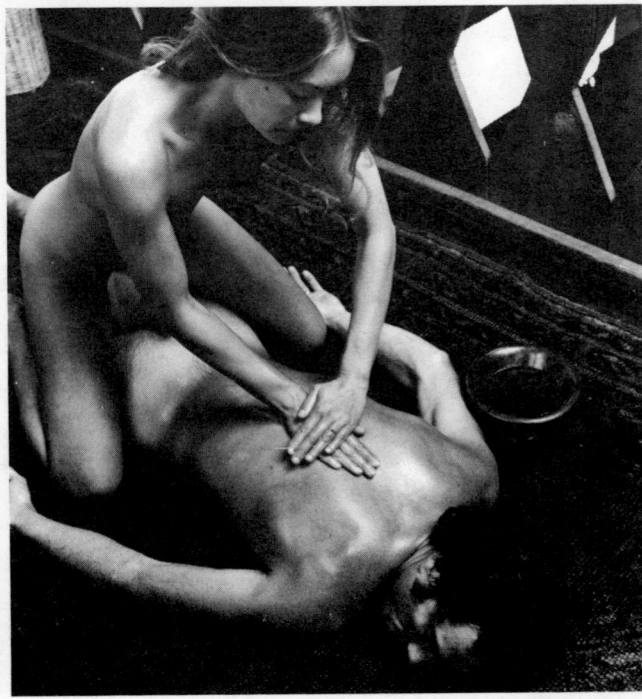
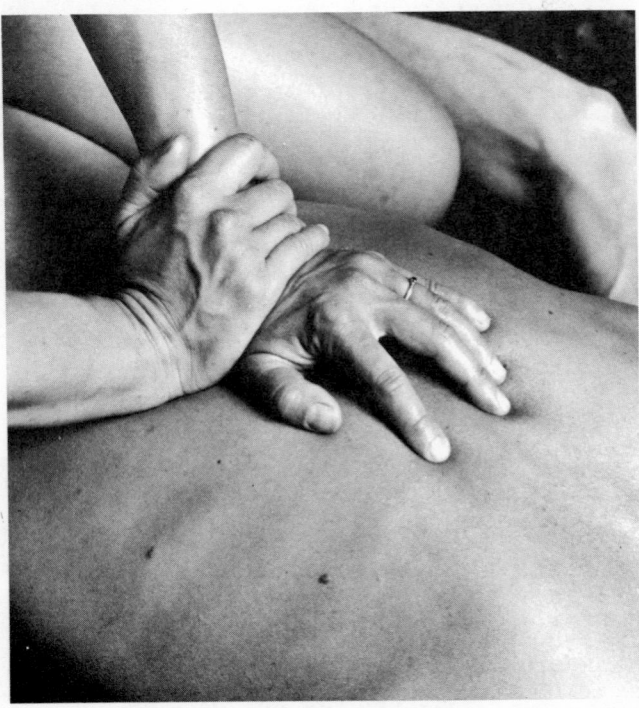

Pull down the spine with a hand-over-hand pressing movement. At the base of the spine bring your hands together so they merge into a ten-finger mandala.
Concentrate on breaking this contact very slowly: with first the heel of the hand, then the palm, then the fingers, and finally the middle finger of the top hand, which should rest right on the spine. Move your hands up to your partner's shoulders one final time without touching his body. The hands are held just an inch above the skin during this final pass.

When you're working on your partner's back, there's a whole range of movements you can get into on the back of the arms. The arms can be rotated (as shown), kneaded, and stroked from one end to another. You can certainly knead parts of the arm that were difficult, if not almost impossible, to reach from the other side of the body. Friction movements, particularly around the elbow, are very effective from this side of the body. You can, if you like, work out a whole sequence for the back of the arms. Be sure to duplicate all your movements on both arms and to give support, whenever you move an arm, above and below the elbow.

Use the full surface of your fingers to brush your partner's body from head to toes. At the toes final contact between ten fingertips and ten toes should be broken very slowly. Your partner will float up from that final moment as though his feet and body had actually left the ground. Mind and body merge at the end of a massage, and many people prefer not to be disturbed for some time. Withdraw from the massage area quietly. Be silent. Let the feeling go on.

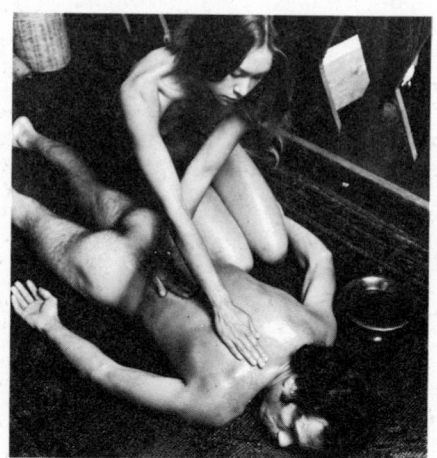

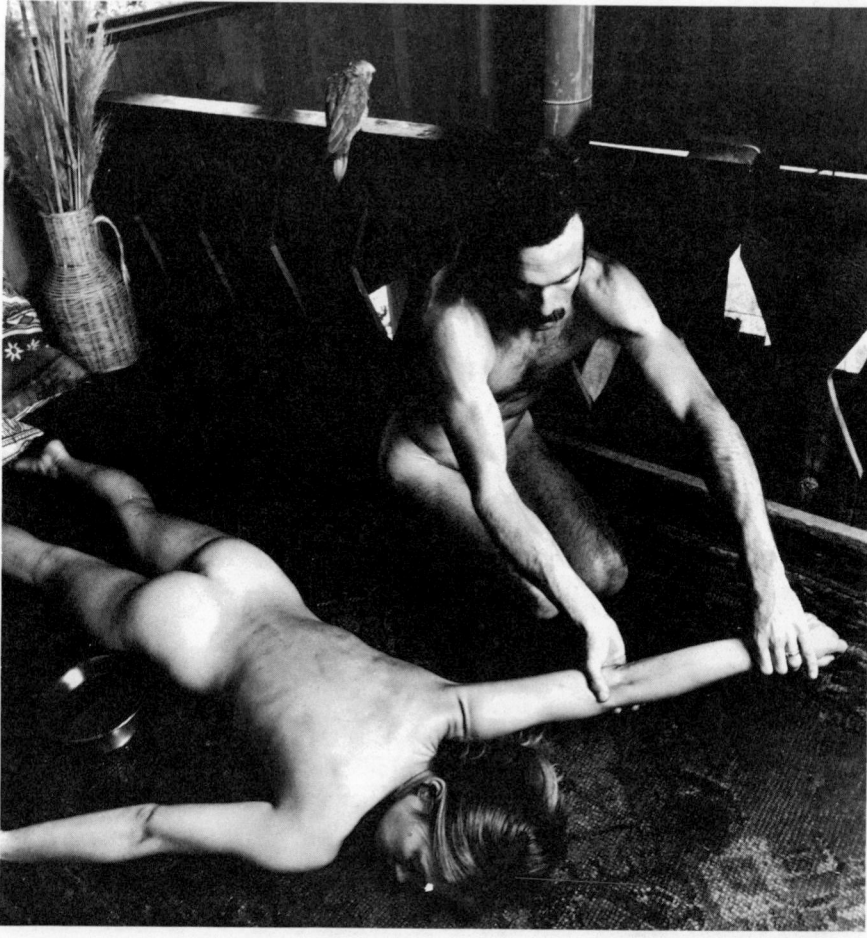

Exercise and Massage

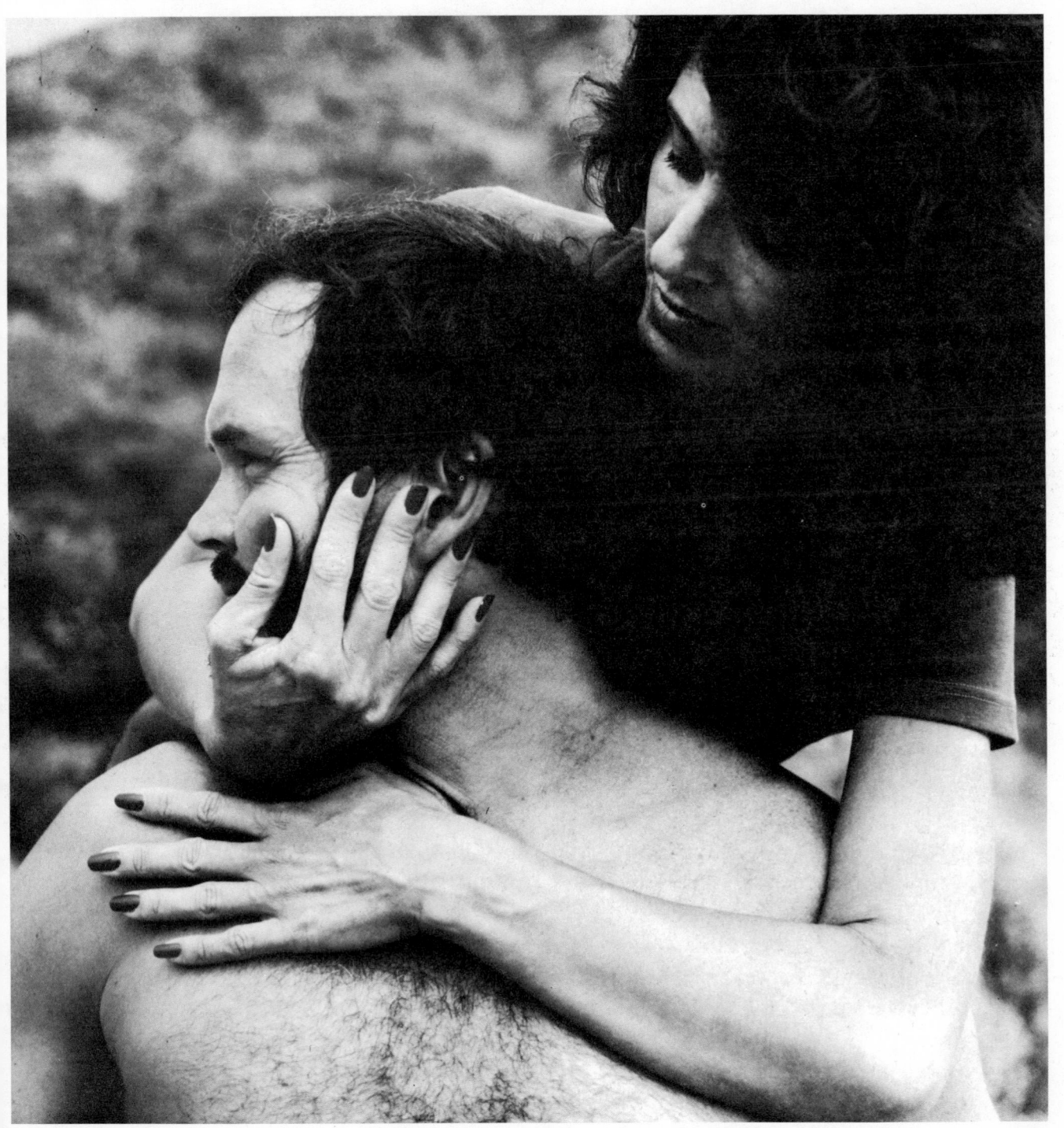

Exercise and Massage

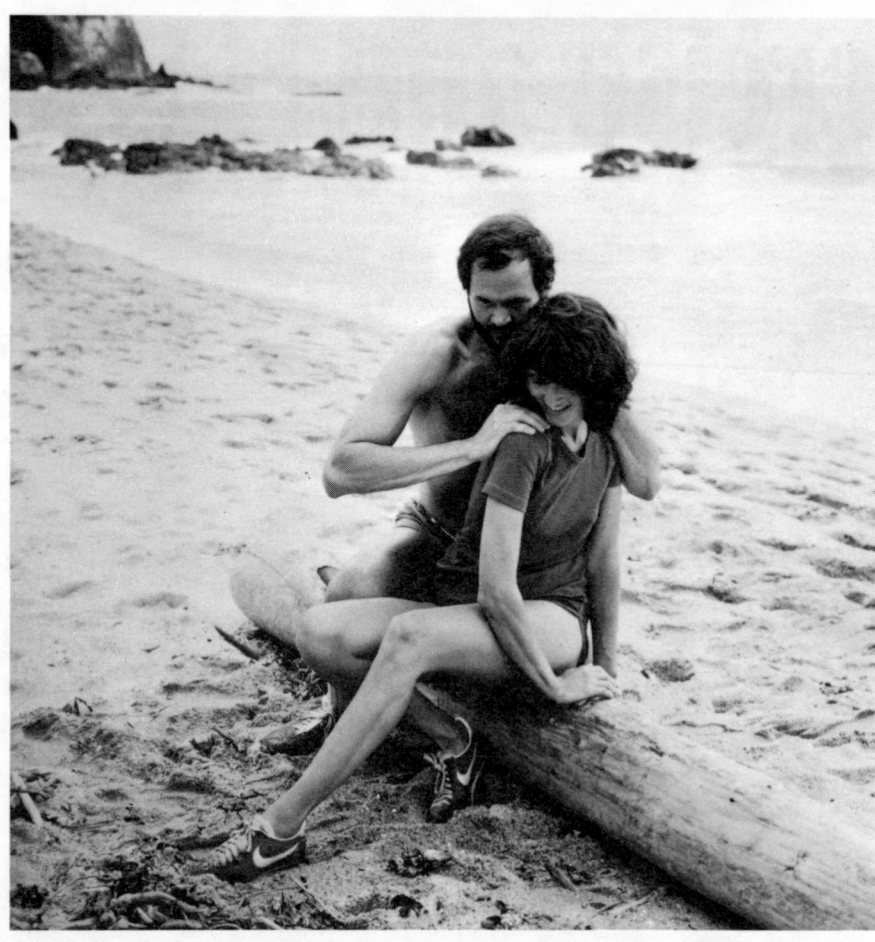

People who exercise are usually very practical-minded and insist on knowing exactly what is going on inside the body. On one level they regard exercise as basic preventive medicine and constantly seek ways to make the machinery of the body work more efficiently. To this end, the overall effects of many health aids are sometimes very difficult to gauge. Diet changes, for example, can take months to register physically. The internal effects during and after massage, however, are immediate and apparent and have been measured.

A ten-minute abdominal massage will decrease, by as much as one hour,

the decomposition time of food in the stomach. The assimilation rate of nutritious elements in the intestines rises significantly. This is particularly important to people who are fastidious about diet and want to get the greatest possible benefit from food. The whole digestive process is massively stimulated, and constipation can usually be dealt with quickly. Production of gastric juice, saliva, and urine is increased. Nitrogen, inorganic phosphorus, and sodium chloride levels in the urine are substantially higher. Many of these benefits have been observed one full week after a single, thorough body massage.

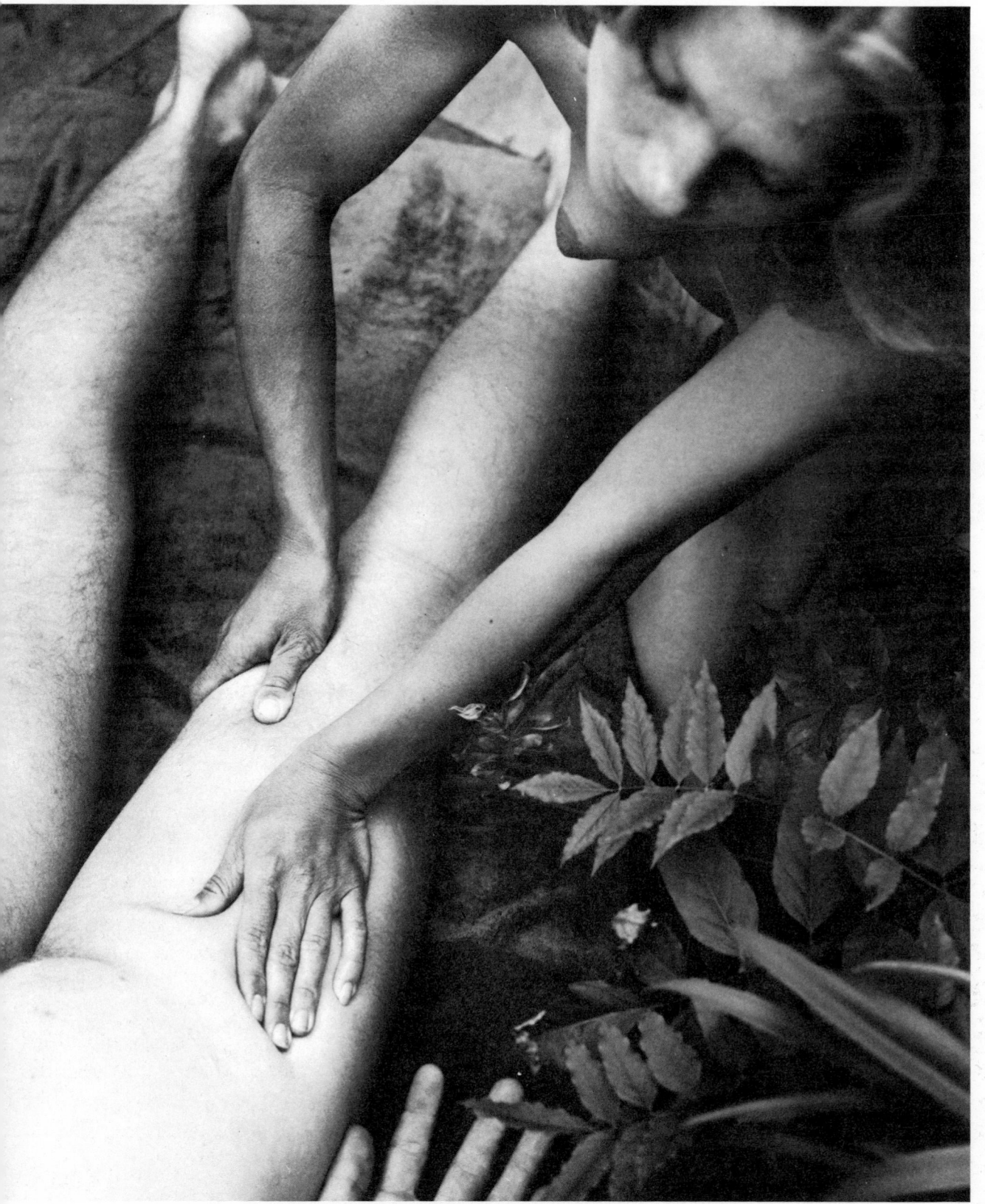

Massage removes dead brittle skin from the surface and allows the living tissue beneath to breathe more easily. Tough, inflexible skin will become softer and far more supple after regular massage. Facial wrinkles, often merely the result of nervous tension, begin to disappear even if the face itself is not massaged. The effects of regular back massage, for example, will be apparent on the face. This is simply a result of the renewed vitality and overall health that massage can bring. Scalp massage stimulates the sebaceous secretion. Here again, the results are often actually visible. Afterward the hair looks glossy and moisturized.

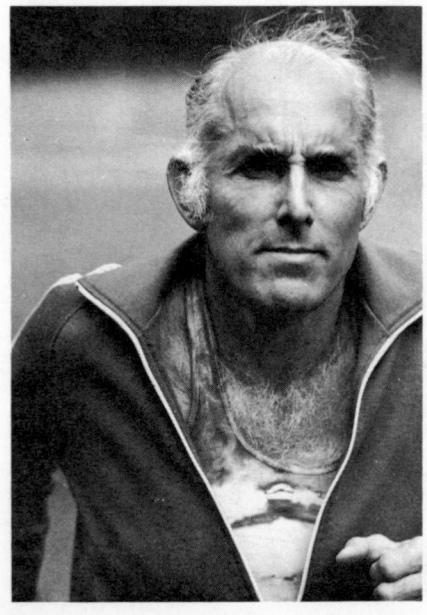

Blood and lymph pass three times more rapidly through a part of the body being massaged than when it is not. While this happens, the pulse rate drops and the heart slows. Movements specifically intended to aid circulation momentarily empty the surface veins. Deep kneading strokes have a similar effect because the valves of the venous system will allow blood flow only toward the heart. Although these movements will speed local blood flow, their overall effect is to lower the blood pressure while they relax the heart and tone the vascular system. Massage cannot manufacture blood cells, but it can put into circulation those that are dormant in the body. Massage can be used to direct red and white blood corpuscles to specific parts of the body. Massive increases in the white blood cell count have been recorded after just five minutes of each of the following common movements: circulation, 85 percent; vibration and friction, 60 percent; percussion, 45 percent; and kneading, 30 percent. Enhanced blood supply will also act as a natural analgesic—that is, it will decrease pain. After massage the oxygen content of the tissues is up 10 to 15 percent, allowing for more efficient combustion of stored energy.

* Douglas Graham, M.D., *Massage: Manual Treatment; Remedial Movements*, J.B. Lippincott Company: Philadelphia, 1913, p. 83.

† Hermann Bucholz, *Therapeutic Exercise and Massage*, Lea & Febiger: Philadelphia and New York, 1920, p. 122.

Although the extraordinary Fluid Release effect was documented at the turn of the century, it has been ignored by antitactile societies for the past seven decades. Nevertheless, if you're interested in health, pay close attention to these astonishing ergographic tests which were designed to measure the work capacity of muscles before and after massage:

. . . after severe exercise a rest of fifteen minutes brought about no essential recovery, whilst after massage for the same period the exercise was more than doubled. One person experimented upon lifted a weight of one kilo (2.2 pounds) eight hundred and forty times, at intervals of one second, by extreme flexion of the elbow-joint, from a table upon which the forearm rested horizontally, and after this he could do no more. When the arm had been massaged for five minutes, he lifted the weight more than eleven hundred times in the same manner as before without fatigue.

*Professor Maggiora, of the University of Turin, has shown the restorative effects of massage upon his own muscles when weakened by physical or mental labor, by electricity, by hunger, loss of sleep, and slight fever. For this purpose the fatigue curves of the right and left middle fingers in maximum voluntary flexion were taken every two seconds with a weight of 3 kilograms. The average results showed that the muscles concerned in this movement could do about twice as much work after a few minutes of massage as they could without.† *

The effects of massage on the nervous system depend on your partner's sex and the intensity of the pressures you use. A woman's nerves are more easily stimulated than a man's. Light to mild pressures will stimulate the nerves while heavy pressure will sedate them. In any case, everything that you do to the nerves will have a direct effect on the muscles they control. There is, in fact, a subtle but significant reciprocal effect between the muscles, nerves, and brain. If any of the three are irritated, the other two will quickly show the effects.

Muscle wastes will irritate the nerves, and that irritation is often enough to cause the muscle to cramp. Nervous people who suffer frequent cramps can often be helped by constant direct pressure on the nerves that supply cramped muscles.*

Ligaments that hold the vertebrae together are small and tight. Because very little rotation is permitted, the tendency is to allow the spine to remain rigid and inflexible. This tendency can become very costly by the age of forty when people discover that tying their shoes has become difficult and painful. Athletes, dancers, yoga students, and folks who just want to feel good can use the following three movements to flex the tiny joints, called vertebrae, that run up and down the spine. If you use those movements regularly as part of your exercise routine, the ligaments between the vertebrae will begin to stretch out, and the entire spine becomes more supple.

In all three movements you will push away from your body and pull toward it at the same time. All three movements are also reversible—that is, you will pull on the side of the body where you pushed and vice versa.

In flexing the neck, you're dealing with vertebrae on the back of the neck. Your partner should assume a stable sitting posture for these adjustments; usually keeping the legs crossed over in front of the body is about right. Cup your partner's chin in one hand, and lay your fingers along the cheekbone. You will be pulling toward your body with this hand. Use the palm of your other hand to press away from

*The effects of massage on the body: L. L. Despard, *Textbook of Massage* (London: 1916); James Cyriax and Gillean Russell, *Textbook of Orthopaedic Medicine*, vol. 2, 9th edition; and Kathryn L. Jensen, *Foundamentals in Massage* (New York: Macmillan, 1932).

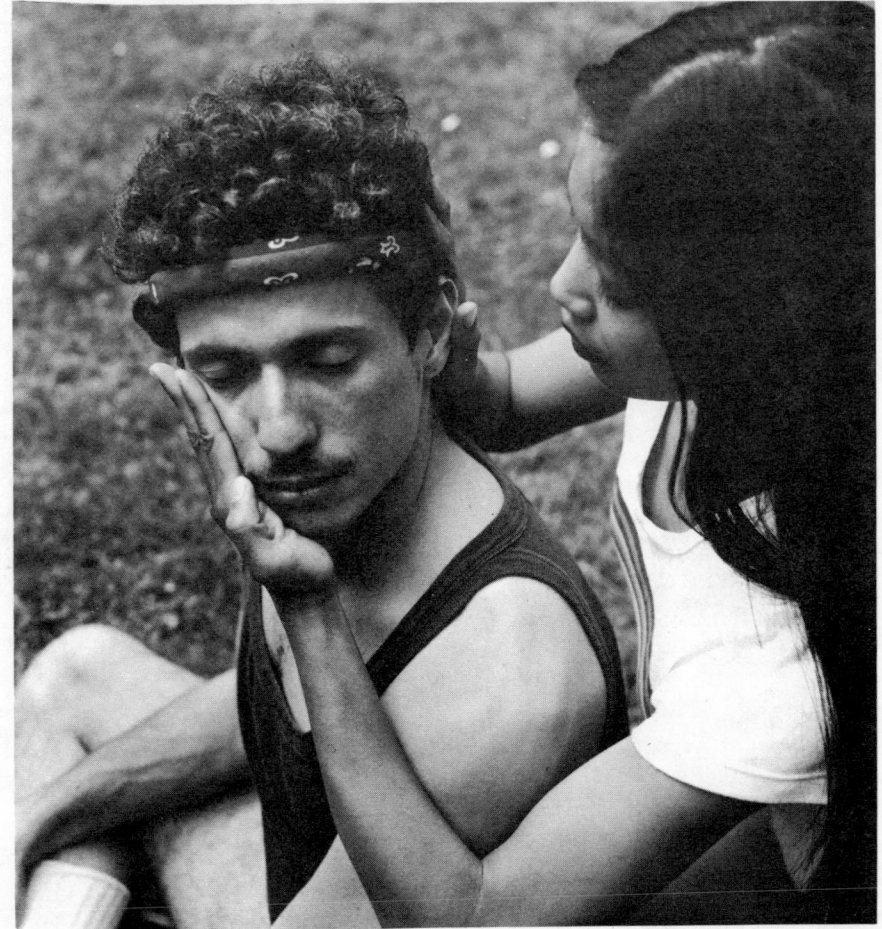

your body on the back of your partner's skull. Press the head right to the point of tension. Be gentle, work slowly, and get some feedback from your partner while you're learning. A neck adjustment is definitely not the place to test your strength and speed. If you use it that way, you both could be very sorry very quickly.

Press to the point of resistance three times, and then simply turn your partner's head to face the opposite shoulder. Reverse your hands, and repeat the movement.

Your partner's shoulders provide you with the best possible lever for stretching the middle of the back. Wrap one hand around one shoulder (as shown) for pushing out. Pull back with your forearm on the other shoulder. There's more pressure required here than on the neck. Again, work with feedback from your partner until you get used to the range involved. The two shoulders should move about the same distance. That means you have to exert equal amounts of pressure with both arms. Resist the temptation to push harder than you're pulling. Stretch to the point of resistance three times, and then reverse the movement.

Has America finally reached the point where physical labor is so distasteful that people no longer know how to do it? The Space Age is rapidly becoming the age of the bad back. Ordinary labor that was once a part of everyone's life is now regarded as so exotic that people are willing to pay health clubs for the privilege of doing physical work. If they would take this physical work to the hills and plant trees, the rest of us might have something to show for it, and masseurs would be spared the shrieks of pain that accompany a gently flexed leg.

The main joint at the base of the back, the one that allows you to bend over, is called the sacro-iliac. This is the joint that invariably suffers when someone lifts a refrigerator without bending the knees. A strained lower back (as though to emphasize the mistake that caused the strain) makes lifting almost anything impossible *unless* you bend the knees.

Like every other massage movement, passively exercising the lower back should cause no pain. Because lower-back problems are not always immediately apparent, there's a simple way you can begin this movement without putting too much pressure on this area. It involves enlisting your partner's aid just a bit, a rare exception to the rule generally followed in massage.

Ask your partner to lie on her side, and lift the lower leg as high as possible. She should then hold the leg in place by clasping her fingers under the knee basket-style (as shown). This will hold the pelvis steady against the lower spine. Hold your partner's leg just under the buttocks and just above the knee (as shown). Press toward your partner with the hand on

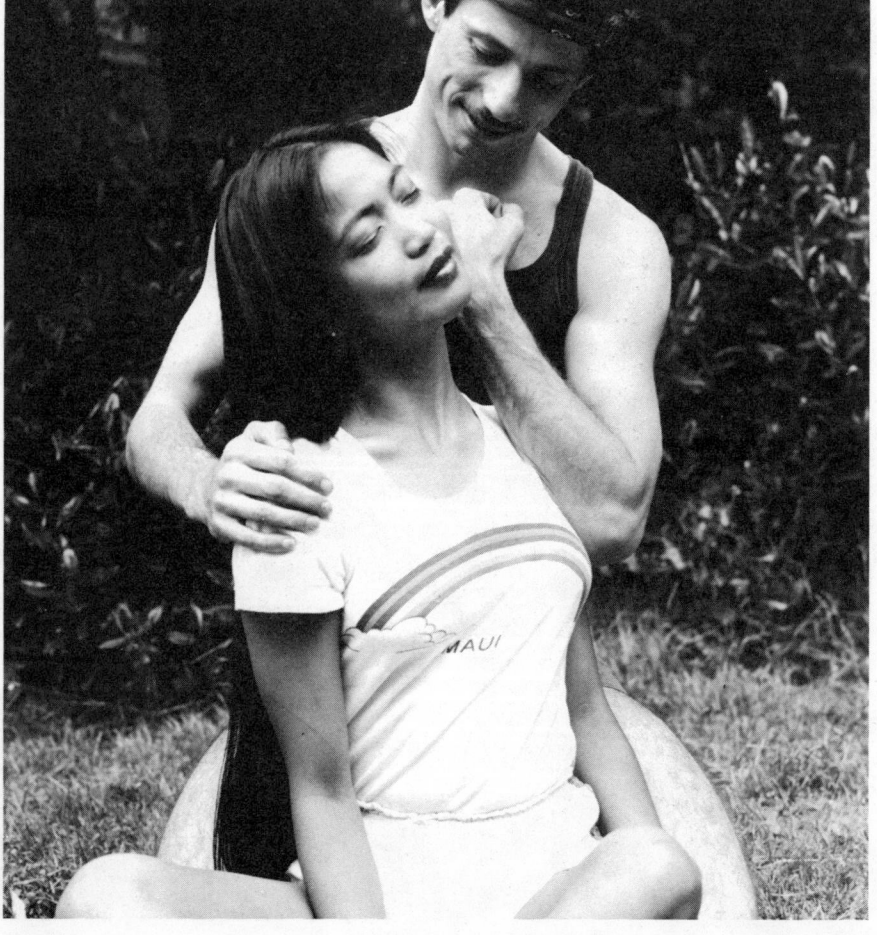

the upper leg while pulling toward yourself with the hand above her knee. If you use light gradual pressures at first, this will put moderate pressure on the lower back. If there's no pain, there should be no lower-back problems to prevent you from going on with this dramatic movement.

Begin again, but this time ask your partner to release her knee when she feels pressure building.

This will allow you to carry the leg all the way back to the final position you see here. Remember that this final position will vary, and you should stop when you feel resistance. Once your partner

releases the knee, the sacroiliac joint is flexed along with the entire lower spine. This movement should be repeated three times and is usually followed, each time, by a deep sigh.

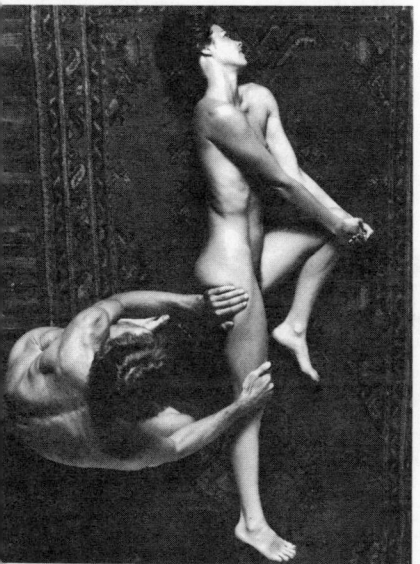

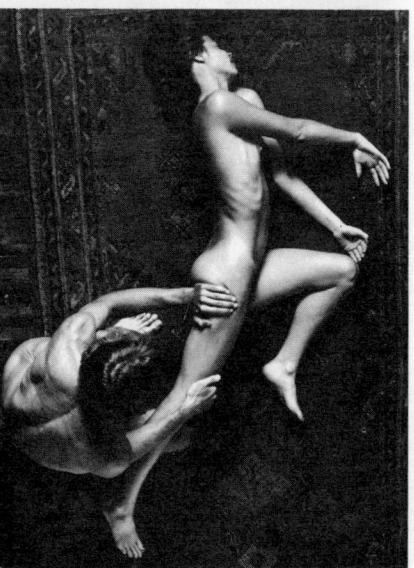

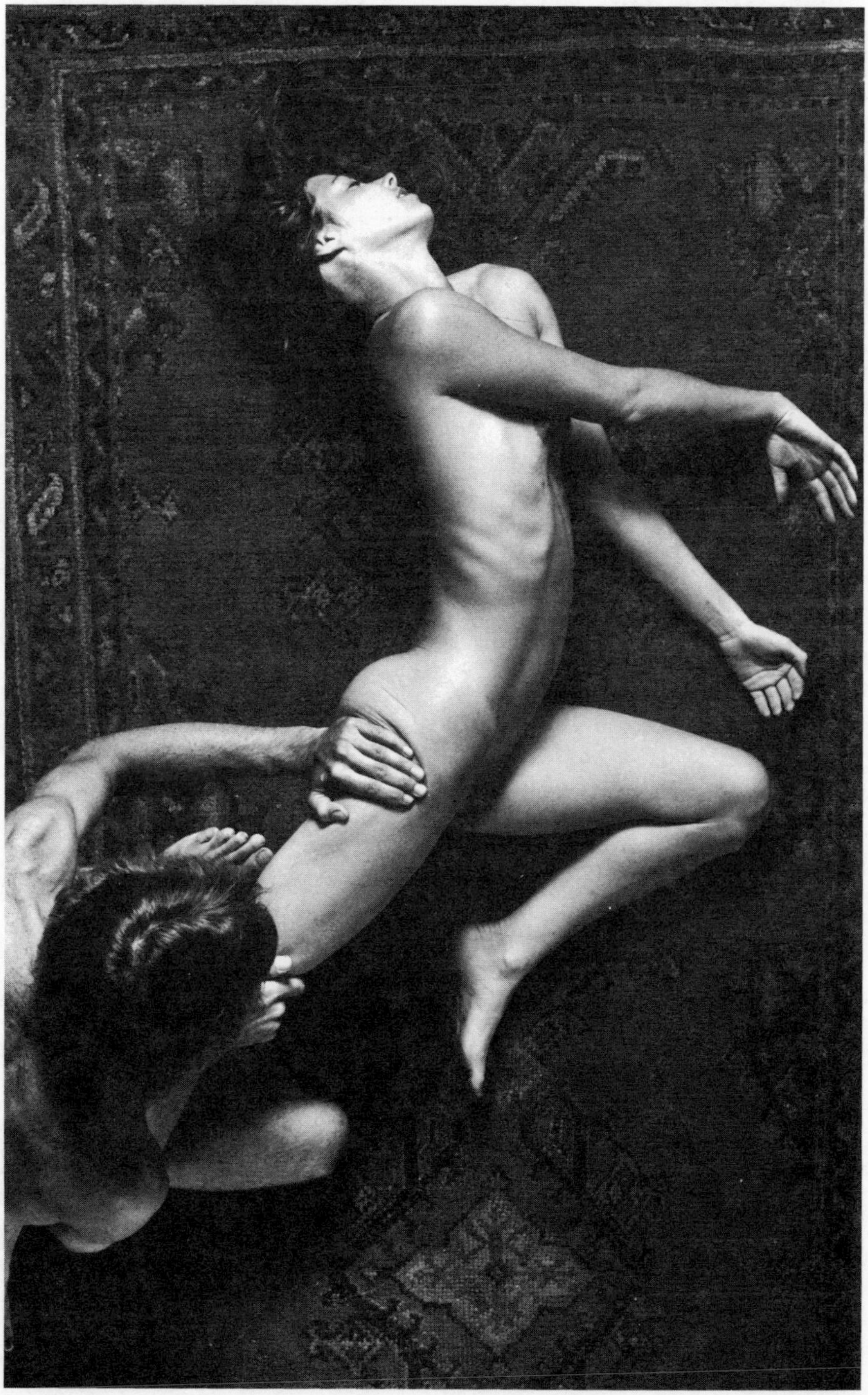

159

Another thriller almost guaranteed to bring forth a few more hearty sighs from your partner is the voluptuous back cracking movement. The large sacroiliac joint connects the vertical spine to the pelvis in a right-angle turn. Even under the most fluid conditions, this joint rotates in a limited arc, and sometimes a sudden movement will push the interlocking surfaces so far that the sacroiliac simply locks up. This movement will free it along with all the other joints of the lower and middle back. It also stretches the muscles throughout that area.

There are two ways to crack the back: one with your partner facing you and the other with your partner facing away. You'll probably want to try them both. And if you hesitate, your partner may beg you to try them both. In each position most of your pressure should go toward twisting at the hips while you steady your partner's shoulders.

With your partner facing away from you, steady the shoulder, pulling it back a bit with your elbow, and press forward with your other hand on the crest of the pelvic bone. Holding the shoulder steady allows the joints of the lower back to turn. Your movement here should be slow and smooth. Stop when you encounter substantial resistance. Sometimes when you reach the point of resistance, you will hear a faint popping caused by the tops of the vertebrae moving across each other.

With your partner facing you, it's possible to move these joints all the way in the other direction. Steady the shoulder by simply pressing against it (as shown). Pull back on the crest of the pelvis with your bent forearm (as shown), or you can lean in farther and use more of your arm right up to the elbow. Once again you may hear that subtle pop. But whether you hear it or not, press right up to the point of resistance and release the back slowly. Back cracking allows your partner to experience one of those delicious postures that occur only during massage.

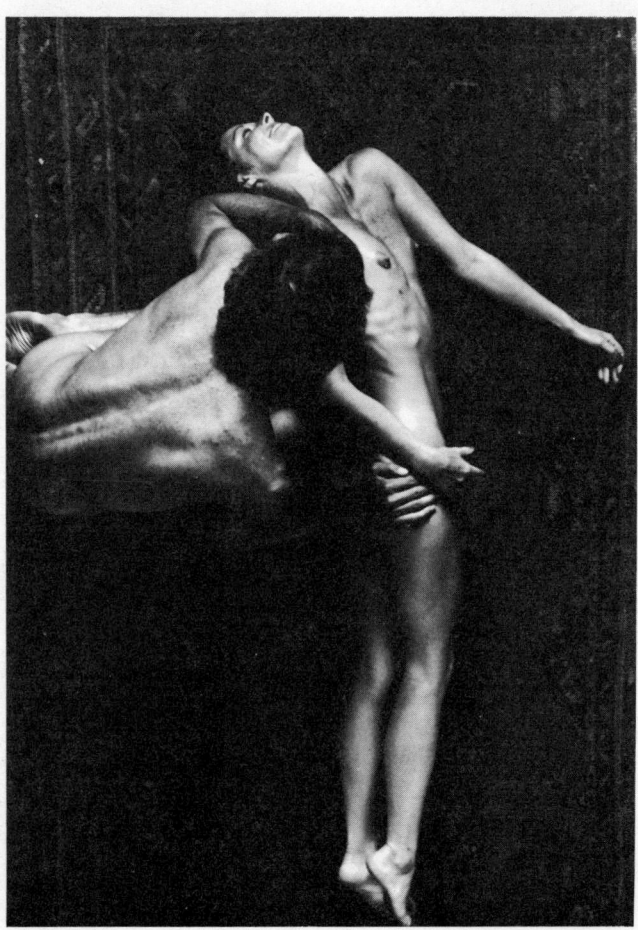 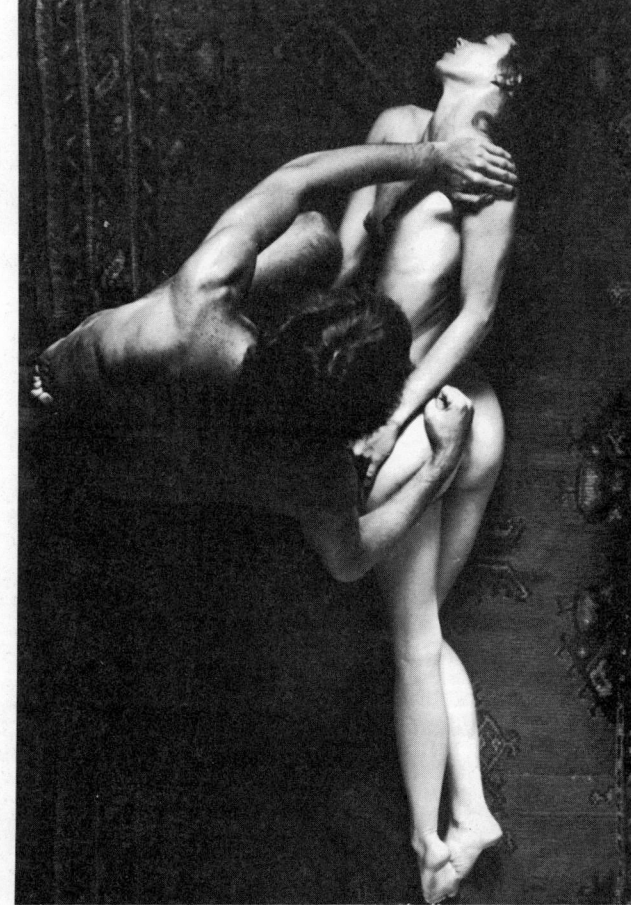

Several thousand years ago Hippocrates commented on the remarkable way massage can be used to mobilize stiff joints. A sluggish, benumbed feeling in the joints discourages a lot of people from exercising, particularly those who prefer to work out in the morning. Every joint is a complicated piece of anatomical machinery, and the interior parts have a way of settling when they are not used. Circulation slows, and the blood vessels contract. Nutrition to the ligaments, tendons, nerves, cartilage and bone inside the joint is decreased. All these changes are confronted quite suddenly by the frustrated athlete who attempts to put a joint into high gear after many hours of inactivity.

The movements that follow are designed to invigorate the joints and get rid of stiffness before exercise. There's a general sequence you can follow at each joint that will get rid of wastes, boost circulation, stretch the ligaments, and lubricate the space where bones meet. Most of the movements in this sequence have been described in the "Full Body Massage" section (see page 38) of the book. A few specialized techniques that were not covered are discussed below.

Begin with a fingertip kneading movement. Whenever possible, this kneading should penetrate deeply into the joint. It's easy to do this on the back of the knee, at the shoulder, and around the hip where there's plenty of flesh.

More delicate joints, like the elbow and wrist, will not accept very deep pressures. Light kneading on these joints will reach the ligaments and tendons at the bone.

Friction movements follow the same sort of pattern as kneading. Use deep pressures on the hip, back of the knee, and shoulder; lighter pressures on the smaller joints. Always be sure to anchor

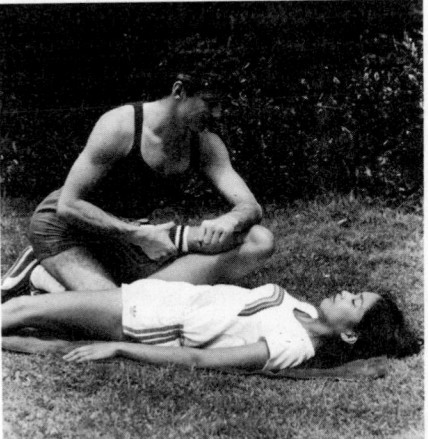

your friction movements close to the joint while you massage so the effects will remain localized.

After you've worked on a joint with kneading and friction, it's time for a more general circulation movement. It isn't necessary to work on the whole limb, but be sure to cover the area above and below the joint you've just massaged. This movement will carry away wastes you've stirred up during kneading and friction. It will also continue the process of bringing nutrients and oxygen to the tissues of the joint.

End your work on each joint by passively exercising it. Work just inside the point of resistance the whole time you're flexing the joint. This entire sequence can be

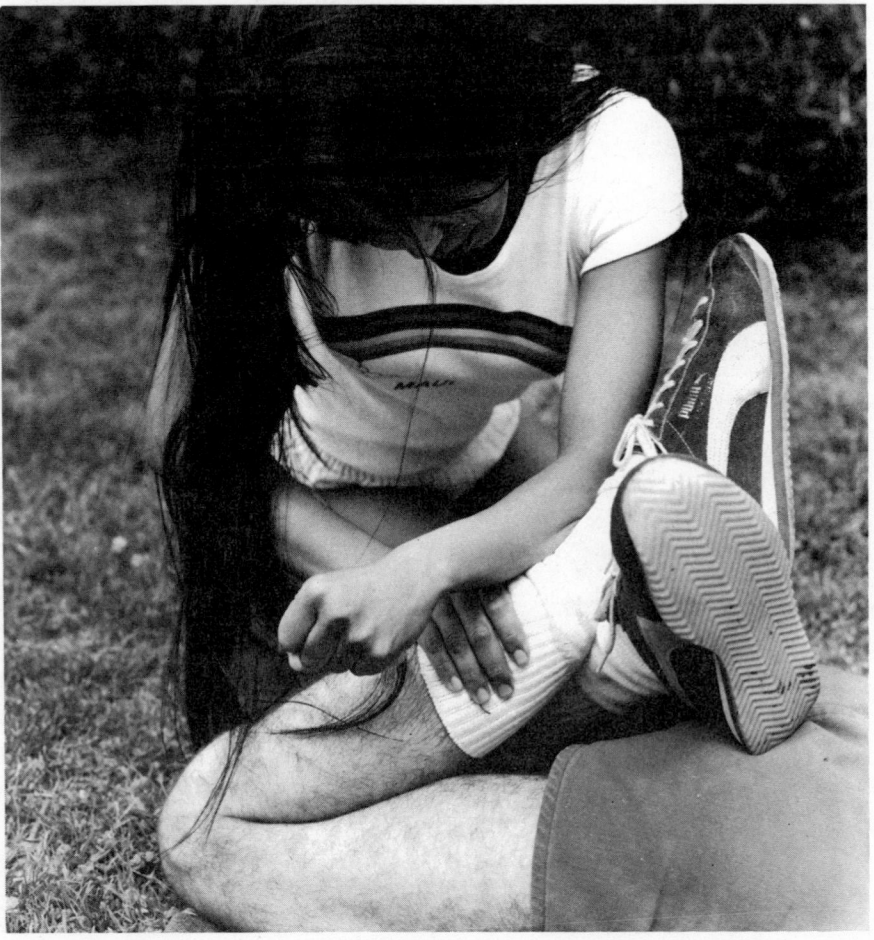

completed in just a couple of minutes on each joint. If you're massaging before a competitive event, you may want to extend this time. Feedback from your partner will help you determine just how much attention each joint will need.

This movement allows you to stretch the ligaments and tendons at all three arm joints simultaneously. At the same time your partner leans forward and pulls away from you quite hard. This puts a healthy horizontal stress on the muscles of the chest. Stretching the chest muscles before you exercise makes it much easier for the lungs to expand.

Grasp both of your partner's hands around the wrists, and let your hands slide up until they make contact with the base of your partner's thumb. Hold the arms fully outstretched (as shown). Lean back slightly. Your partner will then lean forward, but as this happens, you should maintain the same position. This will create a resistance in the arm and chest muscles which will increase as your partner leans forward, farther and farther away from you. Again, do not allow your hands to move.

Here's another movement that acts on the chest muscles. The difference is that instead of pulling out on the arm joints, your partner will flex the muscles of the arm. Again, you'll have to hold your hands steady while your partner leans hard away from you.

Kneel behind your partner, and grasp both hands around the back of the wrist (as shown). Your partner then leans forward and, at the same time, attempts to bring the arms straight out. If building aerobic capacity is one of your partner's goals, this movement will definitely be appreciated.

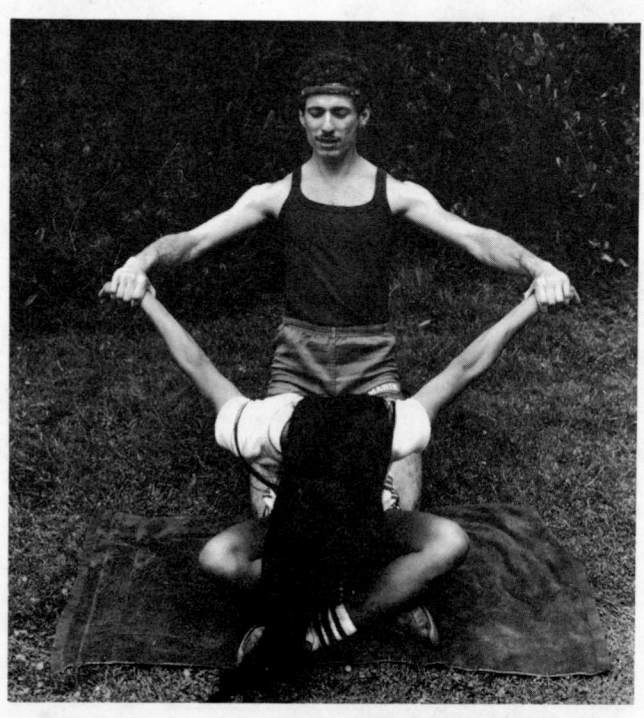

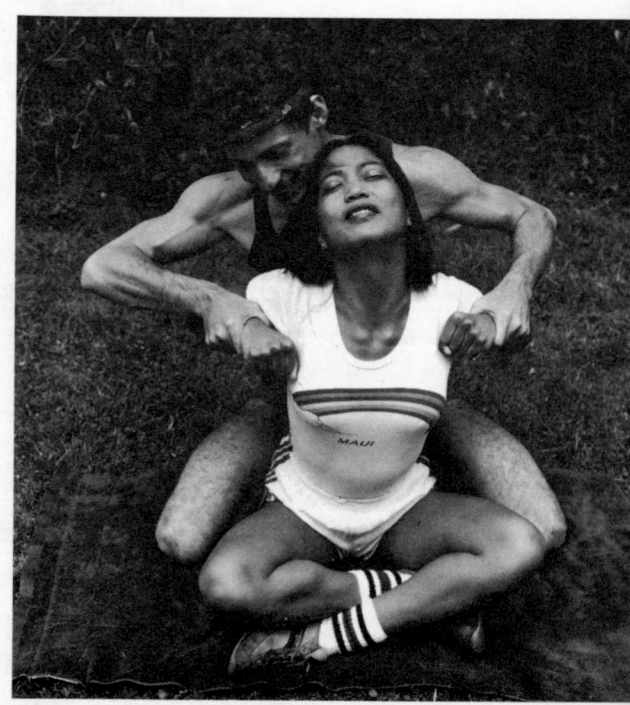

f your partner is involved in a racket sport or any game that involves throwing, you will want to pay special attention to the elbows. Follow through on all the elbow movements in "The Arm" chapter (see page 59), and then have your partner turn over. This will give you very easy access to the back of the elbow and the important ulnar nerve. Some people find it a bit easier to work on the opposite arm by simply reaching across the back (as shown). If you prefer to have the elbow closer when you work, you can, of course, move around the other side of the body. Try it both ways, and use the one that feels most comfortable to you. Be sure to anchor your partner's arm at the wrist, and keep your fingers together even though you're massaging in a limited space. Work on the back of each elbow for at least a full minute with fingertip friction movements.

Thumb friction is a slow movement; it will never move as fast as the four-finger versions of the friction stroke. There is, however, a significant difference in texture between the ball of the thumb and the tips of the fingers. Many people really prefer the thumb and will ask for it if you don't offer thumb friction as part of a massage. The thumb will fit nicely along the side of your partner's knee, and this is a good part of the body to begin experimenting with this movement.

Work on the sides of the knee, and stay off the kneecap itself. Press down a fold of flesh with your free hand, and push up into that fold with your thumb. If circling seems awkward, you can confine the movement to a slow rhythmic up-and-down motion. Work up and down both sides of the knee, pressing the flesh just ahead of your thumb with your free hand.

The familiar rush of excitement that most athletes feel just before the beginning of a competitive event generally helps prepare the body for the exertion that is about to begin. For some very high-strung people any extra excitement is so overwhelming that they turn into nervous wrecks just before a race begins. As these stricken, ashen-faced runners approach the starting line, one is reminded that running is a leisure-time activity and is supposed to be fun. "The saddest thing in the world," said Henry James, "is watching an American trying to have a good time."

Fortunately, if you have four or five minutes and a reasonably warm place to work, it's usually possible to calm down almost anybody. Concentrate on bringing blood to your partner's skin. This will soothe the nerves and effectively lower blood pressure throughout the body. Work on both sides of the body, and try to

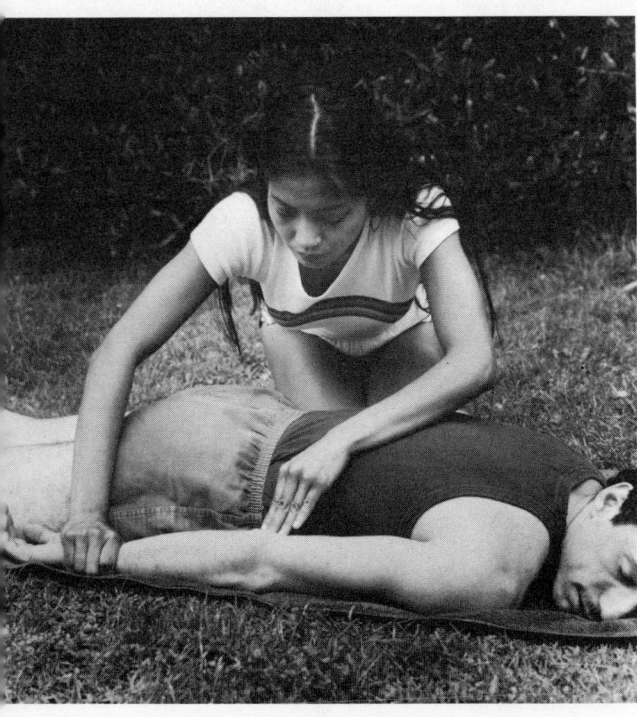

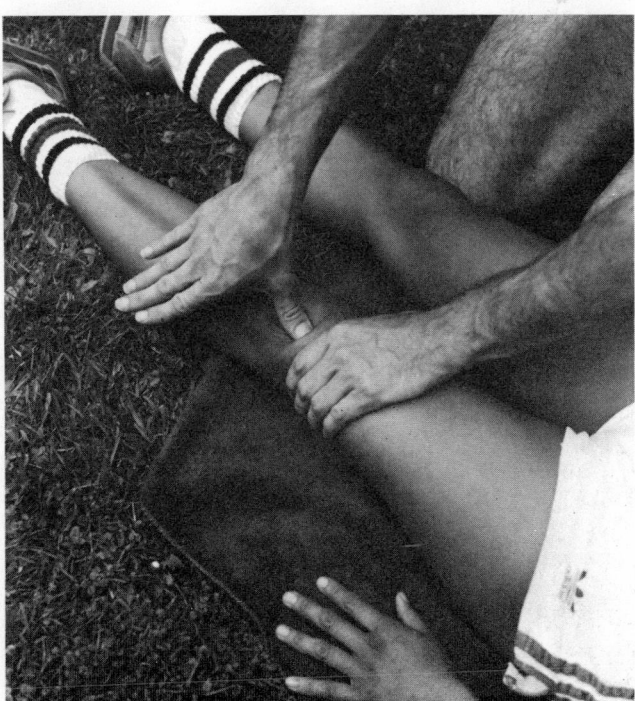

cover as large an area as possible. Use sweeping superficial kneading vibration motions with just enough pressure to maintain constant friction against the skin without actually pulling on it.

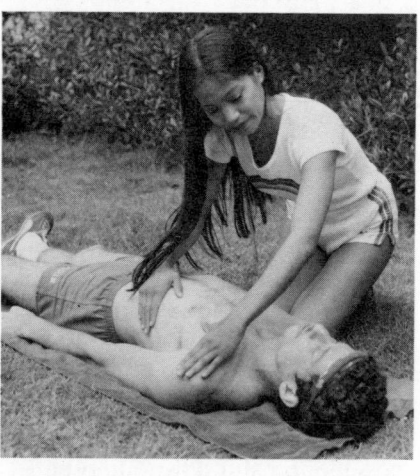

Your stroking should be much faster than a general body massage but not so fast that you will lose control. On the back you can add percussion movements. Quite soon after you begin, the skin will begin to redden visibly as blood is pulled to the surface. Try to finish as closely as possible to the start of the race.

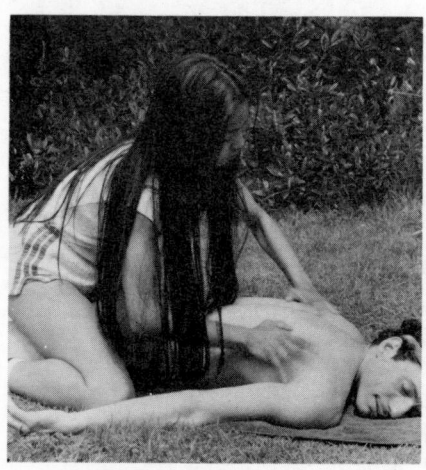

The common misapprehension that one can "work out" tension by exercising may account for the hordes of grimacing runners who seem to have invaded America's parks recently. Masseurs recognize that you cannot relax a tensed muscle by beating on it. If your partner's back feels rigid enough to bounce a ball on, the time has come to get serious about back massage. "The Back" chapter (see page 137) will supply more than enough technique to melt rock-hard backs. But if the tension your partner is experiencing seems

mild enough to permit exercise, you may want to consider the following movement. Since it can relax a large part of the body without oil, it can be used to introduce a friend to the massage experience just about anywhere.

Lean forward onto your forearm, pressing down hard along the two long muscle groups that run parallel to the spine. While you press, rotate your arms, or rub them back and forth so that all movement is beneath the skin. This movement is a giant friction stroke moving slowly against the whole length of these long muscles. That's often enough, by itself, to drain tension from the back and leave your partner feeling relaxed.

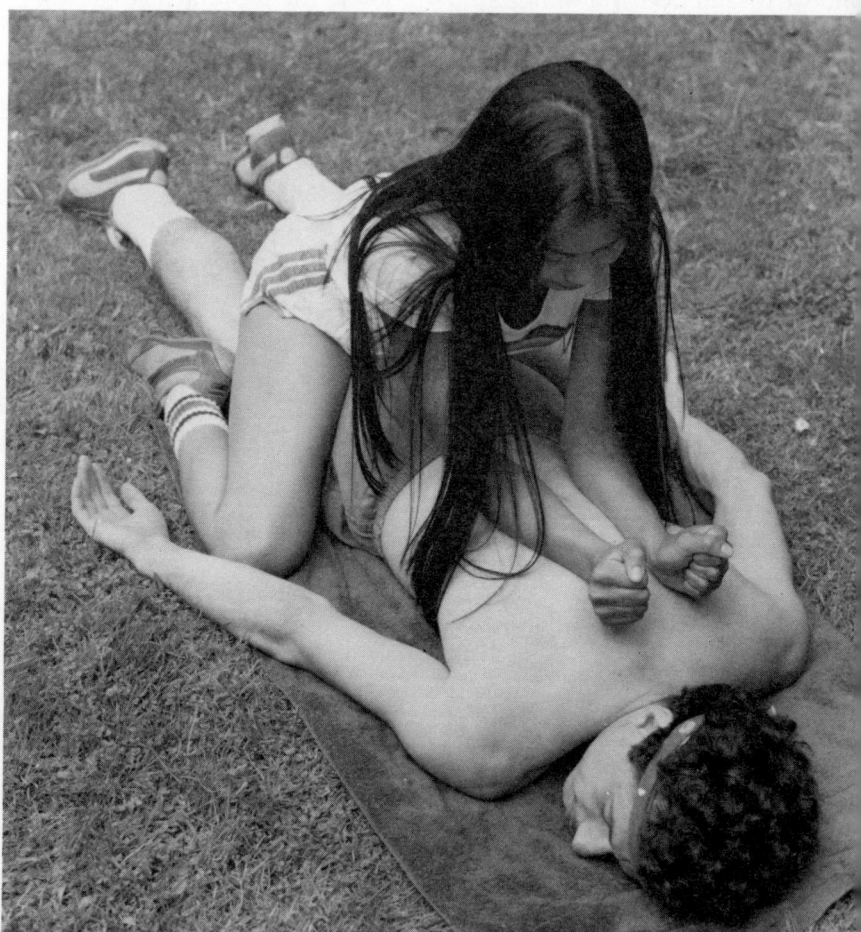

Massage is the original medical tool. A hundred years ago, when the words "massage" and "medicine" were nearly synonymous, detailed massage treatments for specific medical problems were in use throughout the world. At that time, most of the work in this field was done by physicians interested in developing therapeutic movements for a wide range of medical problems.

More recently the medical profession has all but abandoned the practice of massage. Antisensual conditioning, plus the irresistible temptation to prescribe one of the 40,000 drugs now available, seems to have freed doctors from the messy responsibility of actually touching their patients.

"Then too, there is the class of patient who likes massage, and who will fail to own up to recovery, lest, by doing so, he lose all excuse for continuation of the treatment. Massage treatment may thus create a chronic invalid and become a most pernicious form of self indulgence and sensuous enjoyment." *

The very powerful therapeutic potential of massage *has* managed to capture the imagination of certain amateur healers who have breathlessly announced to the world that ordinary massage movements are in the vanguard of alternative medicine. This much is known and can definitely be proved: No medical treatment is older and more thoroughly tested than massage. Have contemporary doctors became so alienated from the bodies of their patients that the practice of massage must be regarded as a medical alternative?

The basic premise in using massage as drugless (or rather predrug) therapy is that pleasure itself is therapeutic. For that reason, every correctly executed massage movement will help your partner. It's always best to massage the entire body and, while doing so, concentrate on the problem area. When a full body massage isn't possible, you can use the movements that follow to deal effectively with specific problems. If your partner is beginning an exercise program and is still basically out of touch with his body, these movements will ease the transition from a sedentary to an active life.

Remember that both massage and exercise can be regarded as drugless therapies. Your partner will get far more out of drugless therapy if he approaches the experience with a drug-free body.

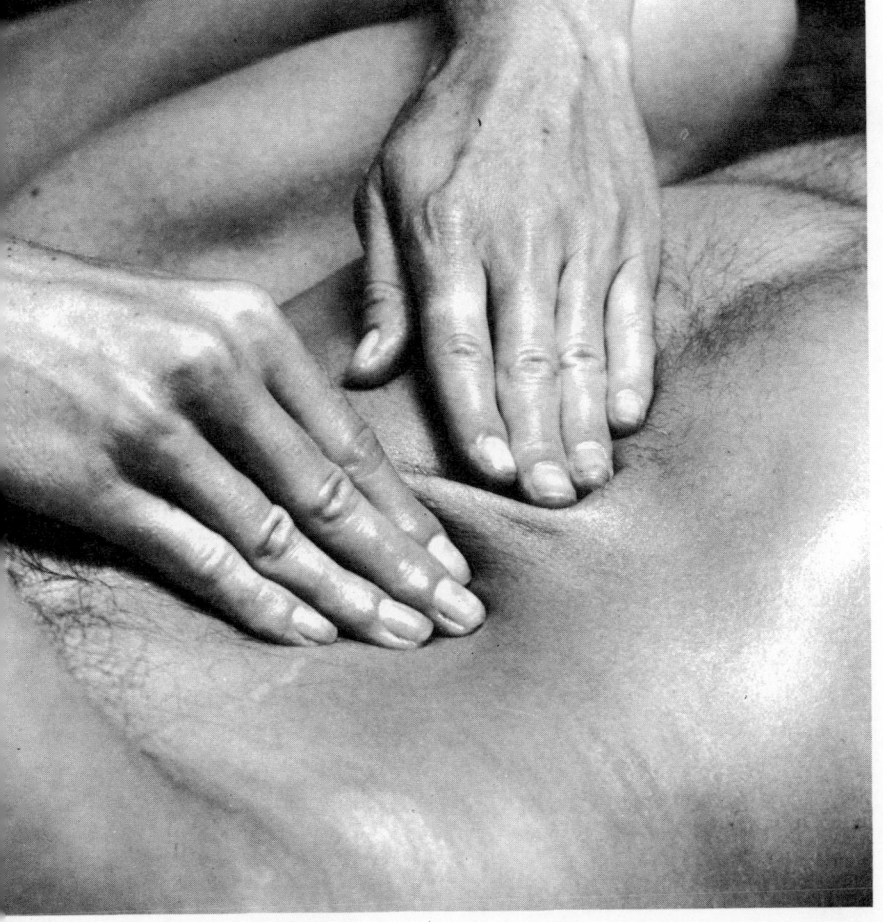

* James B. Mennell, *Physical Treatment by Movement, Manipulation, and Massage* (Philadelphia: P. Blakiston's Son & Co., Inc., 1934), p. 66.

People who begin to use massage as a therapeutic tool realize quickly that they have found a way to eliminate virtually all over-the-counter (and many pre-scription) drugs. Headaches, insomnia, nervous tension, stress, constipation, and all sorts of minor aches and pains respond to strokes that anyone can learn.

Despite the growing popularity of massage, every marathon sees runners suffering needlessly with simple muscle and joint problems that any masseur can deal with readily. It's pathetic to see a good runner collapse with a leg cramp while well-meaning friends advise him to "try to relax" and admonish each other not to touch the cramped leg. How many athletes with minor sprains double the necessary convalescent time by not allowing anyone to touch the sprain until it's completely healed?

Many internal injuries do, of course, require medical attention, and you should certainly see a doctor if you think you've hurt yourself badly. But in common runners' problems involving over-taxed or undersupplied muscles, you can use the massage techniques in this chapter to relieve your partner's suffering substantially.

Many of the same movements which are so valuable to runners who wish to improve their performances can be used to ease the pain of common athletic injuries. Movements in this chapter will show you how to deal with a wide range of problems from chilled muscles, which can usually be corrected in a single session, to muscle and fascia tears, which may require several weeks of daily massage before athletic activity can be resumed.

In almost every case the purely

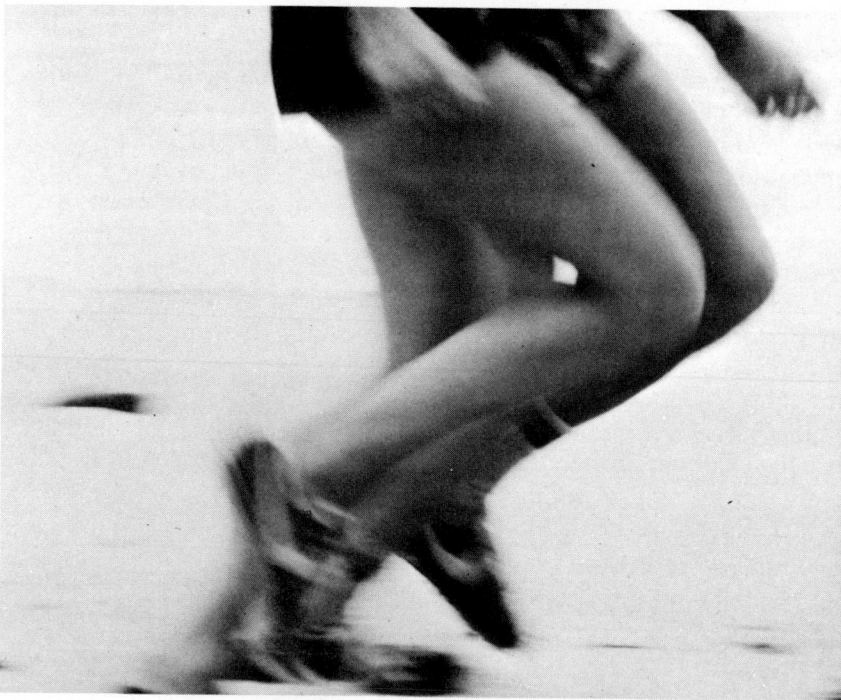

therapeutic effect of localized massage is close to astonishing. You can feel muscles soften while you work and actually see swelling begin to shrink. When muscles are torn or the lower back is badly wrenched massage can not only relieve your partner's suffering but actually shorten the usual recovery time by days or even weeks. No drug or combination of drugs can supply nutrition, remove metabolic wastes, and relax a muscle all at the same time. Greeks, Persians, Romans, and other pre-Darvon cultures certainly recognized this fact and used massage to enrich the lives of their athletes. There's no reason you can't do the same. Remember, too, that every injury brings with it a certain amount of stress.

Incapacitated people who are accustomed to leading active lives discover new things to worry about hourly. The inevitable nerve and muscle tension that results from all this worry will

readily dissolve if you incorporate the therapeutic techniques that follow into a full body massage. One of the nice things about being temporarily incapacitated with a sprain or wrenched back is that it allows people to justify spending the time to receive a complete body massage. Afterward it's usually quite some time before they can remember what they were worried about.

The first rule of massage is that you have to keep your partner warm. Remember that when you run, the body turns into a kind of furnace generating much more heat than usual. The movements in this chapter are designed to be used in the field to provide immediate relief, but there's an important consideration: You should never lay your partner down on a cold, damp surface after exercise. If it isn't at least 70 degrees Fahrenheit where you're exercising, it's best to hold off on the massage until you get indoors.

Including a partner in your exercise routine gives both of you a quick and effective way of dealing with muscle cramps. Muscles usually cramp (or spasm) when their blood supply is reduced or interrupted. A basic consideration in relaxing these muscles is simply the boosting of the blood supply to the area. This, of course, is familiar territory to masseurs. All the movements you've learned that supply nutrition to internal body tissues can be used to improve circulation around a cramped muscle. Begin by working directly on the muscle itself.

Although it's true that any muscle in the body can spasm, most sports-related cramps occur in the arms and legs. A cramped muscle is overcontracted, and it's always helpful to stretch it out while you massage. Stretching a cramped part of the body is certainly not like any other massage movement you've worked with in the "Full Body Massage" section (see page 38). When you stretch the muscle, there's lots of resistance, and it's necessary to hold the cramped muscle in a stretched position while you massage it. The best way to do this is to have a third person hold the limb in place while you concentrate on massage.

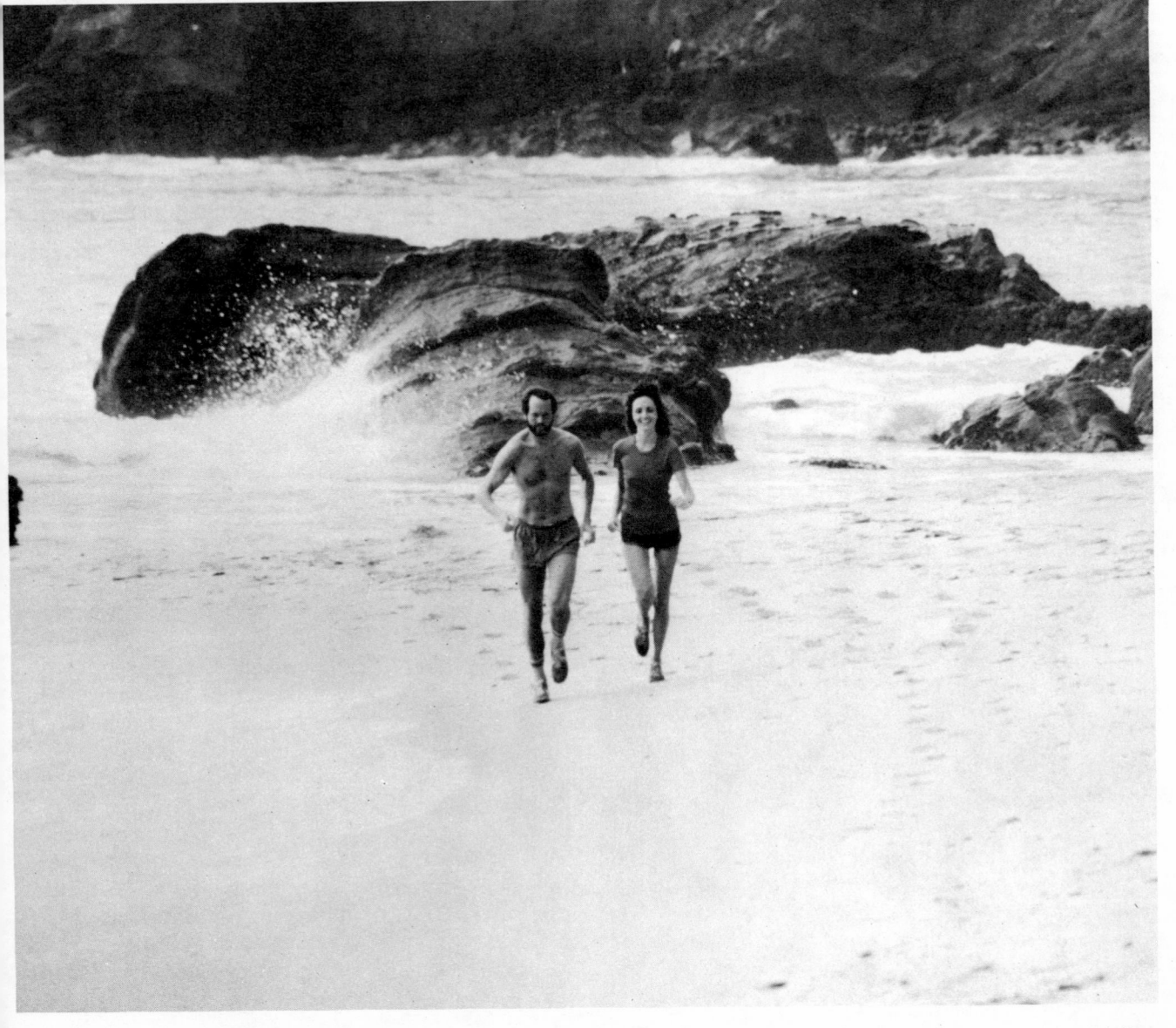

If you and your partner are alone, there are several ways to use your own body as a support for a cramped limb, thus freeing both your hands. Run through them a few times now, and when an emergency occurs, you'll be ready. Remember that panic is usually half the problem, and a cool head will help everyone stay calm.

Leg cramps are all too familiar to runners and dancers. A cramped calf can be stretched by bending the foot with your knee (as shown). This stretches the calf muscle into a position that resembles its relaxed state. Once you increase nutrition to the muscle, it will usually stay that way by itself. Oil the calf if oil is available. If there's no oil, let your hands slip a bit as you work so the skin isn't jerked around too much. Begin by vigorously knead-

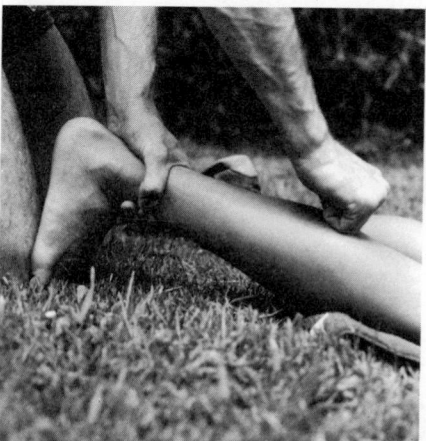

ing the calf (see page 130).

Kneading strokes directly over a cramped muscle should always be firm. Work up and down the leg moderately fast. The slow rhythms of a full body massage are not appropriate until the cramp relaxes. Alternating between full-hand kneading strokes and knuckle kneading (see page 135) will reach deep within the leg. Both these movements are penetrating. Combine them with a full-hand friction to the calf. When you feel the muscle beginning to relax, do fifty firm circulation strokes from the ankle to the lymph centers at the top of the leg. For some curious reason, pain can never be specifically recalled once it is over. By the time you reach the fiftieth circulation stroke your partner's cramped leg may be just a distant memory.

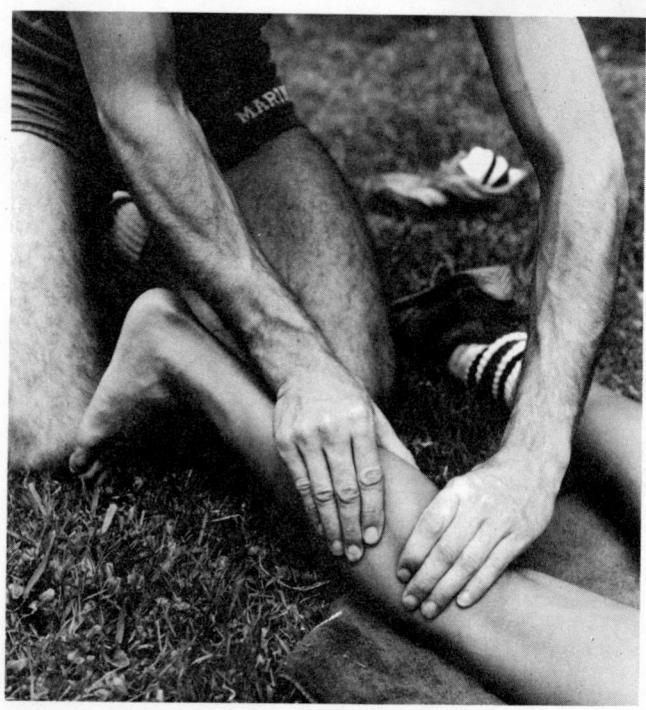

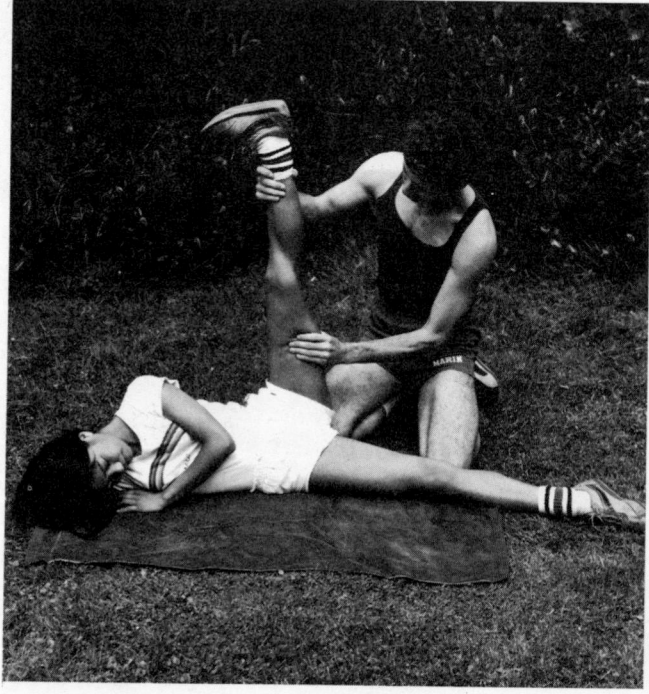

Depending on where an arm cramp occurs, you may want either to flex or to stretch the limb. If the cramp isn't serious, it may do simply to support the wrist with one hand while you knuckle knead the spasm with your free hand.

For bad cramps that require more intense massaging, you will need both hands. Your partner's arm can be easily supported by your kneeling across it (as shown). When you kneel, be sure

you don't come down on the arm with your knee, but rather, fit the arm snugly into the slight arc created by your foot and knee. This will easily hold the arm straight out while you knead up and down the tight muscles. The forearm can be steadied at the hand or wrist if the sprain is below the elbow.

After heavy exertion, racehorses are rubbed very vigorously away from the heart. The idea is to slow down the flow of blood and the heart itself. You can do this in humans as well as horses by literally pressing blood away from the heart. Runners and other athletes who have just completed a strenuous workout (like a race) may have pushed the heart just as far as it will go. Slow everything down by oiling the limbs and stroking rapidly away from the heart. Use the same cupped hand movement that works so well for ordinary circulation movements. Move quickly down all the limbs out toward the hands and feet. Pay particular attention to the legs because they hold a larger quantity of blood and carry it farther from the heart. Keep your partner warm and quiet while you stroke.

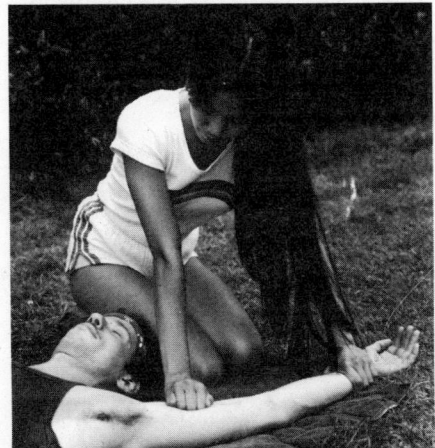

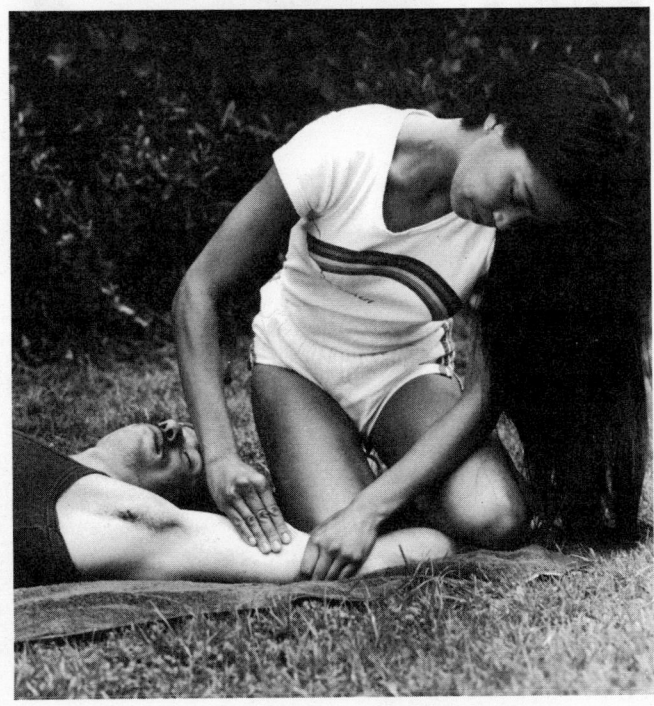

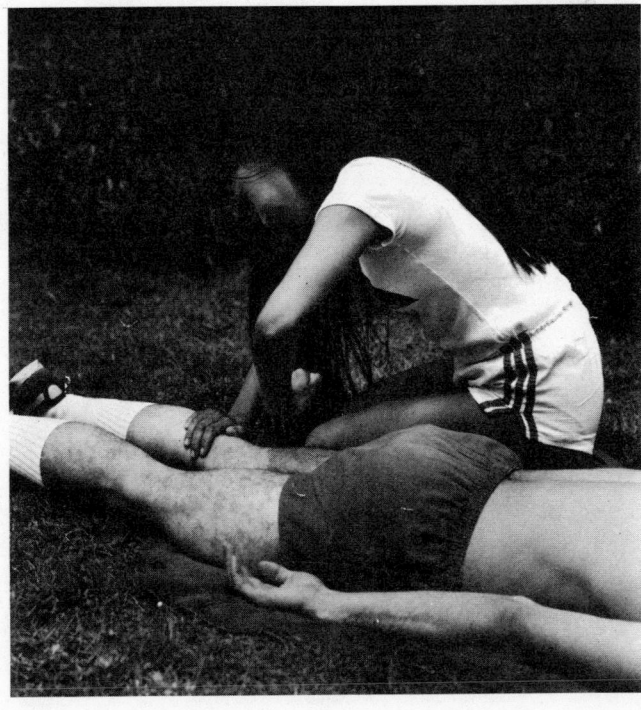

The muscular tension that occurs automatically when the body is chilled is a serious problem if your partner has been running in cold weather. Metabolic wastes which are normally excreted by the muscles are stored in the tissue sheets between muscle groups. When this happens, the fatigue that normally follows a long run is multiplied many times. Painful muscle cramps can ruin the day.

To warm your partner quickly, drape both legs with hot dry towels (see page 20). Remember that the towels need to be pre-heated for only about ten minutes. If you are far from home and hot towels, use massage to warm the body. If your partner's muscles are hard and unyielding,

begin by flexing the leg and rotating it at the hip joint. These movements will free crucial joints and allow you to begin on the leg itself.

Begin with a series of percus-

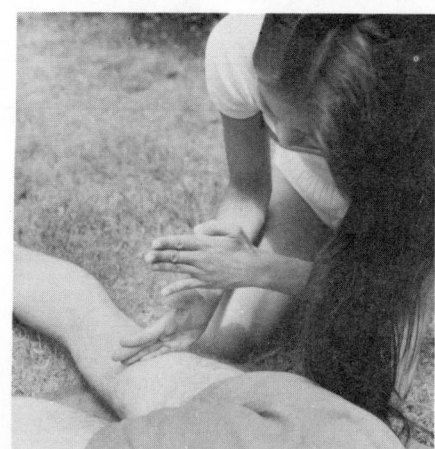

sion movements to stimulate your partner's leg muscles. Continue with at least twenty circulation movements (see page 130) to get the blood moving freely and to begin waste dispersion. Whenever you're working on chilled muscles, it's a good idea to encourage your partner to give you some feedback. After the circulation, move up and down the legs, alternating friction and kneading movements wherever they feel good to your partner. End with a series of at least six more circulation strokes to remove metabolic wastes which have been released by your massage.

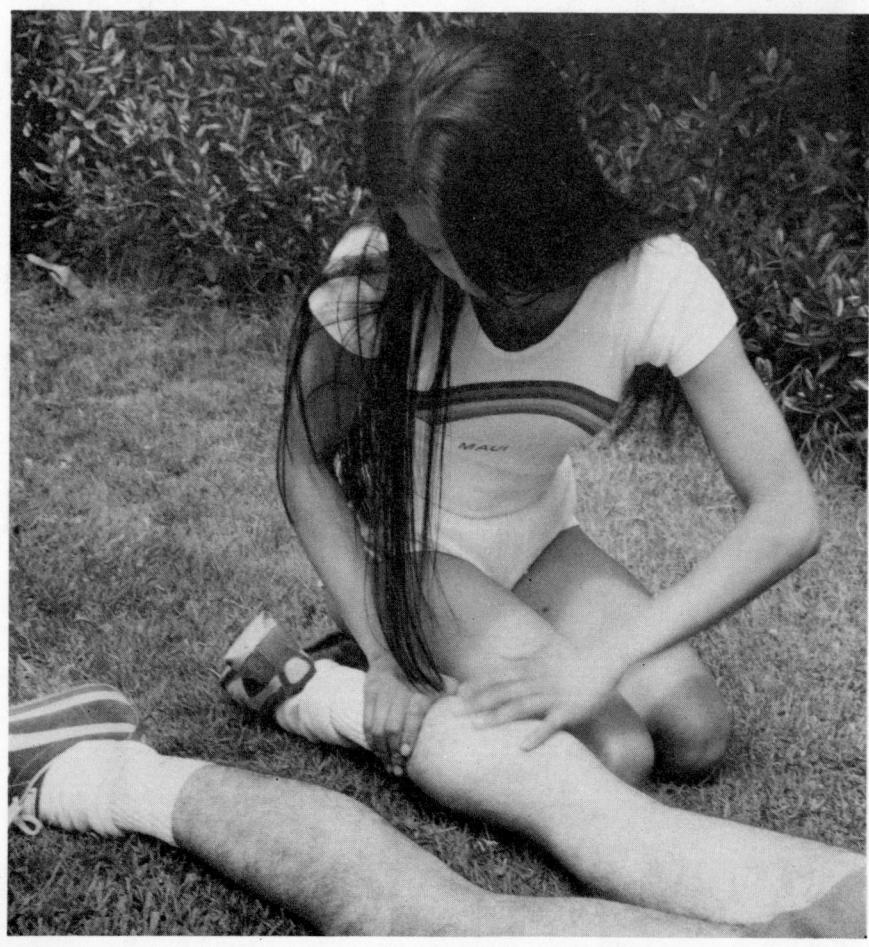

The lubricating fluid present at every joint in the body is normally replenished when the joint is used. One reason people who exercise move well throughout the day is that the joints are well

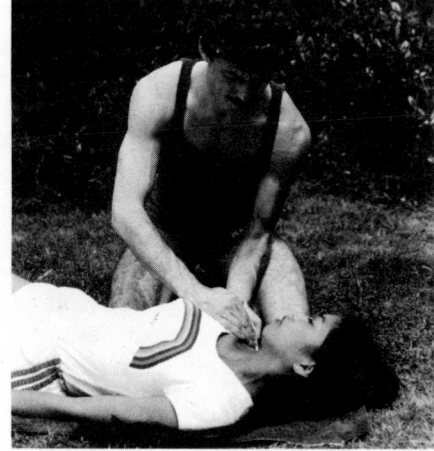

lubricated. After a serious injury like a broken bone, complete inactivity is forced on a part of the body while healing takes place. Depending on your partner's condition before the injury, healing will affect not only the muscle tone but the mobility of the affected joints. Unless the joint has been immobilized for a very long time, you can use massage to restore mobility and make it possible for your partner to begin exercising once again. Massage will provide a convenient bridge between total inactivity and vigorous exercise.

Friction movements coupled with rotation of the injured joint can usually begin just as soon as the bandages and cast come off. Because the range of possible injuries is so great, it's worthwhile here to point out that massage should be used on an injured person only after consultation with a physician. Remember to rotate only to the point of resistance; as soon as you feel tension or your partner experiences discomfort, back off just a bit. To stimulate the area thoroughly, you can work on it for fifteen minutes twice a day, alternating between fingertip kneading, friction, and rotation.

So many people begin exercise programs with the most fantastic expectations. They may have spent thousands of hours prone and motionless before the TV after fat-studded dinners. They may reach without hesitation, for uppers to get going, downers to relax, tranquilizers to stay cool, and sedatives to fall asleep. Still, these same sugar-thrilled snackers tremble with sweet excitement when the new jogging shoes with extra-wide marathon training heels and built-in arch supports are tested on the living-room rug. Somewhere deep inside, the white-hot primeval flame of physical fitness ignites.

Crossing and recrossing the living room, finally rushing out into the backyard and down the street, our new runner instantly joins ranks with the tanned well-jogged types who seem to radiate vitality and vitamin C. You can suddenly become attractive and popular. Next week you will feel like a million bucks. Complete strangers are going to be irresistibly drawn to you. These are not the claims of a new toothpaste, but rather just a few of the bizarre fantasies which are wrongly embraced by neophyte runners who want badly to soar effortlessly into the land of good health and good looks. How sad to watch them fall suddenly to earth just a few blocks from home when one of the beautiful new running shoes twists on some loose gravel underfoot. A few hours later, having abandoned the exercise route to salvation forever, we find our ex-runner sprawled, once again, in front of the TV with a sprained ankle.

Sprains, like torn ligaments, are often the result of poor training. Consequently, beginning athletes are frequent sufferers. No matter how carefully you organize and plan your exercise program, it can eventually result in a sprained muscle somewhere in the body. There is no reason to panic when this happens or to assume that a sprain has somehow negated the benefits of exercise. The discomfort of a sprain, as well as the sprain itself, is only temporary. Massage can be used to reduce substantially the convalescent period that follows:

Graham records patients with severe sprain under his care recovering the full use of the sprained joint in five days when massage was begun at once. In seven hundred cases of sprains and joint contusions treated by French, German, and Scandinavian army surgeons, comparative statistics reveal that we can reasonably expect that sprains treated by massage will recover in one-third the time that those will where the part is kept immobile. [*]

Most of the discomfort of simple sprains is caused by blood and other fluids that have moved into the area. If there's a great deal of pain, your partner may want to check with a doctor to be sure the tip of a bone has not been fractured. If not, you can begin massage immediately after the standard first-aid cold compress has been removed. Cold inhibits further swelling, while massage presses excess fluids out of the injured joint.

---

[*] Kathryn L. Jensen, *Fundamentals in Massage* (New York: Macmillan, 1932), p. 128.

Ankle Sprains: These sprains have a way of happening in inconvenient places, requiring your partner to walk right after an accident. If that seems necessary, it's worthwhile to consider supporting the ankle and foot with bandages until you get to a place where massage can begin. The sequence below, known as basket strapping, will also prevent your partner from aggravating a sprain between massage sessions. It's easy to learn and can be completed in a few minutes with the use of one-inch adhesive bandages.

Basket strapping

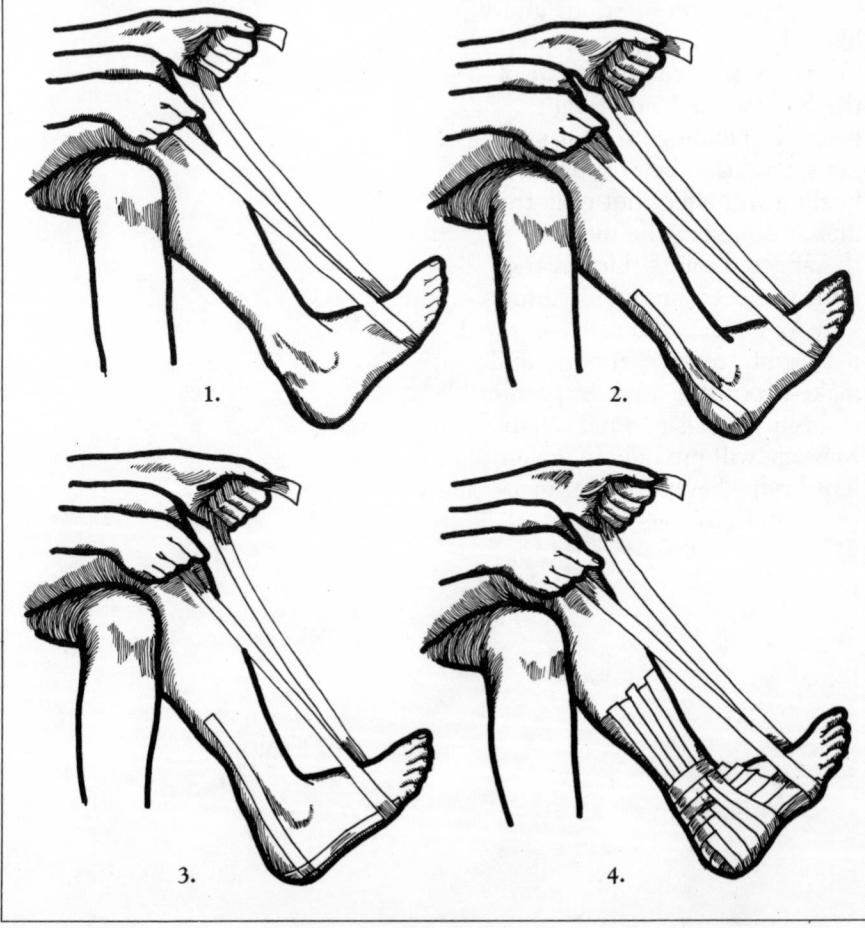

1.   2.   3.   4.

These bandages will give merciful support to the foot and ankle but should definitely be considered a temporary measure. Total support can begin to weaken the supporting structures of the foot after a time. Use basket strapping to get your partner back from the middle of a marathon or off to work the next morning. Bandages should be removed once a day during an extended ankle-and-foot massage and dispensed with as soon as possible.

Parallel fingertip kneading from ankle to knee works best for ankle sprains. Be sure to stay on the fleshy part of your partner's calf and off the bone. If the massage causes no pain, it can be followed by moderate active exer-

172

cises of the foot like walking or by passive exercises like foot rotation (see page 124). Again, feedback from your partner while you work with this sort of injury is particularly important. The feedback will help determine your pressures. Generally it's best to begin with light, gentle strokes. As the swelling recedes and the sprain begins to heal, your movements can become more vigorous. Ideally you should work on the sprain twice a day at first and then increase the frequency of your massage to three or four times a day as healing progresses.

Knee Sprains: Knee sprains always take longer to heal than ankle sprains. Bandages are used,

even in simple sprains, because the web of ligaments at the knee is so complex. Work with a medic, and learn exactly how to unwrap and bandage the knee before and after massage. Muscles around the knee are especially susceptible to atrophy if they are bandaged and kept immobile for long periods. Massage will strengthen these muscles and, of course, reduce swelling at the knee. Fingertip kneading (see page 000) in careful parallel lines on the back of the knee is particularly important. Follow the complete knee massage sequence in "The Front of the Legs" chapter (see page 103). End with friction to the appropriate lymph centers and a full leg circulation.

Shoulder Sprains: Unfortunately shoulder sprains are often aggravated by the movement of powerful muscles on the chest and back. There's no way to prevent this short of massaging the entire chest and back every time you work on the shoulders. It's much more work for you than a sprained ankle, but shoulder movements can be much more troublesome to your partner. It can help your partner relax if you heat the areas around the shoulders with hot towels or a heat lamp before you begin massage (see "Hot Towels," page 20).

Light parallel kneading strokes and friction work best here. Passive shoulder movements will help your partner regain mobility in the joint. Remember that the range of the shoulder joint is often much smaller on older people. If there's discomfort during your passive exercise of the joint, it's best to stop. Get feedback from your partner, and be especially sensitive to the point of tension in the arm when you turn it. Work just a bit farther inside that point than you would during ordinary massage. As in all sprains, stroking toward the heart away from the injury will loosen adhesions and prevent the formation of fibrous deposits during the healing process.

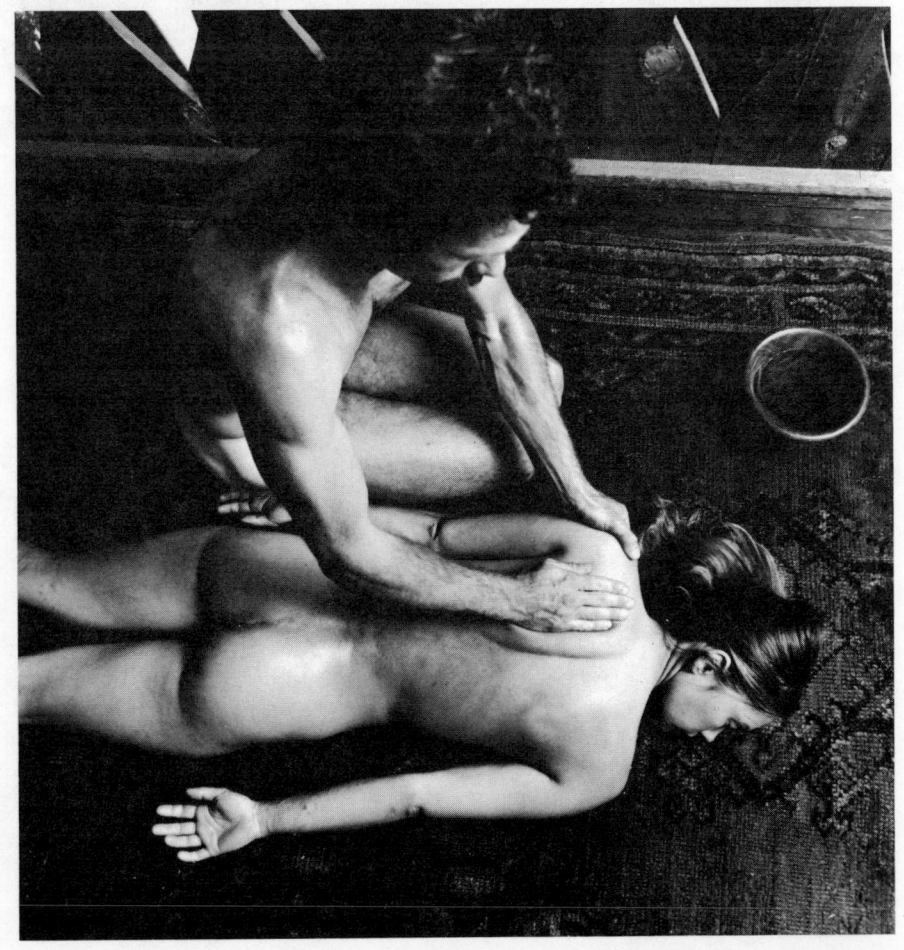

In a number of sports, a practiced flick of the wrist at exactly the right moment will accomplish far more than a simple lunge at the ball with the whole arm or body. Unfortunately those not accustomed to flicking the wrist often tend to flick the entire forearm instead.

While your partner is relearning the correct way to hold a golf club, tennis racket, or bowling ball, you can be massaging the overstretched tendons of the forearm. All these tendons begin at the elbow and should be massaged down from the point of insertion all the way to the hand. Since the elbow joint is so well defined, it's easy to feel the tendon insertion point when you're kneading. But because some of the tendons that begin at the back of the elbow sweep around and *under* the tendons of the front of the arm, it's best to work on both sides of the forearm whenever a tendon is pulled. Begin by clearing the lymph nodes at the top of the arm (see page 61), and follow that stroke with at least ten circulation movements for the entire arm (see page 68).

Once you've stimulated circulation throughout the arm, you're ready to begin fingertip kneading the overstretched tendons. Begin at the elbow, and work down toward the wrist slowly. Pick up the tendons with your fingertips as you work. If the strain seems to be on the back or bone side of the forearm, remember to raise the arm over your partner's head to make that side of the arm more accessible. Knead up and down the arm ten times twice a day. Keep your rhythms slow and steady, and finish with friction movements to the lymph centers at the top of the arm.

Runners and other athletes who push themselves too much are often victimized by muscles that simply refuse to relax. Not even the most devoted marathoner wants to take rock-hard legs to bed. Muscle hardening is not always caused by overexercise. Badly fitted shoes can put an excessive strain on certain foot and leg muscles. Poor posture will create extra work for runners. In addition, past injuries to the spine and feet can cause athletes to favor certain muscles. Whatever the cause, muscle hardening comes about through habitual overexertion of the affected muscles.

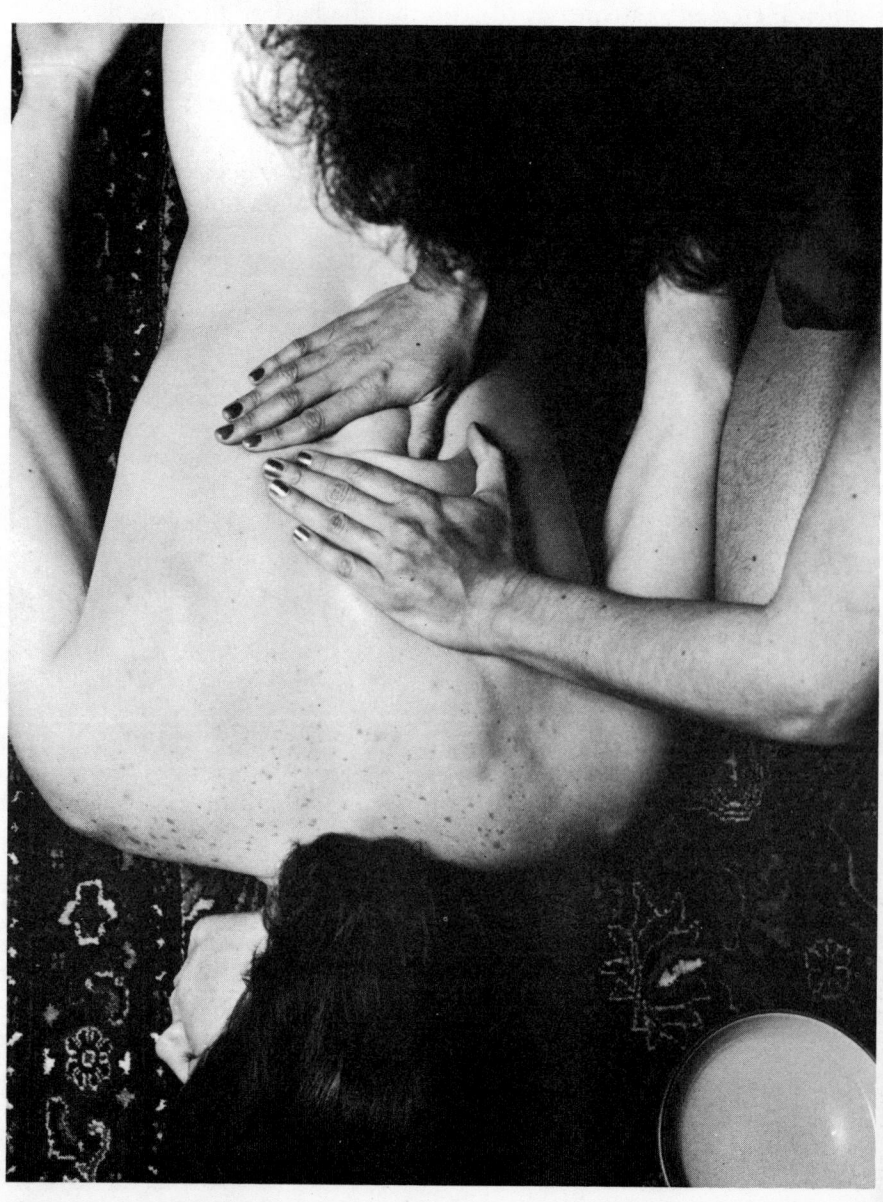

Muscle rolling, loose finger kneading (see page 52), and friction (see page 44), followed by ten circulation movements (see page 156), will generally have dramatic results on hardened muscles. You can often feel your partner's muscles begin to relax as wastes are dispersed and internal circulation is restored. Use firm pressures, and keep your rhythm steady and even. When you're dealing with hardened muscles, be extra sure your massage area is at least 75 degrees Fahrenheit because all muscles will contract when they're chilled.

Prompt medical attention is always necessary when muscles or ligaments are torn. If the muscle is completely severed, surgery is called for right away. Unless there has been a particularly violent-ski accident, it's likely that torn muscles will involve merely the wearing of cumbersome bandages around the shoulder or knee for a few weeks. Treatments vary depending on the severity of the injury, but once the affected part is wrapped with an elastic bandage, careful daily movement and massage will greatly accelerate the healing process. Begin massage as soon as bruised tissues are healed.

When you're massaging around an injury, always be very careful not to cause pain. Feedback from your partner is particularly important, and signs of tenderness should warn you to work a bit farther from the tear. As healing progresses, you can gradually move in closer without causing pain. Gentle fingertip kneading and pressing movements above and below the tear usually work best.

Tears usually happen when poorly coordinated muscles are unexpectedly contracted. The more a dancer or athlete trains, the less likely he is to tear a muscle. Neglecting warm-ups, intense fatigue, and severe chilling during exertion will increase the possibility of a tear. When all three of these careless practices are combined, a dancer or runner is almost inviting some kind of serious problem. At how many marathons have you seen runners who have never attempted twenty-six miles push themselves beyond all reason in the worst kind of weather? These are the runners who frighten novices away from marathon running and keep the medical crews busy all day.

By 50 everyone has the face he deserves.
—GEORGE ORWELL

Because the primary aim of massage is relaxation, the close relationship between stress and illness is of special interest to masseurs. Since the blood supplies nutrition to every part of the body, anything that interferes with blood circulation will damage the entire body. That's why the characteristic venous and arterial shrinking called vasoconstriction, which occurs during stress, is so dangerous. This condition not only forces the heart to work much harder but decreases the supply of nutrients to every part of the body. The familiar bloodless, utterly pale appearance of shock victims provides an extreme example of the outwardly visible effects during stress.

Beneath the skin these effects are just as apparent and often quite devastating. Breathing becomes rapid and shallow; digestion, slow and incomplete. Every body process is degraded. Blood pressure rises, and ultimately the oxygen supply to the brain itself is decreased so that judgment and thought become erratic. That millions of people are now accustomed to living with intense stress is tragically evident in yearly figures which reveal the same grim fact: The three major causes of death in the United States all involve the circulatory system.

Perhaps because of the increased adrenaline flow during stress, the condition is addictive, and some people actually seem to seek it out. There is a peculiar kind of anxiety that seems to characterize certain high-powered types who operate as though anxiety plus pressure equals meaning. Exercise alone doesn't always accomplish much for these people simply because it becomes yet another competitive event. If they exercise alone, they will compete against yesterday's score, distance, or time—exercise followed by stress.

After a while the effects of stress are cumulative, and parts of the body begin to carry tension from day to day. This phenomenon, labeled body armor by Reichian psychologists, simply means that tension has been stored in the muscles for so long that the muscles seem to freeze. Shoulders that tighten up under pressure begin to tighten up every morning automatically. The bloodless complexion that accompanies great stress yields to a kind of permanent pallor.

Finally, the face itself seems to freeze, and people actually lose the ability to smile. What was once an easy natural grin becomes a grotesquely twisted sort of leer. Even worse, after some rubbery contortion that passes for a smile, the mouth seems unsure which expression to assume next and may flicker through a half dozen mood changes before returning to a "normal" state so rigid it would look contrived on the face of a mannequin. Once established, all these unhappy effects seem terribly permanent.

But the effects of body armor are not permanent and will gradually yield to skillful massage. This means that not only can you change the way people feel, but you can sometimes actually change the way they look. One of the great joys in massage is watching your partner regain the use of his very own smile. Throughout the body, the effects of body armor are visible and offer masseurs valuable clues. They can be used to localize and reduce the debilitating effects of stress.

Body armor, of course, is only a surface indication of internal stress. Decreasing stress levels throughout the body allows your partner to experience his body in its natural state—a rare experience to be sure—and a powerful antidote to the anxiety habit. In the "Full Body Massage" section of the book you learned to increase circulation without speeding up the heart. Massaging overstressed individuals, you can go one step farther and actually increase circulation *while you slow the heart* (see "Heart Massage," page 151). Combine pressing movements on each limb with heart massage and general back strokes.

If your partner has a cold, you can use this movement to reach beneath the ribs and vibrate the lungs. It will break up congestion and boost internal respiration, the process in which carbon dioxide is traded for oxygen in the lungs. In the back massage chapter you learned to reach the heart via certain nerves. This movement will go directly to the heart and actually shake it.

Position the flat part of your elbow, not the point, over the center of your partner's back. Be sure to stay off the spine with this movement. Other than that, you can move around the back freely, aiming your percussion effect with your elbow. Strike the heel of your hand with your free fist. One to two blows per second are about right. Speed is not nearly as important as pressure. This is a very powerful movement. Start lightly, get some feedback from your partner, and build up slowly to a pressure that feels good.

It is astonishing how quickly relief and sleep can be effected to seemingly sleepless patients. Time and again I have been called in the middle of the night by men of high standing and great mind. Indeed, during my practice in Washington I frequently had to shut off the light in the White House, telling the officers at the door, as I left, that the President was asleep.
—HARTVIG NISSEN, *Practical Massage and Corrective Exercises*

If insomnia is merely a state of mind, it is hardly alleviated by sleep-aid commercials which are strategically aired just after the eleven o'clock news. Whether the source of your partner's anguish is personal or commercial, persistent worry will soon register as persistent nerve and muscle tension. Masseurs generally seek to go around the source of anxiety and work to quiet the mind by relaxing the body.

Massage-induced sleep is usually so profound that people in it seldom move at all. It is difficult to imagine anything sadder than an insomniac who has just been awakened after a massage and asked to move to a bed. Insomniacs (or anyone else you want to put to sleep) should be massaged on the exact spot where you expect to find them the next morning.

Unless there is a specific problem area like sore feet or a stiff neck, it's usually best to concentrate on your partner's back. By relaxing the muscles around the spine, you reach the trunk of the entire nervous system. A good bit of the tension insomniacs experience is often localized in the rows of muscles that parallel the spine and in the large muscle group that spreads across the shoulders.

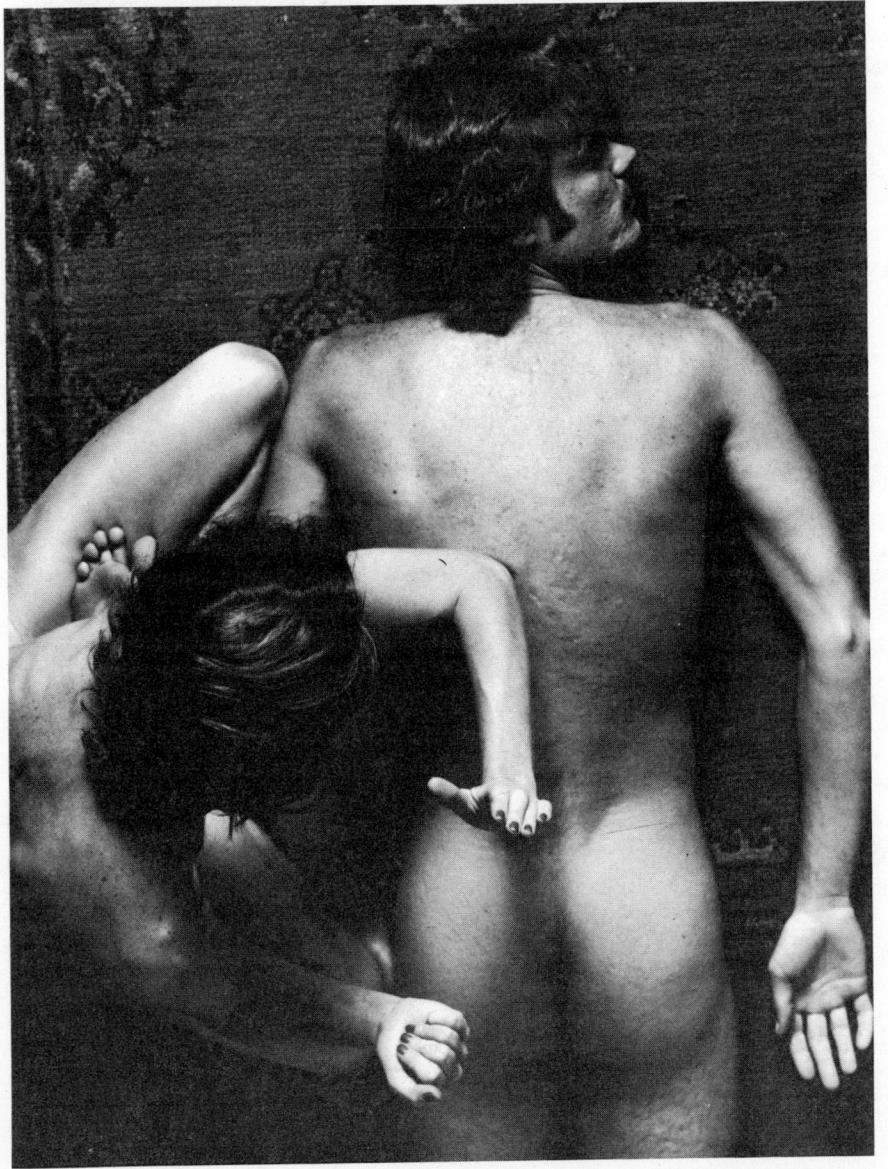

Relaxing these muscles soothes the nervous system.

The magnificent long relaxation stroke for the back (see page 140) repeated 100 times at the same speed is very often enough by itself to do the job. If there are still signs of wakefulness after this movement, continue by kneading the long muscles that parallel the spine (see page 146). Follow the general outline for a complete back massage, but concentrate on the spine, the shoulders, and the base of the neck. It's also helpful to watch your partner's breathing and to pay particular attention to movements that seem to deepen respiration.

Be sure to cover your partner afterward, ventilate the room, and remove yourself quietly. Like the chemical sleep aids, massage is somewhat habit-forming. Expect to be asked back by a most grateful friend.

Regular massage will lower stress levels and can virtually transform the lives of hypertension victims. On your first massage concentrate for a few minutes on the abdominal area. Vigorous kneading over this part of the body will drop your partner's blood pressure by about ten millimeters right away. Then, as you continue with the rest of the body, use light pressures on the far ends of the limbs. Too much pressure here will bring the blood pressure back up again very quickly. People who suffer from hypertension are under constant stress and should seriously consider making massage a permanent part of their lives. Even if this means hiring a professional masseur, the cost, in the long run, will be far less than the teams of specialists who prescribe terrifying drugs and hope for the best.

If your partner's blood pressure problem hasn't become so serious that drugs are the only solution, you may wish to explore this twenty-minute massage "prescription" developed many years ago by Dr. H. V. Barclay of New York:

Begin with your partner lying on his back and elevate the shoulders with a small pillow. The head and neck will fall back slightly. This will passively stretch the upper torso muscles. Every sequence should be repeated at least three times.

Work up and down both sides of the throat with a very light circular friction movement, then knead the upper part of both arms. When you're kneading the arms be sure to cover the fleshy sides as well as the biceps on top. Use the flat part of your hands to stroke out from the middle part of the abdomen to the sides of the torso. Work up and down the abdomen until you have covered both sides at least three times. This brings massive amounts of blood to the large abdominal veins without straining the heart the way overeating does.

When you've finished with the abdomen have your partner lie on his left side facing you and pull the right arm directly over his head. The arm should be perfectly straight and not bent at the elbow. Bend your partner's hand backwards and hold it in place with one hand. Use your free hand to do a circular compression movement from the shoulder to the wrist. Be careful not to use too much pressure over visible veins. Once you've covered the entire arm three times lift it with both hands and set it down straight out under your partner's chin. This stretches the extensor muscles while you knead from the center of the back all the way down to the hand. Finally, raise the arm over the head once again and knead the lower back down to the spine.

Bend the right knee well up against your partner's body and knead the buttocks and back of the thigh. Pull the leg backward and knead the front of the thigh. Bend the knee and knead the front of the leg. Straighten the leg, bend the foot and do one hand compression on the calf.

Have your partner turn over onto the right side and repeat the entire procedure.

When you've finished both sides of the body have your partner lay flat on his stomach and end with friction movements up and down the back. Concentrate on the muscles near the spine.

Appendix

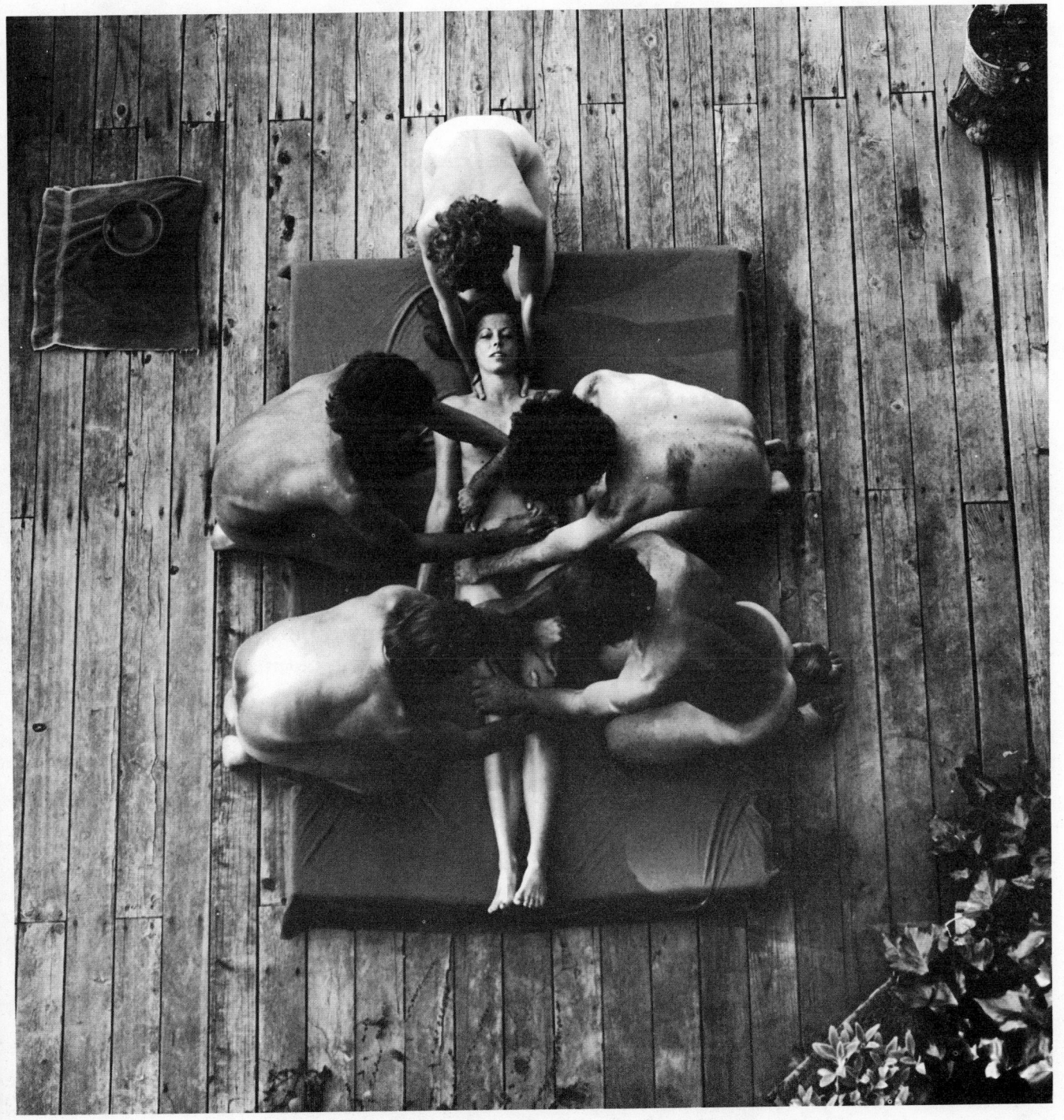

Appendix

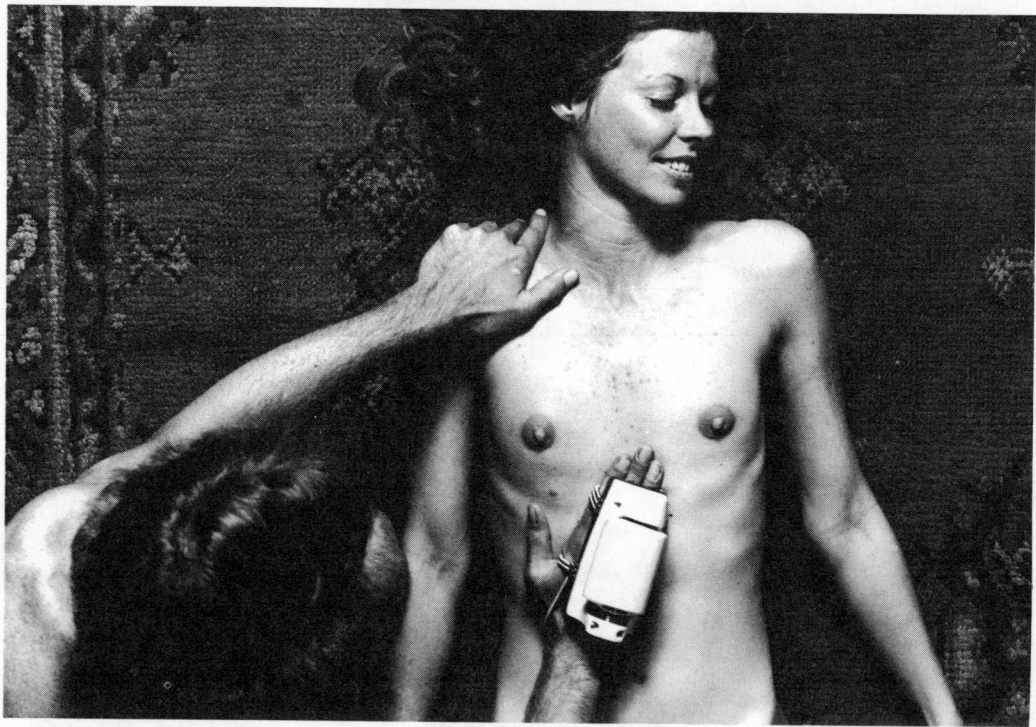

Not 1 person in 10,000 has been massaged by 9 people at once. That situation has simply got to change. Once you have been through this utterly delicious experience, it seems difficult to believe that anything in life could possibly be more important. If this book accomplishes nothing else, I would hope to convince the reader and a few friends to try an evening of group massage sometime soon.

Does it seem strange to imagine groups of diplomats massaging each other? Senators? Generals? In what impossibly futuristic society will we see group massage integrated as a social form along with cocktail parties, dances, weddings, and graduations (your first group massage)? Unlike cocktail parties, where alienation is always in the air, dances with their inevitable wallflowers, weddings where jealousy threatens to

spoil the day, and graduations where somebody doesn't graduate, everybody gets just what he wants out of a group massage. Even if you're not the one receiving the massage this time, your turn cannot be far off. Your immediate reward will come when you see your partner's face assume the kind of expression usually reserved for saints and swamis.

The maximum number of people who can massage together is usually about nine—"usually," because human beings come in a great many sizes and not as many large ones will fit around a very small one. The minimum number for group massage is, of course, two. You see five in the photographs simply because that number is a kind of happy medium and convenient for small parties. For the most part, though, nine is about the limit.

Nine People with Four Hot Towels and Three Electric Vibrators

Nine people massaging together are almost always tempted to speak at some point. Music will distract your partner from inadvertent conversation and the occasional sound of bodies thumping about. It will also relax everyone doing the massage. If you're using a cassette or record player, one of the group should be ready to make changes on the machine when necessary. You might want to scent your massage area before you begin and arrange things so that there are no interruptions from the outside world.

Like many other group activities, group massage requires a certain amount of organization so that traffic jams do not develop. The sequences and body assignments that follow will help prevent confusion while the nine of you are massaging. Still, they are merely suggestions. You may have your own ideas about this sort of thing, and of course, you and your friends are free to roam about the body at will. Do try to stay in rhythm and stick with your territory until somebody else has taken over.

Nine people equals eighteen hands and ninety fingers. When was the last time you were massaged by ninety fingers? These ninety-finger massages are truly smashing gifts and should definitely be considered for your next special occasion. It's all the better if the nine of you get a chance to rehearse a bit first.

The best way to begin a group massage is simply to assign different parts of the body to different people. If everyone sticks with his area for a while, every part of your partner's body that is facing the nine of you will get massaged simultaneously. Two people can massage the legs from just below the knees to the toes, and two people concentrate on the legs above the knee, working from the waist to the knees. Two people sit on either side of the chest, massaging from the neck to the waist. One person massages each arm, working from the fingertips to the shoulder, and one person works on the head.

Two or three plastic squeeze bottles can easily be shared when you oil your partner. Remember to squirt the oil into your palms, not directly onto your partner's body. Begin by oiling your partner's entire body, and try to keep your squeeze bottles handy. Massage by nine people means that oil will be picked up continually, and it will probably be necessary for some of you to add oil from time to time. If a plastic squeeze bottle isn't nearby, you can always get somebody's attention by simply tapping an arm or leg. Whether it's an oil bottle, a towel, or a brush that you want to locate, try to do it without speaking. Occasionally these objects are placed out of reach, and you may have to break contact momentarily to reach for one. That leaves eighty fingers still working while you're gone.

Once you all have oiled your partner, it's easy to go on to simultaneous electric vibration, kneading, and friction movements for the entire body. This is probably not the place to argue the case for owning more than one vibrator. If you have nine friends who are interested in massage, the chances are good that you can come up with several vibrators for group sessions. Try to keep your power cords out of the way. This usually means several electric outlets or extension cords near your massage area. Checking the location of your oil, towels, and vibrators before you begin group massage is particularly important if you want to avoid confusion later.

Group massage will use all the movements in a full body massage. The difference here is that many of these movements happen at once. Even when nine people work together, it's still possible to coordinate things so that your partner will experience specific waves of sensation all over the body. Sometimes it helps to have one person in the group act as an informal sort of leader. A leader can begin and end movements like percussion, kneading, and circulation that can be copied everywhere on the body. This is certainly not to suggest that group massage must become a close-order drill. Your partner will not want to miss the utterly random feeling of nine different sensations happening at once.

Although one person can lift another, there's no way to support every part of the body while lifting. Arms and legs hang down and pull at the joints. Unless there's a big difference in size, the situation is often unsteady, even dangerous. Nine people have the advantage of being able to lift one person while simultaneously supporting every part of the body. The person being lifted feels utterly secure and will gratefully surrender to the joys of group massage afterward. In fact, once you have been lifted this way, you may wonder where these nine people have been all your life.

Every group massage should begin with one of these magnificent lifts. Lifters should keep their fingers together, attempt to be silent, and work in unison. Be sure that the people on the torso are strong enough to support it.

They will have the most weight to bear. Five people should position themselves and lift as in the diagram. Come up slowly, stay together, and be ready to turn your hands as you lift. When you begin the lift, your fingers will be facing away from you. As you press your partner up over your head, let your hands turn slowly until the fingers come all the way around and point toward you. If you aren't lucky enough to have nine people on hand, try the following positions which work well with smaller groups:

Eight. Changes from nine below the waist. Two people lift from the thigh, contacting the legs at the hip joint and just below the knee. One person stands at the feet, facing the head, and lifts the lower legs just above the ankle. Let the knees bend just a bit.

Seven. Changes from six below the waist. Two people stand at the knees and lift the legs at the calf and at the thigh.

Six. Changes from five below the waist. One person stands at the feet, facing the head, and lifts both legs above the ankles. Allow the knees to bend slightly.

Five. See photos.

Four. Changes from five at the head. Let the head fall back slowly as you lift.

Three. Changes from five at the head and below the waist. One person stands at the feet, facing the head, and lifts the legs

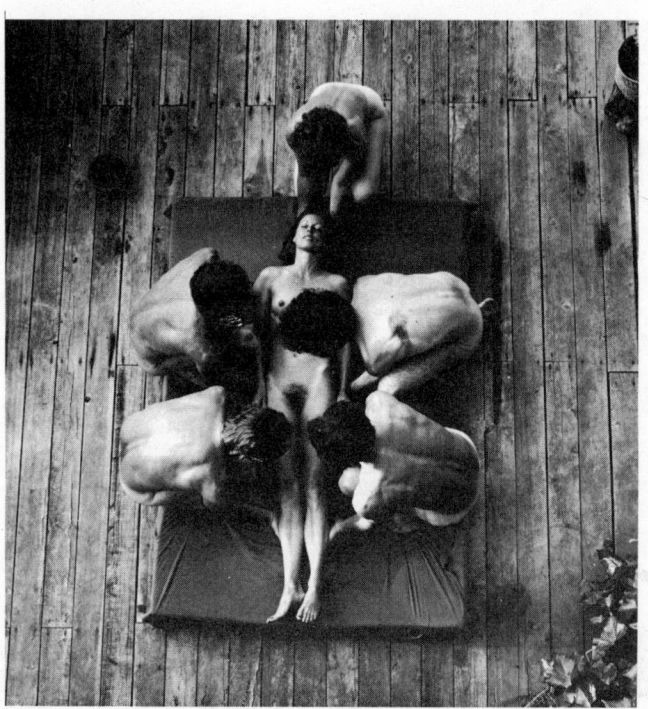

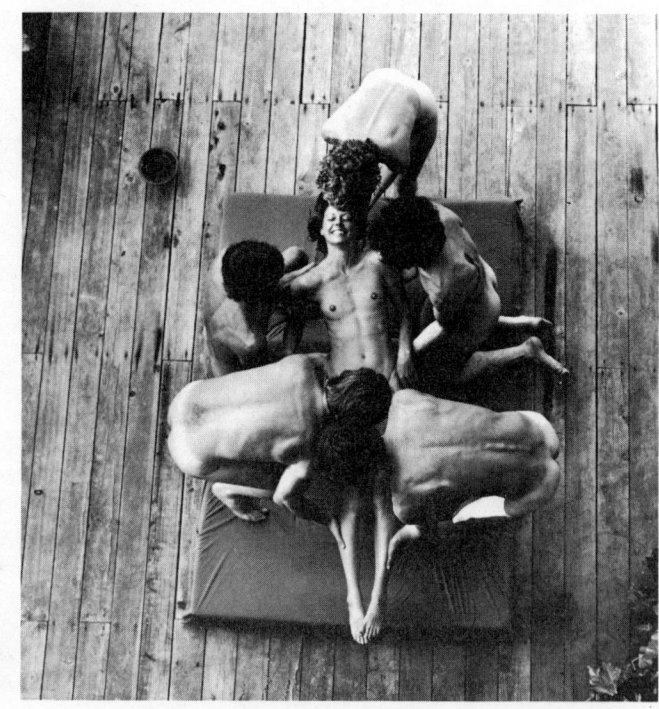

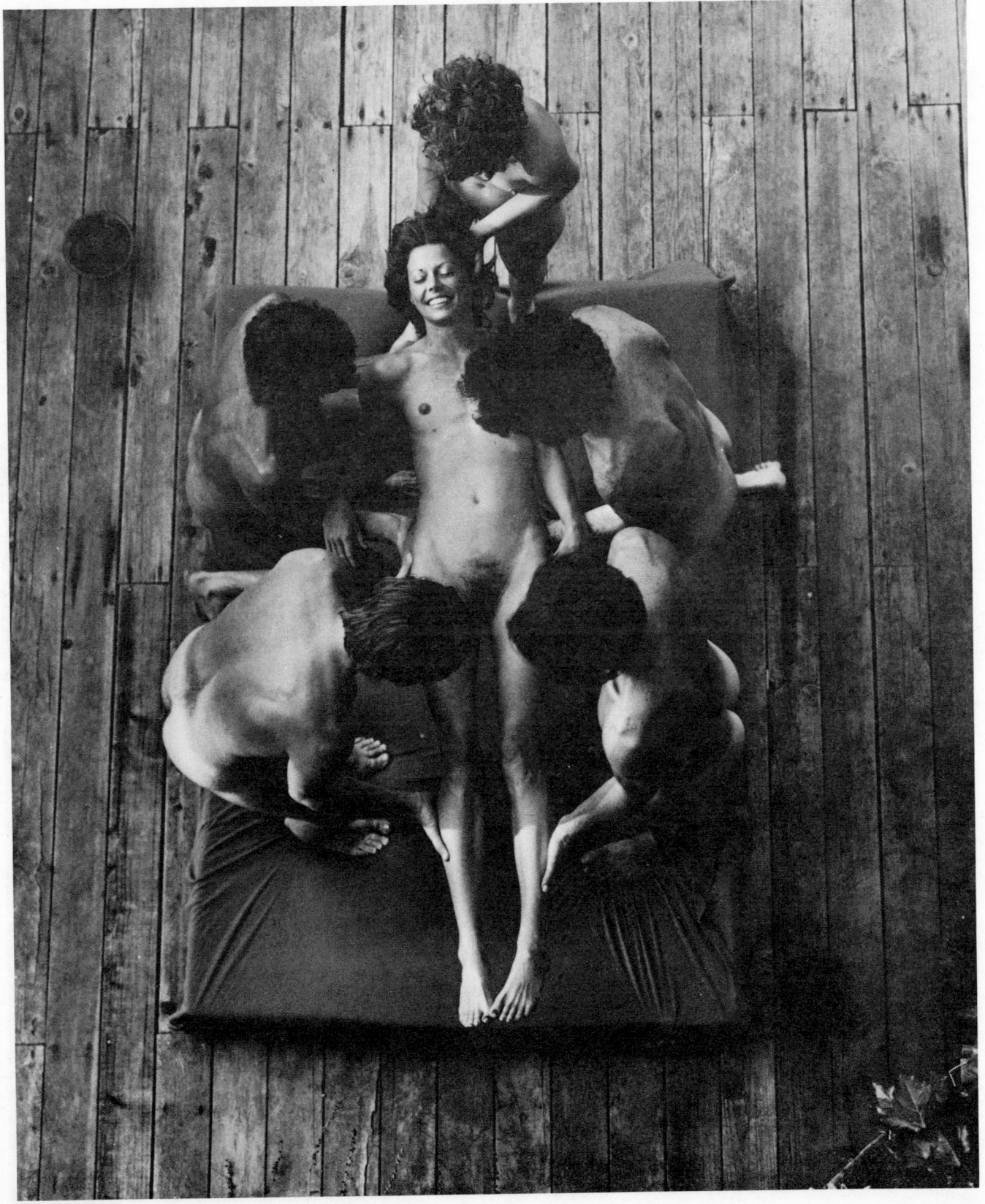

just above the ankles. Be sure to allow the knees to bend slightly if possible. Be sure that the three of you are strong enough to lift smoothly. If you're not, get help, and see above.

Two. Each of you should be strong enough to lift your partner alone. That way, if one of you slips or stumbles, the other can give the necessary support. Lift at the rib cage and at the hip joint

or, if you're not interested in pressing above your head, at the rib cage and behind the knee.

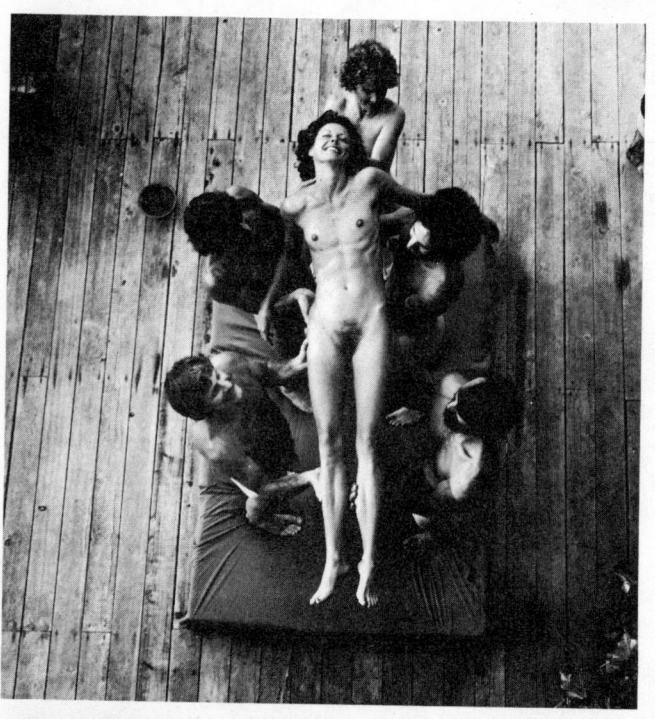
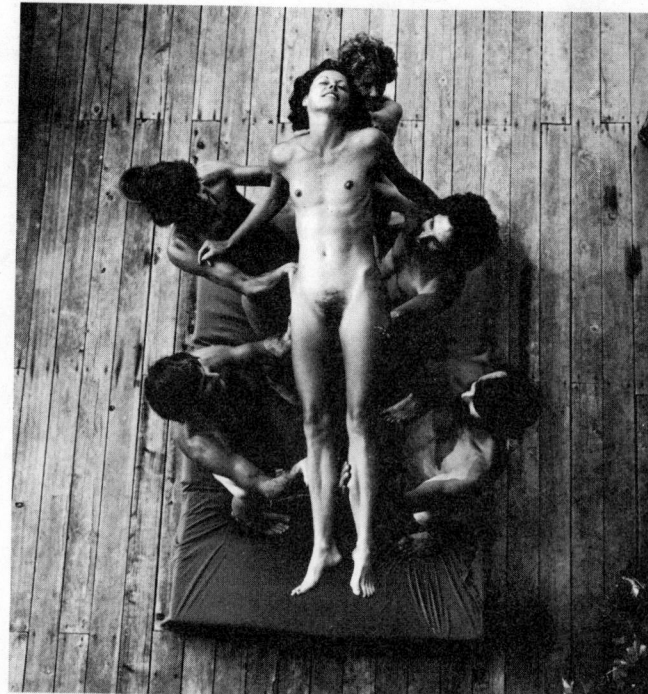
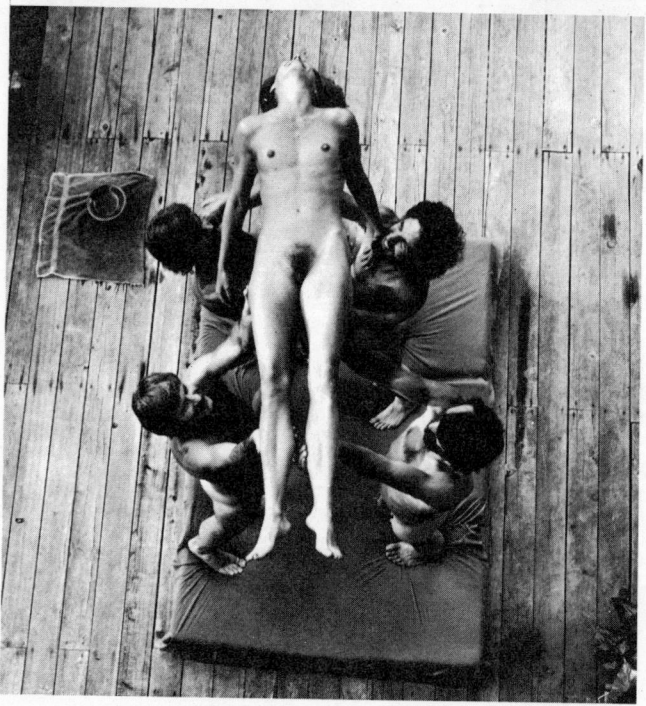
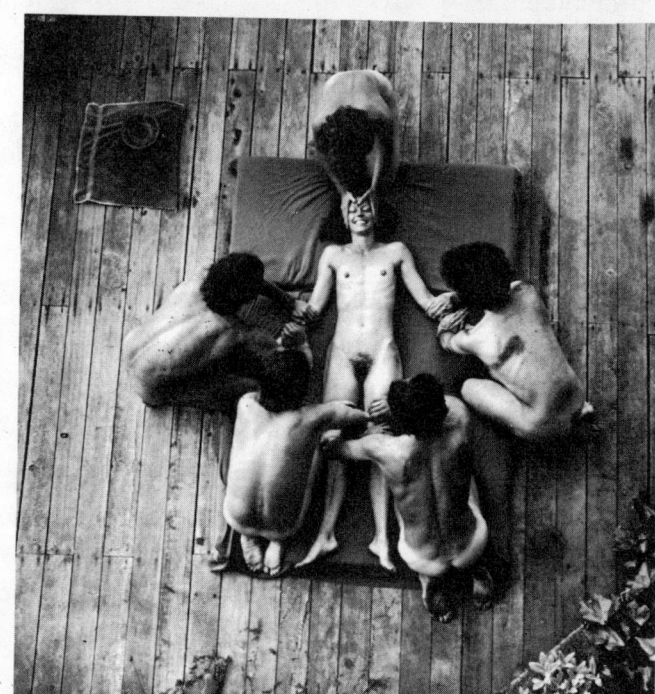

Pedicure was immensely popular in ancient Rome, the world's last great civilization that really appreciated the toe. Since it's easy to spend several minutes on each toe, a pedicure should be either treated as a separate experience from a full body massage or incorporated into group massage. The procedure combines beneficial health aids with optional nail painting, a beauty treatment that has no practical value. Unlike massage, pedicure *is* something you can do for yourself. Most people, however, have never spent twenty minutes on their toes, and that's why a first pedicure can be very satisfying.

Pedicure always begins with a foot bath. If you're using a bath table, simply concentrate on the feet for a few minutes with loofah, sponge, and towel. Otherwise, foot bathing can easily be improvised without resort to a full bathtub or shower. Lift your partner's calves with a large pillow, and place each foot to be bathed over a large pot or enameled bowl. Use a flexible bath hose or a damp sponge to rinse the foot with warm water. Since the skin on the bottom of the foot is the thickest anywhere on the body, a loofah or brush will be far more stimulating than a soft cloth. Don't be afraid to use plenty of pressure. You can always see dirt that ordinary bathing has failed to remove. Wrinkle marks left by nylon socks and high-fashion shoes are usually quite apparent. Rhythmic scrubbing will remove all the dirt and restore the foot's natural complexion.

Use your free hand to support the foot so it doesn't flop around aimlessly while you scrub. Rinse and dry the feet. Sponge them with alcohol, and wait one minute before drying a second time. All this scrubbing and sponging will prepare your partner for the large amount of attention you are about to lavish on his toes.

Toe care should begin by your sponging all the toes with alcohol and, if necessary, removing old nail polish with a polish remover. Grasp each toe between your thumb and forefinger, and clip or file the nails straight across the top. On pointed toes you may want to vary the shape of this cut slightly to conform to the shape of the toe, but be sure not to make a rounded cut. Clip off the excess cuticle with sharp-pointed scissors. Use your forefinger to rub cuticle oil into the nail and against the cuticle. Then press around the cuticle with a small metal pusher (available at any drugstore). Nail polishing is much easier if you separate the toes with balls of cotton. Press eight cotton separators between the toes of both feet, and apply whatever polish your partner prefers. Remove the separators when the polish dries and powder the feet.

If you want to make new friends on your next vacation, try packing a vibrator along with the camera and binoculars. There's no society anywhere on earth that will fail to appreciate this wonderful little toy. People in California enjoy vibrators so much that it's fair to say civilization as *we* know it would collapse without them.

Vibrators that are supposed to be applied directly to the body should not be used for massage. Some of these knobby, unfriendly devices bristle with multiple speed settings, high-low heating elements, and reversible heads. But no matter how many bells and whistles a vibrator offers, the machine should fit on the back of your hand to allow you, not a rubbery disk, to maintain body contact.

Since your partner will rarely protest, it's really up to you to decide just how long you want to maintain the contact. Vibrators are fatiguing, and most people are tempted to switch them off after a few minutes. For that reason many professional masseurs use two electric vibrators at once and move down opposite sides of the body from the scalp to the toes. Whether you use one vibrator or two, be sure the electric cords are arranged so that you can reach every part of your partner's body. Vibrators will massively stimulate circulation and are particularly effective on extremities like the hands, feet, and scalp. The stretch bands that fit around your hands will allow you to bend your fingers and follow the contours of your partner's body.

Move slowly. If you're going to include vibrator movements as part of a full body massage, it's best to do the whole body at the very beginning of the massage before you oil. The easiest way to avoid missing parts of the body is to concentrate on the head first, working up and down both sides of the face in long sweeping movements. Once you've finished the head, go on to the arms. Do each arm and each hand the same way, and then move onto the torso. From the torso it's easy to glide down onto the front of the legs and work down slowly to the feet. Press each foot between your two hands. This will send vibrations right through the foot, whether you're using one machine or two.

If you plan on doing both sides of your partner's body, it's best to begin on the back so that your partner has to turn over only once. That way you will end on the front of the body, ready to begin a full body massage without asking your partner to turn again.

The vibrator, of course, is an excellent way to amplify friction and vibration movements throughout the body. Even so, try to resist the temptation to introduce this high-powered little machine halfway through a full body massage. It will shatter the mellow vibrations you've worked so hard to maintain.

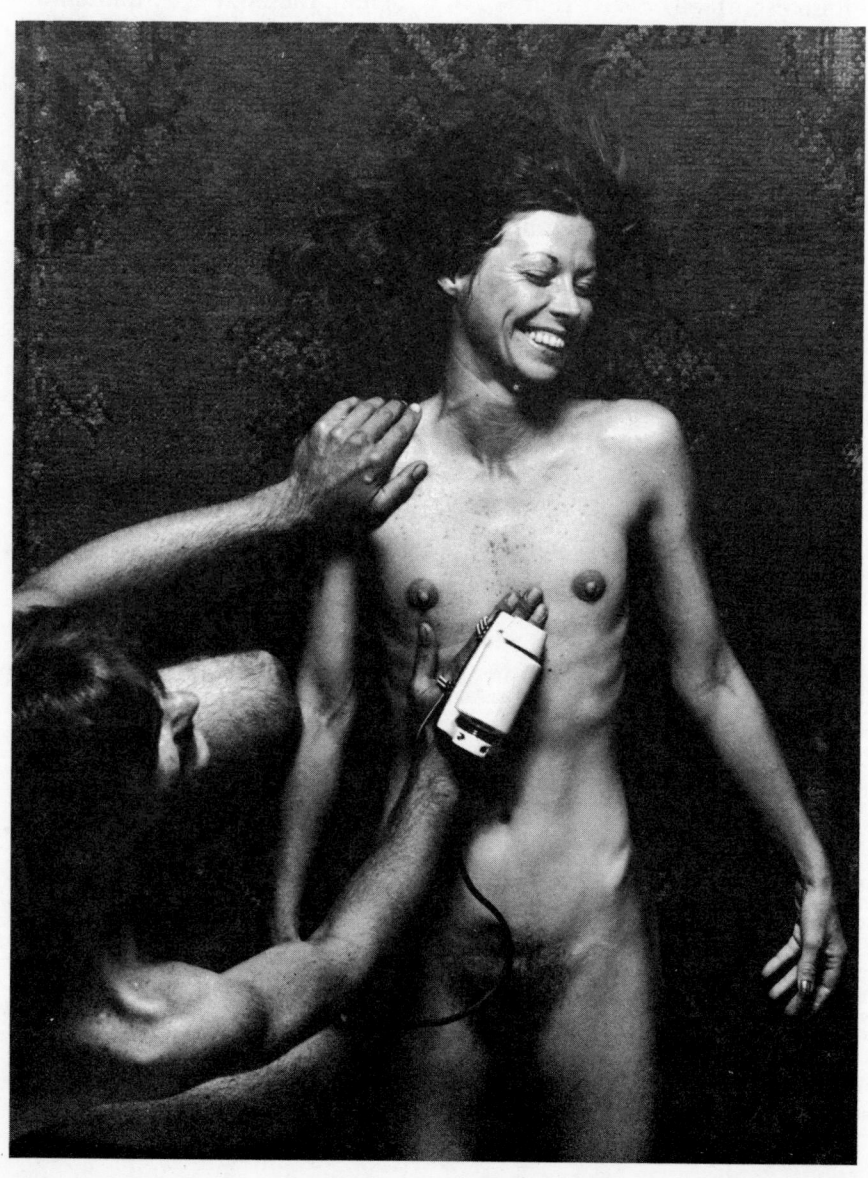

Fat is "burned" or metabolized by the body. Dieting will prevent the formation of new fat deposits, but no matter how serious your partner is about reducing, getting rid of existing fat depends on internal combustion rates. Burning fat requires oxygen, and massage will boost the oxygen consumption of the body 10 to 15 percent. Dieters who are massaged can expect an improvement in fat combustion rates throughout the body, and the effectiveness of *any* diet (measured in weight loss) can be immediately increased by 10 to 15 percent.

If your partner is interested in spot reducing, you can focus this increased fat combustion anywhere in the body by concentrating your massage efforts on a specific area. Deep kneading movements will reach all the way through a limb or inside the torso to fat deposits around the vital organs.

Overweight people often have negative images of themselves that massage can help to change. They have learned to view the body as a terrible burden that must be tolerated every day; massage teaches them to enjoy the body and love the flesh while they lose it.

. . . it was a thrill to me to distance myself from Yvette, to try to see her as a stranger, and then look through that stranger to the other woman I knew.
—V. S. NAIPAUL, A Bend in the River

Modern society's obsession with sex may have come about because lovemaking is the only form of tactile pleasure available to adults. What other experience offers two adults an opportunity to share extended physical contact and feel good about it? Massage satisfied that crucial need for thousands of years in societies where sexual freedom was unknown. Sex therapists can use the movements in this book to

provide patients with a new perspective on what it means to be touched.

The most recent sexual revolution which supposedly liberated all of us somehow ignored most of the body. Liberated lovers usually concentrate on the so-called erogenous zones and all but ignore the remaining 95 percent of the body. You have sexual or genital liberation without a more general *sensual* liberation. Nowhere is this sensual frigidity more apparent than in some of the new sex therapy centers, where massage is taught simply to allow bored,

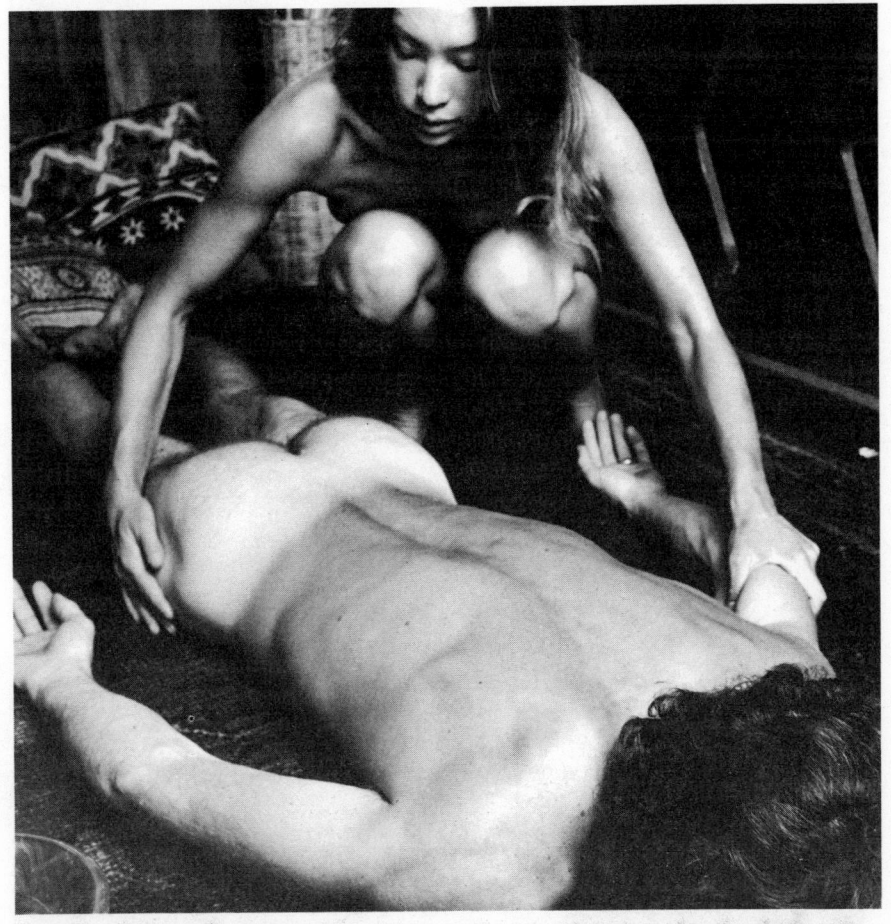

frigid, and alienated lovers to discover each other's bodies. How many lovers have lived together for years without ever stroking the infinitely tender sides of each other's fingers and toes?

Every therapist has worked with people who will not permit themselves to enjoy sex. They may be so frightened that the whole body will tense up during the most casual physical contact. This unhappy phenomenon is called pleasure censorship and can be effectively neutralized by sex therapists with massage training. Patients learn to relax and then begin massaging each other. Usually it's best to begin with the hands (see page 70) and gradually, over several sessions, extend your massage to cover the entire body.

Sex therapists who work with massage invariably discover people whose pleasure censors take over the moment massage begins. They sometimes talk on and on, they may stiffen from head to toe, or they may seem to be uncontrollably ticklish. (Many of these same folks will lie perfectly still while the dentist plows into a molar.) The best way to calm them is with a little music and some quiet talk. But be sure to let the conversation taper off when your partner begins to relax.

Complicated lectures during massage function only as distractions that take the mind away from the body. They encourage sensual frigidity by offering the mind concepts instead of feelings. Any effort to bring your partner to a specific point of view during massage is a very personal violation.

If one learns anything during massage, it is to be silent and become one with your feelings. It is this exquisite moment, when mind and body merge, that the sensually frigid deny by substituting emptiness for well-being and pain for pleasure. In a sensually frigid society where pain is practically the only sensation people allow themselves, pleasure becomes a revolutionary act.

Masseurs work hard and usually make pretty good money for their time. The work is very satisfying because they're giving people something tangible and real. Complaints are rare. Since customers tend to be loyal, it's possible to build a decent-sized clientele without advertising. If you insist on advertising, be ready for some strange phone calls. You can try prefacing your ad with a slightly defensive qualification like "nonsexual." (How many dentists do you know who call themselves nonsexual?) But even if you spell it out the bizarre phone calls will probably come. Unfortunately the word "massage" has become a popular euphemism for prostitution, and until a new code word is chosen, massage ads will be misunderstood.

Most parts of the country now require that you be licensed to practice massage professionally, and licensing requirements vary from county to county. Getting licensed usually means that you have to spend several hundred dollars attending a state-approved massage school. Some of the most brutal attempts at massage that I've ever seen have been self-righteously executed by state-approved massage school graduates. On the other hand, a decent massage school will allow you to learn from your mistakes so that your clients do not become your victims. One of the most valuable things about the experience is the feedback you can get from other students. Shop around before you pay your dues, and keep both eyes open.

If you're going into professional massage work, it's worthwhile to consider purchasing a portable massage table. One of these tables will put an end to the constant stream of customers tramping through your home. It also allows you to bring massage to sick and injured people who simply cannot get to your place. As long as bureaucrats insist on licensing masseurs, perhaps they will get around to licensing the manufacturers of portable massage tables. Some of these tables are built like Chinese boxes. When unfolding the legs, one is confronted with a maze of perplexing wood struts, wire buttressing, and loose plastic connectors. The worst of them will collapse without warning midway through a massage, hurling your partner to the floor three feet below. That kind of experience doesn't do much to foster the kind of trust masseurs work to build. If necessary, you should be able to climb on your massage table, straddle your partner's legs, and lean forward to work on the back. A good portable massage table will remain perfectly steady while you do this. Very light tables may be easier to get into a taxi but can eventually prove quite embarrassing. If you're on the table working on your partner's back when the legs decide to fold, that's two of you plummeting to the floor.

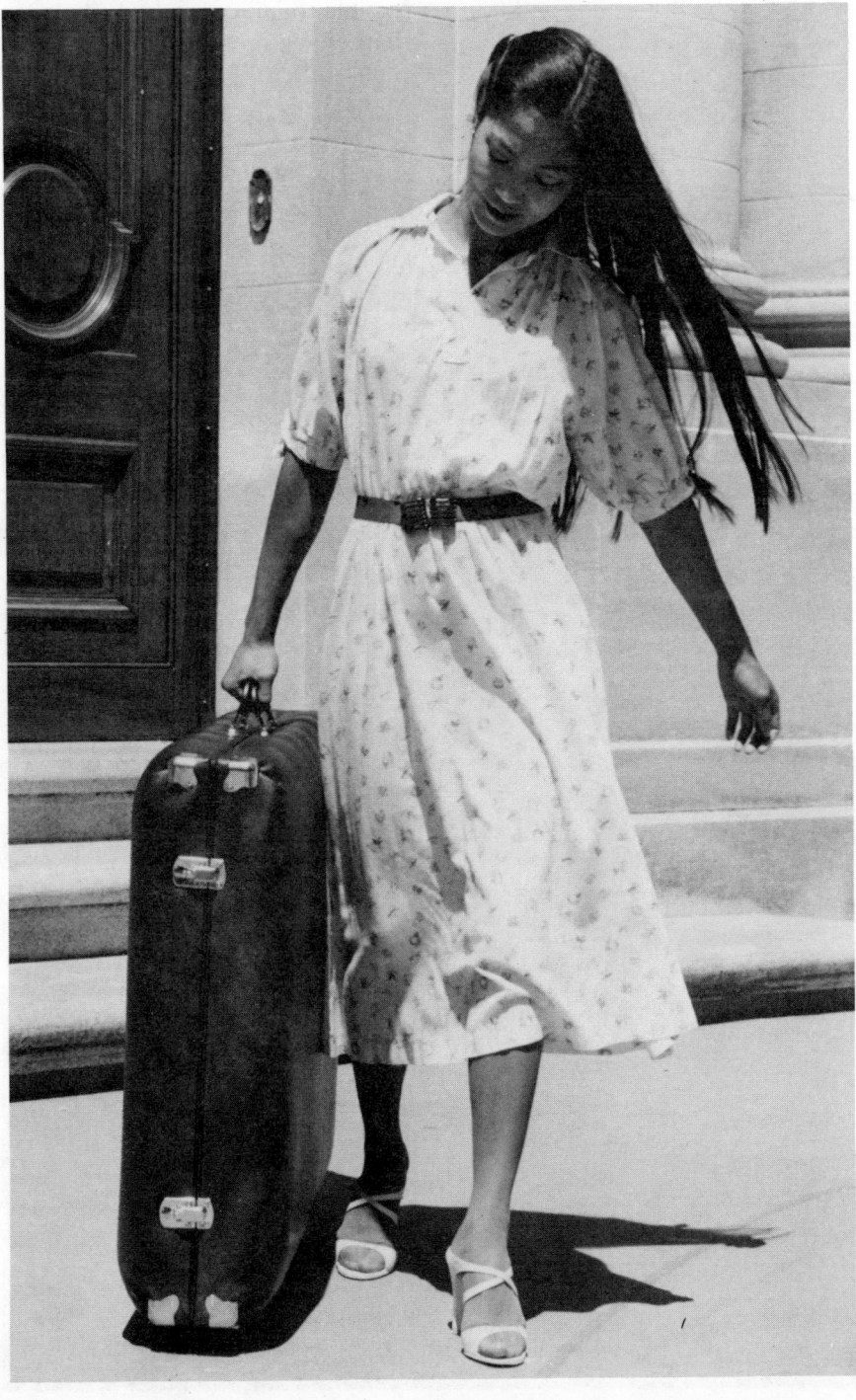

Having survived several such crashes, I was most grateful to discover the Astra massage table, for my money the best portable massage table on the market. The manufacturer now supplies these tables with wheels and a traveling case. Thus equipped, you can actually check the Astra onto an airplane and take it with you the next time you visit your maiden aunt. Astras are made by Frank and Marie Petticord (4236 Grove Street, Oakland, California, 94609) who guarantee the table for as long as you own it.

Above all things one should remember that regularity of breathing is of special importance.
—BERNARR MACFADDEN,
Building of Vital Power

There are more than 600 muscles scattered throughout the body, and somewhere in fitness literature is a specific exercise for just about every one of them. White rats will spin a wheel endlessly because there's really not much else happening in a cage. We humans do have our diversions, but perhaps they are not particularly apparent to certain overzealous marathoners. Who are these fanatical runners who disappear into the sunset day after day, leaving behind no good deeds? Have they managed to escape from Father Time? Do they need friends or family? How can we know these speedy devils? Perhaps the only way is to study those who are left behind to wait. The runners' widows. You see them pacing back and forth at the finish line as though the line itself were a kind of widow's walk. And the runners they wait for never come home.

The perpetual stiffness that seems to plague many exercise addicts is probably due to a condition known as work atrophy. When muscles are repeatedly overstrained, the dilated blood vessels are finally unable to bring in sufficient nutrition to cover expenditure of energy. Often, in dancers who have overtrained, work-atrophied leg muscles will harden just short of actual cramping. Cyclists who overextend themselves frequently have the same problem. Appropriate friction and kneading movements will, of course, bring sufficient nutrition to the muscles to relax

them. A far better approach is to relax the whole person.

Exercise addiction can be cured. Treatment should begin in the morning, before the urge to exercise blots out all communication. People who begin the day with a full body massage will hesitate to run away from the person who gave it to them.

There are so many pressing social concerns that it's easy to forget the outrageous treatment handicapped people must put up with every day. Despite the admirable progress that has been made toward justice and equality, we still live in a society that finds the handicapped embarrassing or, worse still, chooses to ignore them altogether.

Massage is one of the surest antidotes to the loneliness most handicapped people must endure. Being touched gently and carefully by another human being is tangible proof we are not alone.

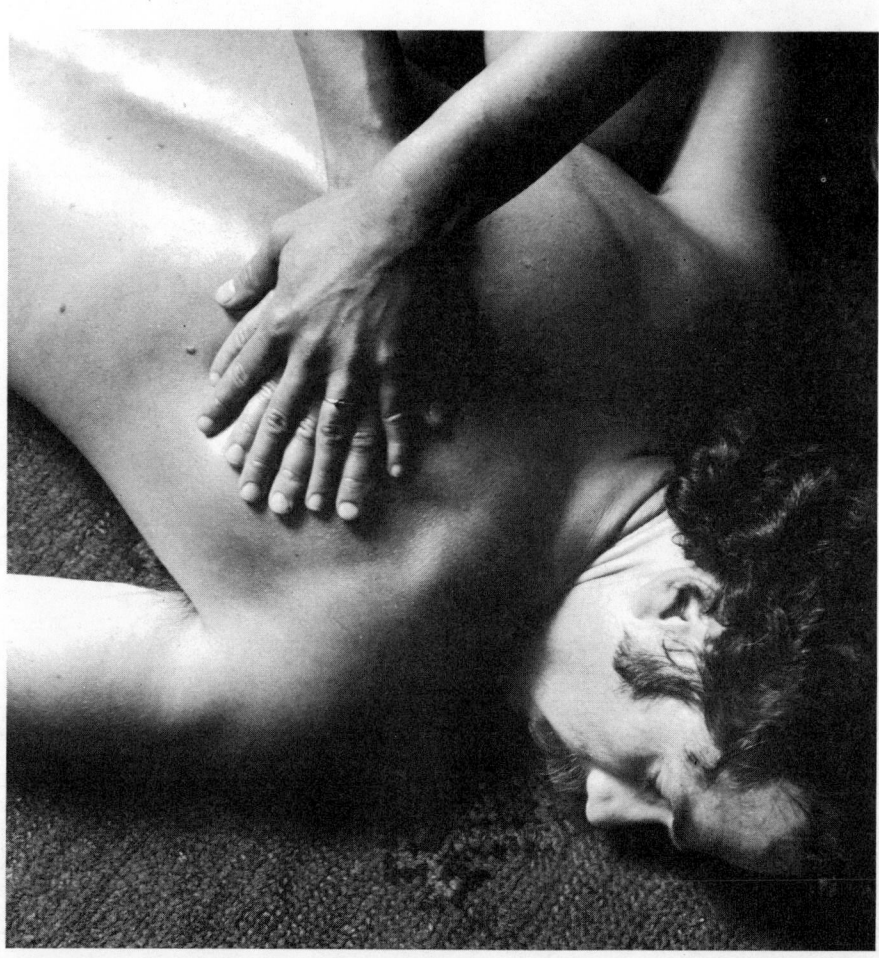

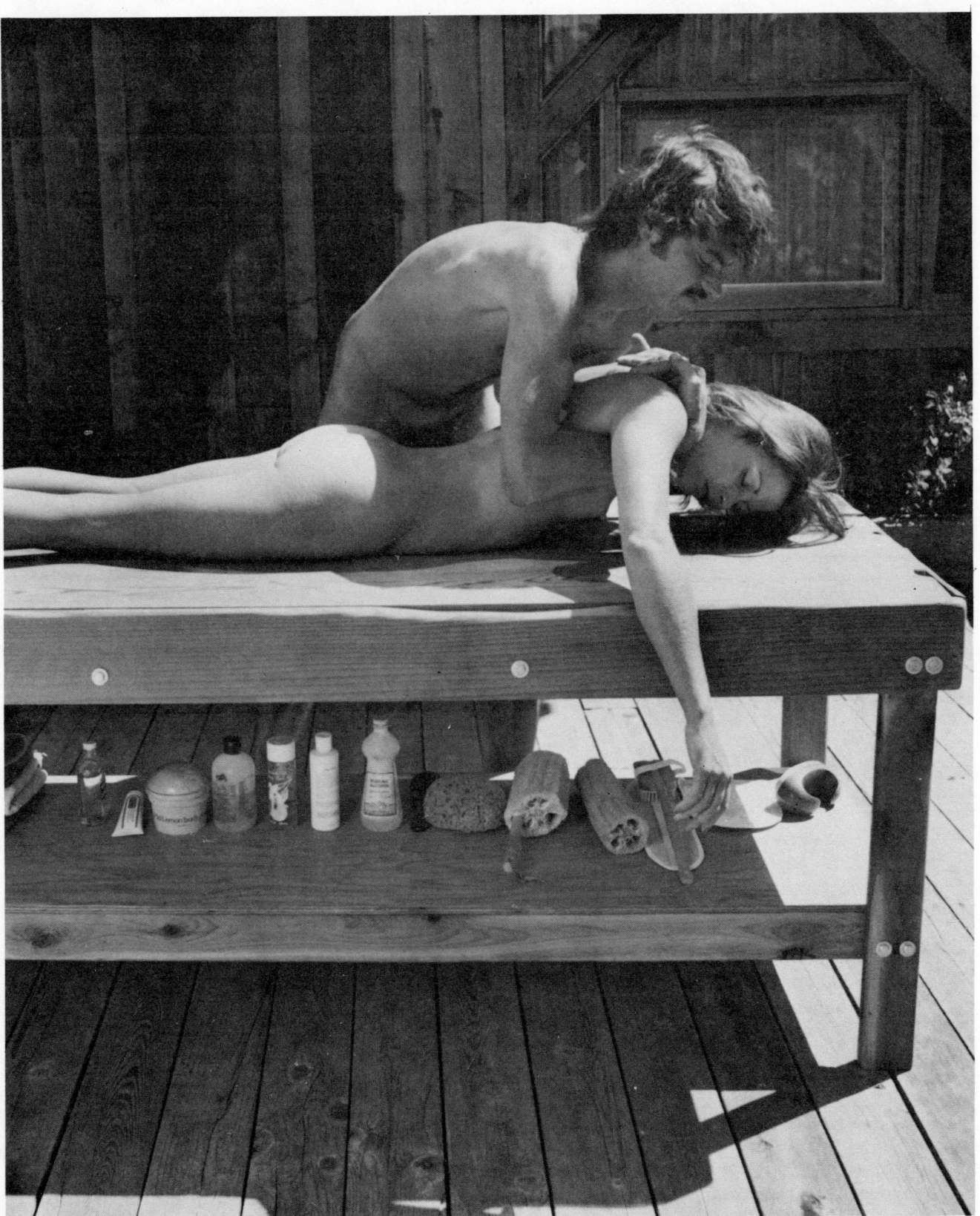

Flesh Lovers
Bath table design and illustration:
Dave Mohrmann
Homemade bread and brandy: Lee
Wakefield
East Bay Boogie: Brian Erickson
Eleventh Hour News: Dr.
Robert Payette

Most of *The New Massage* was
photographed during the hot
California summer of 1979.
Inside: Isom Buenavista, Steve
Colwell, Peggy Davis, Donna
Fahri, Howie Gordon, Linda
Herman, George Huck, Gordon
Inkeles, Sharon Kane, Randall
Krivonic, Little, Don Long, Mimi
Love Morgan, Victoria Organo,
Suzanne Paisley, Elaine Schelb,
Damien and Jude Sharp, Adele
Sloan, Bruce Strowbridge, Bruce
Walczyk, Carla Winter, Jerzy and
Kamiko, Kaisha and Soto, Ron
and Louise.

Special thanks to: Donna
Cohen, Bob Gordon, Elaine
Markson, Holly Sweet and Kitty
Wallis